Molecular Mechanisms and Pathophysiology of Sepsis

Molecular Mechanisms and Pathophysiology of Sepsis

Guest Editor

Vlad Pădureanu

MDPI

Basel • Beijing • Wuhan • Barcelona • Belgrade • Novi Sad • Cluj • Manchester

Guest Editor
Vlad Pădureanu
Department of Internal
Medicine
University of Medicine and
Pharmacy of Craiova
Craiova
Romania

Editorial Office
MDPI AG
Grosspeteranlage 5
4052 Basel, Switzerland

This is a reprint of the Special Issue, published open access by the journal *International Journal of Molecular Sciences* (ISSN 1422-0067), freely accessible at: https://www.mdpi.com/journal/ijms/special_issues/1BY03Z4JDX.

For citation purposes, cite each article independently as indicated on the article page online and as indicated below:

Lastname, A.A.; Lastname, B.B. Article Title. *Journal Name* **Year**, *Volume Number*, Page Range.

ISBN 978-3-7258-7206-0 (Hbk)
ISBN 978-3-7258-7207-7 (PDF)
https://doi.org/10.3390/books978-3-7258-7207-7

Contents

About the Editor

Vlad Pădureanu

Vlad Pădureanu graduated in 2011 from the Faculty of Medicine, University of Medicine and Pharmacy of Craiova. In January 2012, he started a specialization in internal medicine after passing the national residency exam. In 2016, he obtained a Master of Science in the Management of Health Units. He advanced through academic ranks by competition and has been a Lecturer in Internal Medicine—Medical Semiology since 2021.

He has participated in numerous national and international congresses with oral presentations and posters, including United European Gastroenterology Week, the Congress of the European Federation of Internal Medicine, and the Falk Symposium. His work has received six national awards from the Romanian Society of Internal Medicine and the Romanian Society of Gastroenterology and Hepatology.

He is a member of several professional organizations, including the Romanian Society of Internal Medicine, the European Federation of Internal Medicine, the Romanian Society of Gastroenterology and Hepatology, the Romanian Society of Cardiology, and the Balkan Medical Union. He has published over 100 papers as first author or co-author in journals indexed in ISI Web of Science, Medline/PubMed, and other databases, including *International Journal of Molecular Sciences*, *Biology*, *Biomedicines*, *Journal of Clinical Medicine*, and *Diagnostics*.

He has been involved in four research projects and is the principal investigator of one competitively awarded grant (approximately €10,000), currently in progress. He holds the title of senior physician in internal medicine, with additional qualifications in cardiology and ultrasound imaging.

He has authored and co-authored four textbooks for medical students and residents. His research interests include genetic polymorphisms, inflammation, oxidative stress, sepsis, acute pancreatitis, diabetes mellitus, liver diseases, and rheumatic diseases.

International Journal of
Molecular Sciences

MDPI

Editorial

Special Issue "Molecular Mechanisms and Pathophysiology of Sepsis"

Vlad Pădureanu

Department of Internal Medicine, University of Medicine and Pharmacy of Craiova, 200349 Craiova, Romania; vlad.padureanu@umfcv.ro

Sepsis was characterized for more than 20 years as a microbial infection that results in blood leukocyte alterations, tachycardia, tachypnea, and fever (or hypothermia). With fatality rates dropping to 15–25%, sepsis is widely understood to be a dysregulated systemic inflammatory and immunological response to microbial invasion that results in organ damage. With in-hospital death rates close to 30–50%, septic shock is still characterized as sepsis with hyperlactataemia and concomitant hypotension that needs vaso-pressor therapy. Sepsis is frequently linked to protracted inflammation, immune suppression, organ damage, and lean tissue wasting, rather than an immediate life-threatening condition, thanks to earlier detection and increased adherence to recommended practices. The post-sepsis time is receiving more and more attention, and the post-acute phase of this devastating syndrome is characterized by long-term effects derived from the acute systemic infection. Patients who survive sepsis also suffer long-term cognitive and functional disabilities and a persistent risk of death after discharge. Although in-hospital mortality has decreased due to earlier recognition and better application of optimal practices, immunomodulatory drug use has so far produced unsatisfactory results. In a similar vein, no biomarker can definitively identify sepsis or forecast how it will manifest clinically. Improvements in sepsis outcomes are expected to remain gradual and gradual due to its complexity.

The exceedingly complicated illness known as sepsis is brought on by a host's reaction to infection, becoming dysregulated. Because of its high mortality and morbidity, sepsis has just been designated a global health priority by the World Health Organization. Sepsis must be identified quickly in order to prevent negative consequences and lower mortality by initiating therapy as soon as possible. In fact, it has been calculated that the death rate from sepsis increases by 7–10% for every hour that treatment is delayed. However, because sepsis lacks distinct signs and symptoms, early diagnosis is still difficult.

At its core, sepsis is an inflammatory illness caused by the innate immune system becoming activated. The innate immune response in sepsis is characterized by two main findings. According to the first study, sepsis is typically brought on by complement and certain cell-surface receptors on cells whose main function is surveillance [1], simultaneously recognizing several infection-derived microbial agents and endogenous danger signals. These cells, which are physically situated where they may continuously sample their local environment, include immunological, epithelial, and endothelial populations. A complex intracellular signaling system with redundant and complementary activities is induced when pathogen-associated molecular patterns (PAMPs) or damage-associated molecular patterns (DAMPs) bind to complement, Toll-like receptors, nucleotide-binding oligomerization domain (NOD)-like receptors, retinoic acid-inducible gene (RIG)-like receptors, mannose-binding lectin, and scavenger receptors, among other receptors [2].

The second important discovery in sepsis is that the expression of several common gene classes involved in inflammation, adaptive immunity, and cellular metabolism is ultimately triggered by the activation of these signaling pathways. To put it another way, the identification of numerous bacteria, viruses, and fungal components, along with host products of tissue damage, results in the recruitment of pro-inflammatory intermediates. These intermediates then phosphorylate mitogen-activated protein kinases (MAPKs), Janus kinases (JAKs), or signal transducers and activators of transcription (STATs), and nuclear translocation of nuclear factor-κB (NF-κB), to mention a few.

Numerous early activation genes, including cytokines linked to inflammation (such as tumor necrosis factor (TNF), IL-1, IL-12, IL-18, and type I interferons (IFNs), are expressed when NF-κB is nuclear translocated and its promoter is activated. In addition to polarizing and suppressing adaptive immunity components, these cytokines start a chain reaction of other inflammatory cytokines and chemokines, such as IL-6, IL-8, IFNγ, CC-chemokine ligand 2 (CCL2), CCL3, and CXC-chemokine ligand 10 (CXCL10).

The endothelium changes from an anticoagulant state (in health) to a procoagulant state (in sepsis) due to changes in the expression of several procoagulant and anticoagulant proteins, such as thrombomodulin, tissue factor, von Willebrand factor, plasminogen activator inhibitor 1 (PAI-1), and activated protein C. Vascular endothelial (VE)-cadherin internalization brought on by pro-inflammatory proteases results in the loss of endothelial tight junctions and an increase in vascular permeability [3].

In this Special Issue (SI) of the *International Journal of Molecular Sciences* (IJMS), entitled "Molecular Mechanisms and Pathophysiology of Sepsis", we highlighted the latest findings regarding immune dysregulation, myocardial dysfunction, adrenal damage, biomarkers, and neonatal fungemia. Five original articles and three critical reviews make up this SI, which is well-balanced. In addition to highlighting knowledge gaps and potential avenues for future research, these papers summarize recent results in the subject of sepsis. The reviews cover important directions such as (i) biomarkers as beacons: sepsis-associated hepato-renal injury [4]; (ii) the role of scavenger receptor BI in sepsis [5]; (iii) neonatal fungemia by non-candida rare opportunistic yeasts [6].

A thorough transcriptome landscape of early-stage sepsis is shown by Taha S. et al., which demonstrates dual-pattern immune dysregulation marked by innate immune hyperactivation and simultaneous inhibition of adaptive immunity, translation, and metabolism [7]. While downregulated programs demonstrated extensive deficits in antigen presentation, protein synthesis, and energy metabolism, upregulated genes and pathways highlighted excessive neutrophil activation, inflammatory signaling, and innate immune priming. Findings that identify actionable gene networks open the door to tailored treatments and point-of-care diagnostic technologies, which could revolutionize the way sepsis is managed in critical care settings.

According to Harvey BI et al., there are sex-based variations in cardiac failure after direct LPS infusion, with male hearts having noticeably lower LV contractile performance than female hearts [8]. Estrogen itself might not have much of an impact on female hearts in response to direct LPS injection, since the proestrus/estrus and metestrus/diestrus groups showed similar amounts of LPS-induced cardiac dysfunction. The mechanisms behind sex-mediated LPS-induced cardiac failure require more investigation, especially the mitochondrial elements causing myocardial variations. New treatments for septic cardiomyopathy may be possible if these significant unknowns are resolved.

In a diverse group of burn patients at high risk of sepsis, Schiavello M et al. [9] propose the possible use of certain circulating EV-miRNAs, including miR-483-5p, -miR-193a-5p, and -miR-188-3p, as biomarkers for the diagnosis of sepsis. Additionally, researchers found that some EV-miRNAs (miR-1-3p, miR-34a-3p, and miR-193a-5p) change depending on how sepsis progresses, while other EV-miRNAs (miR-34a-3p and miR-193a-5p) are linked to the clinical severity of sepsis. These newly discovered circulating indicators may prove to be useful in the future for both prognostic classification and the identification of sepsis in burn victims.

Halimi F et al. used the following sepsis models to compare the transcriptome profiles in the livers of mice and pigs: lipopolysaccharide (LPS)-induced endotoxemia in pigs, which causes sterile inflammation; and cecal ligation and puncture (CLP) in mice and fecal instillation (FI) in pigs, both of which cause polymicrobial septic peritonitis [10]. The pig FI model more nearly reflects the metabolic dysfunction seen in the CLP liver than the pig LPS model, despite the fact that the elevated inflammatory pathways were equally activated in the two pig models. With a typical inflammatory signature among the upregulated genes and metabolic dysfunction among the downregulated genes, the two porcine sepsis models generally resemble the mouse CLP model, according to this thorough comparison of the hepatic responses in mouse CLP versus LPS or FI in pigs. The swine models were unable to reproduce the hepatic ER stress shown in the murine model. The pig FI model is more similar to the mouse CLP model than the pig LPS paradigm when it comes to examining metabolic dysfunction in the liver during sepsis.

Mrozewski L et al. looked into how C5a affected apoptosis and PC12 signaling. In PC12 cells, incubation with 10 nM C5a caused caspase activation via a mechanism that was dependent on C5aR. JNK/MAPK, ERK/MAPK, p38/MAPK, and AKT (PI3K) signaling that is dependent on C5aR was triggered by exposure to sepsis levels of C5a (10 nM). Additionally, after 24 h of exposure to 10 nM C5a, the expression of proteins linked to apoptosis, inflammation, and cell survival increased while that of proteins linked to adhesion, chemotaxis, and anti-inflammatory actions decreased. These findings shed light on the process by which C5a triggers PC12 cell apoptosis and cellular signaling. These results imply that the mechanism of adrenal impairment in sepsis may be significantly influenced by increased complement C5a levels [11].

Early detection and effective treatment are essential for lowering the mortality and morbidity of sepsis, a potentially fatal illness. Numerous putative sepsis biomarkers implicated in various disease processes have been evaluated. Furthermore, new and potential biomarkers such as non-coding RNAs have been developed as a result of recent technological advancements [12]. Given that the only available therapy options for sepsis patients are antibiosis, focus eradication, and critical care support, it is clear that new medicines are required. Characterizing the mechanistic features linked to the onset or course of sepsis would aid in the development of novel therapeutic approaches because the anamneses of sepsis patients are quite diverse. In order to prevent or treat the progression of sepsis, publications that clarify the molecular pathways in vitro or in vivo in preclinical models are invited, as are patient studies that offer insights into novel therapeutic ideas.

This Special Issue, "Molecular Mechanisms and Pathophysiology of Sepsis," published eight papers, including five original research papers and three review articles, all of which addressed different aspects of sepsis, biomarkers, molecular mechanisms and pathophysiology, and animal models.

We would like to express our full appreciation to the authors who contributed papers to this Special Issue. The remarkable quality of these studies will certainly add new content and generate new openings in multidisciplinary research into molecular mechanisms and pathophysiology of sepsis.

Acknowledgments: We would like to express our gratitude to all the authors who contributed to this Special Issue, and to the *International Journal of Molecular Sciences* team for their assistance during the review and editorial process.

Conflicts of Interest: The authors declare no conflicts of interest.

References

1. Takeuchi, O.; Akira, S. Pattern recognition receptors and inflammation. *Cell* **2010**, *140*, 805–820. [CrossRef] [PubMed]
2. Tang, D.; Kang, R.; Coyne, C.B.; Zeh, H.J.; Lotze, M.T. PAMPs and DAMPs: Signal 0s that spur autophagy and immunity. *Immunol. Rev.* **2012**, *249*, 158–175. [CrossRef] [PubMed]
3. Parikh, S.M. Dysregulation of the angiopoietin–Tie-2 axis in sepsis and ARDS. *Virulence* **2013**, *4*, 517–524. [CrossRef] [PubMed]
4. Pasare, M.A.; Prepeliuc, C.S.; Grigoriu, M.G.; Miftode, I.L.; Miftode, E.G. Biomarkers as Beacons: Illuminating Sepsis-Associated Hepato-Renal Injury. *Int. J. Mol. Sci.* **2025**, *26*, 4825. [CrossRef] [PubMed]
5. Hao, D.; Xue, J.Y.; Wang, Q.; Guo, L.; Li, X.A. The Role of Scavenger Receptor BI in Sepsis. *Int. J. Mol. Sci.* **2024**, *25*, 13441. [CrossRef] [PubMed]
6. Mpakosi, A.; Cholevas, V.; Meletiadis, J.; Theodoraki, M.; Sokou, R. Neonatal Fungemia by Non-Candida Rare Opportunistic Yeasts: A Systematic Review of Literature. *Int. J. Mol. Sci.* **2024**, *25*, 9266. [CrossRef] [PubMed]
7. Taha, S.; Bindayna, K.; Aljishi, M.; Sultan, A.; Almansour, N. Transcriptomic Profiling Reveals Distinct Immune Dysregulation in Early-Stage Sepsis Patients. *Int. J. Mol. Sci.* **2025**, *26*, 6647. [CrossRef] [PubMed]
8. Harvey, B.I.; Yoniles, A.M.; Monsivais, A.; Du, J.; Zadorozny, L.; Yu, Q.; Wang, M. Sex-Specific Differences in LPS-Induced Rapid Myocardial Dysfunction. *Int. J. Mol. Sci.* **2025**, *26*, 5963. [CrossRef] [PubMed]
9. Schiavello, M.; Bosco, O.; Vizio, B.; Sciarrillo, A.; Pensa, A.; Pivetta, E.; Morello, F.; Risso, D.; Montrucchio, G.; Mariano, F.; et al. Profiling of miRNAs Contained in Circulating Extracellular Vesicles and Associated with Sepsis Development in Burn Patients: A Proof-of-Concept Study. *Int. J. Mol. Sci.* **2025**, *26*, 1844. [PubMed]
10. Halimi, F.; Vanderhaeghen, T.; Timmermans, S.; Croubels, S.; Libert, C.; Vandewalle, J. Comparative Analysis of Hepatic Gene Expression Profiles in Murine and Porcine Sepsis Models. *Int. J. Mol. Sci.* **2024**, *25*, 11079. [CrossRef] [PubMed]
11. Mrozewski, L.; Tharmalingam, S.; Michael, P.; Kumar, A.; Tai, T.C. C5a Induces Inflammatory Signaling and Apoptosis in PC12 Cells through C5aR-Dependent Signaling: A Potential Mechanism for Adrenal Damage in Sepsis. *Int. J. Mol. Sci.* **2024**, *25*, 10673. [PubMed]
12. Agnello, L.; Ciaccio, M. Biomarkers of Sepsis. *Diagnostics* **2023**, *13*, 435. [CrossRef] [PubMed]

International Journal of
Molecular Sciences

MDPI

Article

Transcriptomic Profiling Reveals Distinct Immune Dysregulation in Early-Stage Sepsis Patients

Safa Taha [1,*], Khaled Bindayna [2], Muna Aljishi [1], Ameera Sultan [1] and Nourah Almansour [3]

1 Princess Al Jawhara Center for Molecular Medicine, Genetics and Inherited Diseases, Department of Molecular Medicine, College of Medicine and Health Sciences, Arabian Gulf University, Manama P.O. Box 26671, Bahrain; munajma@agu.edu.bh (M.A.); ameeraa@agu.edu.bh (A.S.)
2 Department of Microbiology & Immunology, College of Medicine and Health Sciences, Arabian Gulf University, Manama P.O. Box 26671, Bahrain; bindayna@agu.edu.bh
3 Immunology and Microbiology Department, Dasman Diabetes Institute, Kuwait City 15462, Kuwait; nourah.almansour@dasmaninstitute.org
* Correspondence: safat@agu.edu.bh; Tel.: +973-17-237-333

Abstract: Sepsis is a life-threatening condition characterized by dysregulated immune responses to infection. To elucidate early transcriptional changes in sepsis, we conducted a case–control study profiling gene expression in whole blood from 20 early-stage sepsis patients and 9 healthy controls. Using Affymetrix Clariom D Human Arrays and robust preprocessing, we identified differentially expressed genes (DEGs) using standard bioinformatic pipelines. A total of 344 genes were significantly upregulated, while 9703 were significantly downregulated in sepsis patients ($|\log2FC| > 1$, adjusted $p < 0.05$). Pathway enrichment and Gene Ontology analysis revealed activation of innate immune pathways, neutrophil degranulation, and cytokine signaling, alongside suppression of lymphocyte differentiation and antigen presentation. These results suggest a shift toward an innately driven inflammatory state in early sepsis. Our findings provide transcriptomic insights that may support the development of early diagnostic biomarkers and therapeutic targets.

Keywords: sepsis; transcriptomics; differential gene expression; innate immunity; microarray; early diagnosis

1. Introduction

Sepsis represents a complex syndrome of systemic inflammation resulting from infection and is a leading cause of mortality in intensive care units globally [1]. It is increasingly understood not as a uniform disease but as a dynamic continuum of immunological states, ranging from hyperinflammatory responses to immunosuppression [2]. This heterogeneity makes diagnosis and treatment particularly challenging. With current biomarkers like procalcitonin and CRP offering limited specificity and prognostic power [3–7], there is a growing demand for precision tools to characterize the molecular events that define sepsis onset and progression.

Recent advancements in transcriptomic profiling offer a window into these molecular dynamics. High-throughput gene expression analysis enables the identification of unique immune signatures, paving the way for biomarker discovery, mechanistic insights, and stratified therapy [8–11]. Notably, blood-based transcriptomic profiling serves as a minimally invasive yet informative tool that captures systemic host responses in real time [12,13]. By characterizing the transcriptional programs active during early sepsis, we can uncover key regulatory pathways involved in immune activation, metabolic reprogramming, and organ dysfunction [2,14–20].

Previous transcriptomic studies, such as those by [4,6], have characterized host responses in sepsis across diverse cohorts, primarily focusing on broad immune signatures or longitudinal outcomes [8,9]. In contrast, this study specifically targets early-stage sepsis within 72 h of symptom onset, capturing acute transcriptional changes in a Middle Eastern cohort using high-resolution Affymetrix Clariom D Arrays. By integrating advanced network analyses like WGCNA with traditional DEG and clustering approaches, we uncover modular gene networks that reveal novel regulatory hubs, offering unique insights into immune–metabolic reprogramming. These findings extend beyond the existing literature by identifying candidate biomarkers for early diagnosis and potential therapeutic targets tailored to the initial hyperinflammatory phase of sepsis.

In the present study, Figure 1, we used Affymetrix Clariom D Human Arrays to comprehensively profile blood gene expression in early-stage sepsis patients compared to healthy controls. Integrating differential gene expression, enrichment analyses, and machine learning clustering techniques, we identified upregulated pathways related to neutrophil activation and cytokine signaling [3,6,21], as well as the suppression of translational, metabolic, and antigen-presentation machinery [4,7,22]. These transcriptomic alterations mirror the paradoxical immune profile observed in sepsis, where exaggerated inflammation coexists with profound immune paralysis [2,23–25]. This expanded introduction sets the stage for a deeper investigation of the early molecular shifts that may underlie clinical outcomes in sepsis.

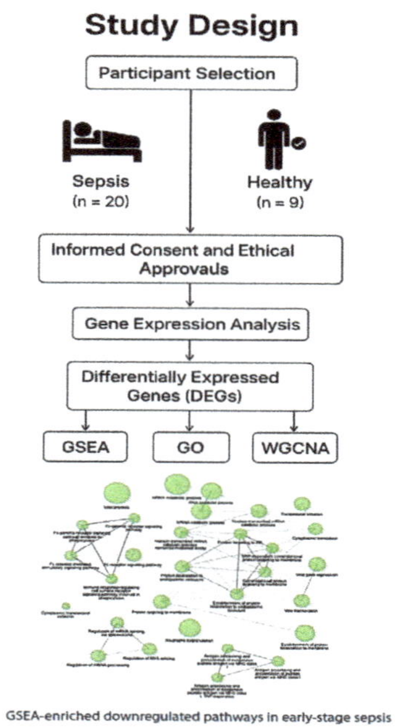

Figure 1. Study Design and Gene Expression Analysis Workflow This diagram outlines the study design and the workflow for gene expression analysis. The study involved the selection of participants, including 20 individuals with sepsis and 9 healthy controls. All participants provided informed consent, and the study received ethical approval. The gene expression analysis was conducted to identify differentially expressed genes (DEGs). Subsequent analyses included Gene Set Enrichment Analysis (GSEA), Gene Ontology (GO) enrichment, Weighted Gene Co-expression Network Analysis (WGCNA), and an examination of metabolic processes. The diagram also highlights the regulation of miRNA processing and the GSEA-enriched downregulated pathways in early-stage sepsis.

2. Results

Below is a schematic representation of the case–control study comparing early-stage sepsis patients ($n = 20$) with age- and sex-matched healthy controls (n = 9). The diagram outlines participant enrollment, consent and ethical approvals, sample collection, and downstream transcriptomic analysis. Visual elements highlight group differentiation and overall study flow.

2.1. Multidimensional Scaling and Differential Expression Analysis

Multidimensional Scaling (MDS) of normalized gene expression data revealed clear separation between early-stage sepsis patients and healthy controls along dimension 1, indicative of distinct global transcriptomic landscapes (Figure 2A). Healthy samples clustered tightly, reflecting high transcriptional uniformity, whereas sepsis samples exhibited greater dispersion, highlighting heterogeneous immune responses among patients, consistent with clinical variability in sepsis outcomes [8,9,26]. This clear segregation validated dataset quality and supported robust downstream analyses.

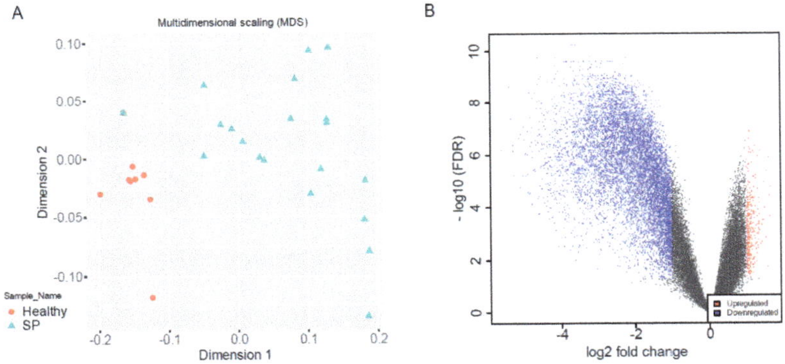

Figure 2. Transcriptomic separation and differential expression in early-stage sepsis. (**A**) MDS plot showing clear transcriptomic separation between sepsis patients and healthy controls along dimension 1. (**B**) The Volcano plot shows the log2 fold change (x-axis) versus the -log10(FDR) (y-axis) for each gene. Genes that are significantly upregulated are marked in red, while those that are significantly downregulated are marked in blue. The gray points represent genes that do not meet the significance threshold for differential expression. This visualization helps to identify genes with distinct immune signatures, highlighting their roles in the biological processes under study.

Differential expression analysis identified a total of 10,037 significantly dysregulated genes between sepsis patients and healthy controls ($|\log2FC| > 1$, adjusted $p < 0.05$), comprising 344 upregulated and 9703 downregulated genes (Figure 2B). The volcano plot visually underscored balanced yet pronounced patterns of immune activation and suppression, reflecting a complex host response characteristic of early-stage sepsis [1,2,8].

Top significantly upregulated genes included PCDHB11 (log2FC = 1.64), MIR1185-2 (log2FC = 1.42), MIR3156-2 (log2FC = 1.41), MIR1185-1 ENSG00000221525 (log2FC = 1.38), and MIR4323 (log2FC = 1.35). These genes have been associated with regulatory roles in immune responses and inflammatory pathways, highlighting their potential involvement in the innate immune activation observed in sepsis [3,6,21,23].

In contrast, significantly downregulated genes included FBXO7 (log2FC = −5.62), EIF1AY (log2FC = −5.41), HLA-DRA (log2FC = −5.36), MKRN1 (log2FC = −5.31), and RPL10 (log2FC = −5.30). Notably, the substantial suppression of HLA-DRA, critical for antigen presentation and adaptive immune responses, highlights significant impairment in adaptive immune function, potentially contributing to immune paralysis during severe septic states [7,17,20,27]. EIF1AY and RPL10 further underscore substantial suppression of protein synthesis processes, aligning with observations from bi-clustering and enrichment analyses [22,26,28].

Functional annotation of these dysregulated genes emphasized significant suppression of pathways related to antigen presentation, oxidative homeostasis, and protein synthesis, indicating a strategic reallocation of cellular resources from adaptive immunity towards innate immune activation and energy conservation during systemic inflammatory stress [2,26,29].

The coordinates of each sample in an MDS plot and a full list of differentially expressed genes are provided in Supplemental Information Tables S1 and S2.

Gene Set Enrichment Analysis (GSEA) confirmed these findings, highlighting significant negative enrichment (NES < -2.4, adjusted $p < 0.0001$) of key translational and biosynthetic pathways such as co-translational protein targeting to membranes, SRP-dependent co-translational protein targeting, protein targeting to the endoplasmic reticulum (ER), establishment of protein localization to endoplasmic reticulum, and cytoplasmic translation (Figure 3). Specifically, crucial genes involved in these pathways, including SEC62, SEC63, SEC61A1, RPL18, RPS20, and HSPA5, showed coordinated suppression, indicating a substantial disruption in protein synthesis and cellular maintenance mechanisms under septic conditions [2,22,30,31].

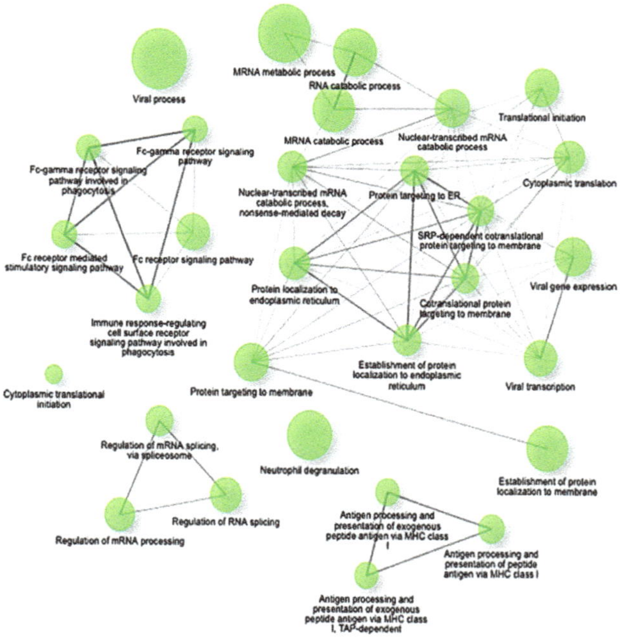

Figure 3. Network View of GSEA-Enriched Downregulated Pathways in Early-Stage Sepsis. This network visualization highlights the downregulated pathways in early-stage sepsis, including mRNA metabolism, RNA catabolism, viral processes, and immune response-related pathways. Nodes represent specific pathways, and edges indicate interactions between them.

Conversely, pathways positively enriched in early sepsis prominently included innate immune activation and inflammatory signaling processes. Notable positively enriched pathways encompassed Toll-like receptor (TLR) signaling, cytokine-mediated interactions, neutrophil immunity, and NF-κB signaling, underscoring a pronounced early inflammatory response [32–36]. These pathways are critically involved in the initial recognition and rapid immune response to pathogens, suggesting that the transcriptional profile in early sepsis prioritizes rapid innate immune activation over cellular homeostasis and metabolism [2,8,37–39].

GSEA output metrics are detailed in Supplemental Information Table S3.

The enrichment network map shows significantly downregulated gene sets (NES < −2.5, FDR q < 0.01) in early-stage sepsis. The nodes represent individual gene sets, and the edges indicate functional overlaps based on shared genes. The clusters highlight key suppressed biological programs, including translation initiation, ribosome biogenesis, oxidative phosphorylation, and mRNA catabolism. The network underscores a coordinated shutdown of biosynthetic and metabolic pathways in response to immune activation.

2.2. K-Means Clustering and Functional Module Analysis

K-means clustering of the normalized expression matrix identified six transcriptional modules, labeled A through F, each representing a distinct biological program associated with early-stage sepsis (Figure 4). The number of genes within each cluster ranged from 22 in Cluster A to 658 in Cluster D, highlighting variable modular complexity.

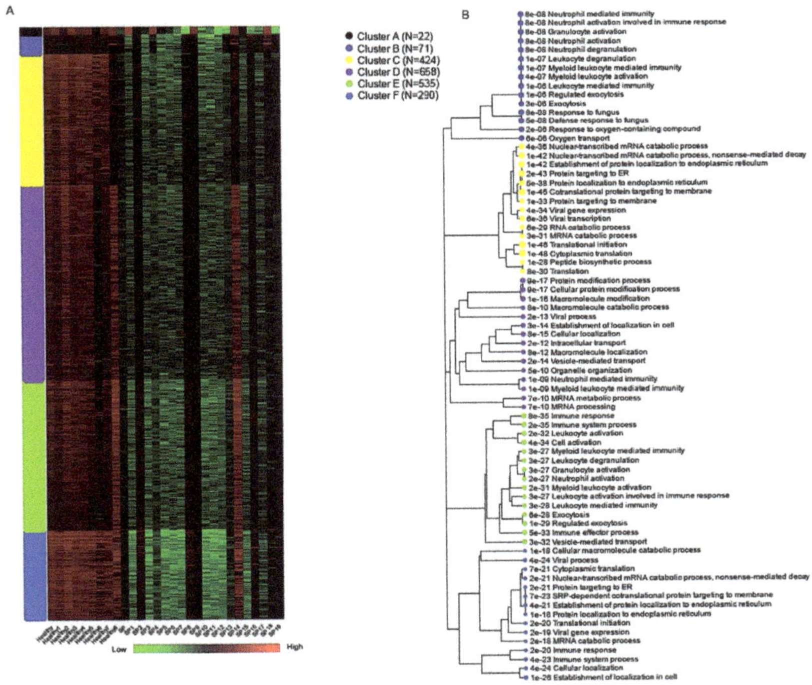

Figure 4. Gene clustering and functional enrichment of early sepsis transcriptome. (**A**) A heatmap showing six k-means gene expression clusters (A–F) across healthy controls and sepsis patients. Cluster B is enriched for neutrophil-mediated immune activation, while Cluster F shows the coordinated downregulation of translation-associated genes. The heatmap is row-normalized, and a scale bar indicates low (green), intermediate (black), and high (red) gene expression levels. (**B**) An enrichment tree map of biological processes associated with the six clusters. Each branch represents a GO term, with node proximity and hierarchy reflecting functional similarity. Prominent enriched processes include neutrophil activation, mRNA catabolism, vesicle-mediated transport, and translational initiation.

Among these, Cluster B (71 genes) showed robust enrichment for immune-related processes, particularly those involving neutrophil activity and innate immune defense. Key genes in this module included SPI1, MMP9, MMP8, S100A9, S100A12, DEFA1, and DEFA1B, all of which play central roles in neutrophil-mediated inflammation, pathogen clearance, and cytokine signaling [3,6,23]. Gene Ontology (GO) enrichment analysis for Cluster B revealed strong associations with the following:

Neutrophil activation involved in immune response (adjusted $p = 8.2 \times 10^{-8}$) Granulocyte degranulation (adjusted $p = 8.2 \times 10^{-8}$); Defense response to fungus (adjusted $p = 4.9 \times 10^{-8}$).

Due to the imbalance in differentially expressed genes (with the majority being downregulated), most clusters show reduced expression levels; however, cluster F is distinct in exhibiting a markedly stronger downregulation. Cluster F (290 genes) was distinguished by the widespread transcriptional suppression of genes involved in core cellular functions such as protein biosynthesis and RNA metabolism. This includes downregulation of components of the translation machinery, mRNA catabolism, and viral gene expression pathways. These signatures were consistent with results from bi-clustering and Gene Set Enrichment Analysis (GSEA), further underscoring extensive translational arrest and metabolic reprogramming during early sepsis [26,30,40–42]. Enriched GO terms for Cluster F included the following:

mRNA catabolic processes (adjusted $p < 1 \times 10^{-50}$);

Translation initiation;

Viral gene expression and antigen processing [7,43–45].

These findings underscore a pronounced transcriptional dichotomy during early sepsis, where acute immune activation coexists with suppression of essential biosynthetic and metabolic pathways. This suggests a strategic reallocation of leukocyte resources to support immediate immune defense, potentially at the expense of long-term cellular maintenance. Such immune–metabolic tradeoffs may contribute to the development of immunosuppression and increased susceptibility to secondary infections commonly observed in sepsis patients [2,8,17].

Details of K-means clustering and Functional Module Analysis are provided in Supplemental Information Table S4.

2.3. Bi-Clustering Analysis

Bi-clustering analysis identified a dominant co-expression module consisting of approximately 1000 genes that exhibited coordinated upregulation in healthy controls and significant suppression in sepsis patient samples (Figure 5). This substantial bi-cluster represents a critical transcriptional signature reflective of systemic transcriptional reprogramming commonly observed in early-stage sepsis.

Detailed functional annotation and literature-supported analysis revealed that genes within this bi-cluster were profoundly enriched in pathways related to ribosomal function, oxidative phosphorylation, and core metabolic processes. Key genes involved in oxidative phosphorylation, including ATP5A1, ATP5B, and ATP5J, and numerous ribosomal protein genes (e.g., RPS20, RPL31), demonstrated consistent downregulation in sepsis samples, supporting the notion of translational and metabolic suppression as a response to acute systemic inflammation [22,46–50].

Additional suppressed genes within the bi-cluster were identified in pathways critical for protein synthesis and cellular maintenance, including EIF4B involved in translation initiation, VAMP3 associated with vesicle-mediated transport, and DCUN1D1 involved in protein ubiquitination. The uniform suppression of these genes highlights extensive cellular reprogramming aiming to conserve energy and limit protein production during severe inflammatory stress, a phenomenon documented previously in various systemic inflammatory states, including sepsis [35,38,39,44,46,49].

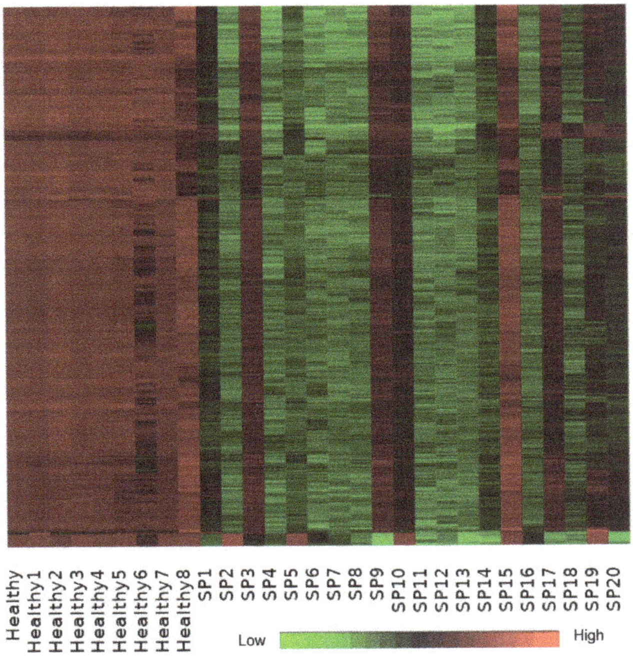

Figure 5. Bi-clustering reveals transcriptional suppression of metabolic and translational programs in early sepsis.

Moreover, the observed downregulation of genes involved in maintaining cellular oxidative balance, such as CYB5R4, highlights impaired antioxidant defenses in septic patients, possibly exacerbating oxidative damage and contributing to cellular dysfunction commonly noted in sepsis-induced organ injury [17,48].

Collectively, this bi-cluster analysis underscores a coordinated transcriptional response strategy characterized by metabolic shutdown, decreased translational activity, and impaired oxidative balance. These processes represent key pathophysiological mechanisms contributing to immune dysregulation and organ dysfunction in early-stage sepsis, offering insights into potential therapeutic targets aimed at restoring cellular metabolism and function [51–54]. A list of 1000 genes identified using bi-clustering analysis is provided in Supplemental Information Table S5.

The heatmap shows a dominant co-expression bi-cluster of approximately 1000 genes across 29 samples, including healthy controls and early-stage sepsis patients. The expression matrix is z-score normalized per gene (row-wise), with red indicating high expression, green low expression, and black representing intermediate expression. Genes in this bi-cluster show consistent upregulation in healthy controls and suppression in sepsis patients, capturing a robust transcriptional signature associated with translational arrest and metabolic downregulation.

2.4. WGCNA Identifies Distinct Co-Expression Modules Altered in Sepsis

To explore higher-order transcriptional relationships, we applied Weighted Gene Co-expression Network Analysis (WGCNA) to high-variance genes [49]. This analysis identified several distinct gene modules significantly associated with the sepsis phenotype, notably the turquoise and blue modules (Figure 6).

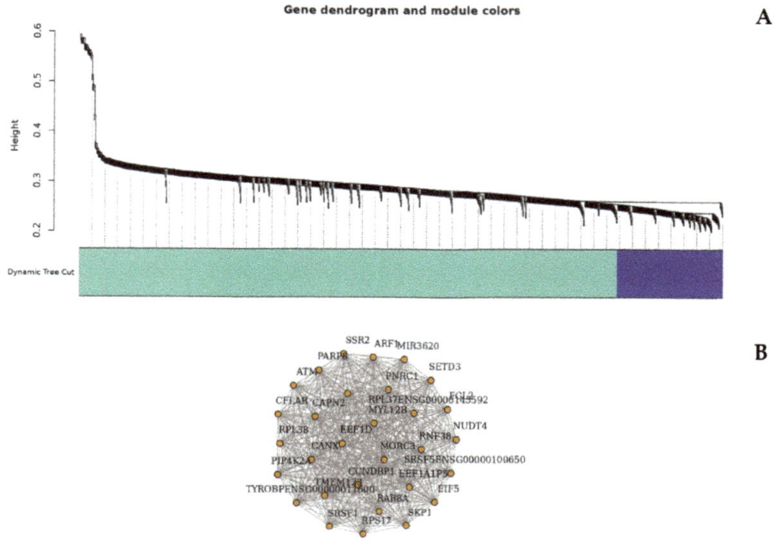

Figure 6. WGCNA-based co-expression modules and gene connectivity in early-stage sepsis. (**A**) Gene dendrogram with dynamic tree cut illustrating module detection by hierarchical clustering. Major modules (e.g., turquoise, blue) represent co-expressed gene sets. (**B**) Network plot of top hub genes from turquoise module within key module. Nodes represent genes, and edges denote co-expression relationships, highlighting tightly interconnected functional sub-networks.

The turquoise module (Module 1), comprising 835 genes, exhibited a strong positive correlation with sepsis status (r = 0.76, $p < 0.01$). Genes in this module, such as 15-SEP, 7-MAR, 7-SEP, and AC011404.1, were enriched in biological processes related to neutrophil activation, cytokine signaling, and Toll-like receptor pathways—aligning closely with differential gene expression (DEG) and enrichment analysis findings [24,37].

In contrast, the blue module (Module 2), containing 164 genes, was negatively correlated with sepsis (r = −0.68). Representative genes within this module included AC013394.2, AP000240.9, and CTD-2370N5.3, which were primarily involved in ribosome biogenesis, oxidative phosphorylation, and protein synthesis pathways [23,41]. This aligns with the observed suppression patterns noted in the bi-clustering and Gene Set Enrichment Analysis (GSEA) [26].

Functional annotation of these modules confirmed significant immune–metabolic reprogramming and translational suppression during early sepsis, with WGCNA highlighting modular gene networks that underpin and extend insights derived from traditional DEG analyses [42,45,48]. A full list of genes with their designated clusters, identified using Weighted Gene Co-expression Network Analysis (WGCNA), is provided in Supplemental Information Table S6.

3. Discussion

Our comprehensive transcriptomic analysis of early-stage sepsis reveals coordinated and multifaceted immune dysregulation characterized by simultaneous upregulation of innate immune responses and downregulation of adaptive immunity, antigen presentation, protein synthesis, and metabolic homeostasis. These findings reinforce the dual-phase paradigm of sepsis, where an early hyperinflammatory response coexists with cellular exhaustion and immunosuppression [1,2,10].

Multidimensional Scaling (MDS) demonstrated clear separation between septic patients and healthy controls, highlighting significant global transcriptomic shifts. Increased dispersion among sepsis samples reflects heterogeneous immune responses, consistent with clinical variability in disease progression and outcomes [10,11,30].

Differential expression analysis identified significant upregulation of genes involved in neutrophil activation and inflammatory signaling, including *OLFM4, LCN2*, and *S100A12*. These genes play roles in antimicrobial defense, tissue infiltration, and cytokine-mediated feedback loops, exacerbating tissue damage during sepsis [3–5,24]. These transcriptional signatures align closely with pathways governed by Toll-like receptor (TLR) signaling and NF-κB activation, emphasizing innate immune activation dominance [24,37].

Conversely, markedly downregulated transcripts included *HLA-DRA*, *CTSS*, and TXNIP, along with broad sets of ribosomal and oxidative phosphorylation genes. Gene Set Enrichment Analysis (GSEA) confirmed suppression of key biosynthetic processes, including ribosome biogenesis, translation initiation, mRNA catabolism, and oxidative metabolism [23,26,34,41]. These shifts indicate immune-metabolic reprogramming of leukocytes, prioritizing inflammatory responses over cellular maintenance functions—potentially serving as an energy conservation mechanism during systemic stress [42,46,47].

K-means clustering and bi-clustering analyses provided complementary insights into the transcriptional landscape of early-stage sepsis. K-means clustering revealed distinct gene expression modules, including Cluster B, enriched for neutrophil-mediated immune responses, and Cluster F, characterized by widespread downregulation of genes involved in translation and protein synthesis. These modules reflect the dual nature of sepsis pathophysiology, where hyperactivation of innate immunity coexists with suppression of cellular maintenance programs.

In parallel, bi-clustering analysis uncovered a dominant transcriptional signature comprising approximately 1000 genes that were consistently highly expressed in healthy controls but markedly suppressed in sepsis patients. This bi-cluster encompassed key components of ribosomal function, oxidative phosphorylation, and mRNA processing. Notably, ATP synthase subunits (*ATP5A1, ATP5B*), cytoskeletal proteins such as VIM (Vimentin), and numerous ribosomal protein genes (*RPS20, RPL31*) exhibited profound transcriptional repression [23,41].

The consistent downregulation of these core homeostatic and metabolic pathways underscores a global transcriptional reprogramming aimed at reallocating cellular energy toward immune defense rather than biosynthetic activities. While this strategy may enable rapid inflammatory responses, it comes at the cost of translational arrest and metabolic shutdown, potentially contributing to immune exhaustion, impaired tissue repair, and organ dysfunction. These findings highlight critical vulnerabilities in septic leukocytes that may serve as targets for therapeutic intervention, particularly strategies aimed at restoring metabolic balance and protein synthesis capacity during recovery from sepsis [42,44].

Extending these findings, Weighted Gene Co-expression Network Analysis (WGCNA) uncovered additional regulatory architecture by clustering genes into co-expressed modules with distinct biological functions correlated to disease status [49]. The turquoise module, highly associated with sepsis, was enriched with genes involved in neutrophil-mediated immunity, cytokine signaling, and TLR pathways [24,37]. Conversely, negatively correlated blue and green modules contained genes responsible for ribosome structure, translation, mitochondrial respiration, and antigen presentation, mirroring the suppressed pathways observed in GSEA and bi-clustering [23,26,41]. These insights underscore that immune and metabolic systems are regulated through highly coordinated modular networks, extending beyond individual gene activation.

WGCNA enhances transcriptomic profiling resolution by identifying functional units beyond DEGs, reinforcing the reproducibility of the immune-metabolic switch observed in early sepsis [42,45,48]. The convergence of MDS, DEG, GSEA, clustering, and WGCNA analyses robustly supports the dual-phase model of sepsis pathogenesis [10,22,42].

The identified transcriptomic signatures, particularly the upregulation of neutrophil-associated genes (*OLFM4, S100A12*) and the suppression of adaptive immunity markers (HLA-DRA), hold significant potential for clinical translation. Unlike existing biomarkers like procalcitonin or CRP, which lack specificity for early sepsis [8,9], our gene signatures could enable precise risk stratification and early diagnosis within the critical first 72 h. For instance, a diagnostic panel targeting *OLFM4* and *S100A12* could identify patients at risk of rapid disease progression, guiding timely interventions such as antibiotics or immunomodulatory therapies. Additionally, the suppression of translational and metabolic pathways (e.g., *ribosomal genes, ATP5A1*) suggests therapeutic opportunities to restore cellular homeostasis, potentially via metabolic modulators or immunotherapies targeting immune exhaustion. These biomarkers could be integrated into point-of-care assays or machine learning models to personalize sepsis management.

These modules offer practical translational potential, containing candidate hub genes that could serve as early biomarkers or therapeutic targets for stratifying sepsis patients and modulating inflammatory-metabolic balances. Future studies should validate these signatures across broader longitudinal patient cohorts to assess their diagnostic and prognostic efficacy [40,45,48].

Together, our findings illustrate a complex transcriptional landscape in early-stage sepsis, highlighting immune escalation and suppression of cellular homeostasis. Integrative network-based methods like WGCNA offer new interpretative avenues for immune dynamics, identifying actionable gene regulatory nodes.

A limitation of this study is the reliance on microarray-based transcriptomic profiling without orthogonal validation of key differentially expressed genes (DEGs) such as *HLA-DRA, OLFM4,* and *S100A12*. While microarray data were rigorously quality-controlled and normalized, future studies should employ quantitative real-time PCR (qRT-PCR) to confirm these transcriptional changes. Additionally, protein-level validation using techniques such as ELISA or flow cytometry for *HLA-DR* and LCN2 could further substantiate the translational relevance of these findings, bridging the gap between transcriptomic signatures and clinical applicability. Such validations are planned as part of our ongoing research to strengthen the identified biomarkers' diagnostic and prognostic potential.

4. Materials and Methods

4.1. Study Design

This study utilized a case–control design to investigate gene expression patterns in early-stage sepsis. We included two groups of adult participants aged 18 years and older: Group 1 comprised 10 patients diagnosed with early-stage sepsis, while Group 2 included 9 healthy controls. Patients were recruited from the Intensive Care Unit (ICU) at Salmaniya Medical Complex (SMC) in Bahrain. Healthy controls, free from infections or inflammatory conditions, were selected from blood donors at the SMC Blood Bank, ensuring that age and sex were matched between the groups. All participants provided informed written consent, and ethical approvals were obtained from the College of Medicine and Health Sciences at Arabian Gulf University, SMC, and the Ministry of Health in Bahrain.

4.2. Early-Stage Sepsis

The clinical diagnosis of sepsis was based on the Sepsis-3 definitions, which require either suspected or confirmed infection alongside an increase in the Sequential Organ Failure Assessment (SOFA) score of 2 or more points. This diagnosis considers symptoms onset within the last 72 h. Patients must exhibit at least one of the following abnormal vital signs:

Fever (≥38.0 °C) or hypothermia (≤36.0 °C), tachycardia (heart rate > 90 beats per minute), tachypnea (respiratory rate >20 breaths per minute), or altered mental status.

Septic Shock: A subset of sepsis characterized by persistent hypotension requiring vasopressors to maintain a mean arterial pressure (MAP) ≥ 65 mmHg and a lactate level >2 mmol/L despite adequate fluid resuscitation.

4.3. Healthy Controls

Controls were individuals without any history of infection or sepsis, matched for age and gender with the patient group. They had no chronic illnesses that could influence immune response, such as diabetes or autoimmune diseases.

4.4. Exclusion Criteria

Patients were excluded if they had undergone major surgery within the last 30 days, were immunocompromised (e.g., receiving chemotherapy or corticosteroids), were pregnant, or had concurrent infections complicating the diagnosis of sepsis. Additionally, individuals under 18 years of age were excluded (Table 1).

Table 1. Inclusion and exclusion criteria.

Criteria	Early-Stage Sepsis	Healthy Controls
Inclusion Criteria	Clinical diagnosis of sepsis (Sepsis-3)	No history of infection or sepsis
	Symptoms onset within the last 72 h	Age and gender matched with patients
	At least one abnormal vital sign	No chronic illness affecting immune response
Exclusion Criteria	Recent major surgery within the last 30 days	Not applicable
	Immunocompromised status	
	Pregnancy	
	Concurrent infectiona complicting diagnosis	
	Individuals under 18 years of age	

4.5. Blood Sample Collection and RNA Extraction

Blood samples were collected using Tempus™ Blood RNA Tubes (Applied Biosystems™, Waltham, MA, USA) and vortexed for 10 s to ensure thorough mixing with the stabilizing reagent. RNA extraction was performed using the Stabilized Blood-to-CT™ Nucleic Acid Preparation Kit, following the manufacturer's guidelines. Initially, 500 µL of each Tempus-stabilized blood sample was transferred to a 1.5 mL microcentrifuge tube. To this, 250 µL of 2X PBS was added, followed by vortexing for 10 s and brief centrifugation. Next, 20 µL of Tempus™ Pellet Enhancer was added; the mixture was vortexed again for 10 s and centrifuged at 5000× g for 10 min. The supernatant was carefully removed, leaving approximately 50 µL behind with the pellet. Washing steps were repeated three to five times: first, 750 µL of Tempus™ (Chicago, IL, USA) Washing Buffer 1 was added and vortexed until the pellet dissolved, then centrifuged at 5000× g for 2 min. The washing buffer was removed, retaining about 20 µL of residual supernatant. Subsequently,

750 μL of Tempus™ Washing Buffer 2 was added, vortexed briefly, and centrifuged again at 5000× *g* for 2 min, after which the tube with the pellet was placed on ice. To eliminate any genomic DNA, a digestion solution mixed with DNase I (1:100) was prepared and added to a microcentrifuge tube. After mixing, 129 μL of this digestion solution was added to the pellet, which was pipetted up and down five times to break it up. The mixture was incubated at room temperature for 8 min. Finally, 10 μL of Stop Solution was added, and the sample was incubated for an additional 2 min before being stored at –80 °C for further analysis.

4.6. Microarray Data Generation and Quality Control

Gene expression profiling was performed using the Affymetrix Clariom D Human Array. The quality of the extracted RNA from peripheral blood mononuclear cells (PBMCs) was assessed using an Agilent Bioanalyzer. The purified RNA was used as a template for first strand cDNA synthesis following the "GeneChip® WT PLUS Reagent Kit" (Thermo Fisher Scientific, Santa Clara, CA, USA). The first amplification was carried out from a total of 250 ng of initial RNA. Subsequently, the second strand of cDNA was synthesized. This double-stranded cDNA was then used to synthesize cRNA, which was purified, and its concentration measured. A second cycle of cDNA synthesis was performed, followed by hydrolysis, purification, fragmentation, and labeling. Finally, the labeled fragmented cDNA was hybridized to the GeneChip® Clariom D Human Array (Thermo Fisher Scientific) at 45 °C for 16 h in the Affymetrix GeneChip® Hybridization Oven 645. After hybridization, the chips were washed and stained using the Affymetrix GeneChip® Fluidics Station 450, following the procedures described in the "GeneChip® WT PLUS wash and stain Kit" protocol. All chips were scanned at room temperature using the Affymetrix GeneChip® Scanner 3000 7G. Data preprocessing steps included importing CEL files into the Transcriptomic Analysis Console (TAC) software. The Transcriptome Analysis Console (TAC) software version 4.0.0.25 by Thermo Fisher Scientific Quality control methods involved visual inspections of boxplots and density plots to assess data distribution and quality. Normalization of the raw expression data was performed using the Robust Multi-array Average (RMA) method, which includes background correction, quantile normalization, and summarization of probe sets. All analyses were performed using R (version 4.4.1) and Bioconductor (version 3.19). The Transcriptomic Analysis Console (TAC, version 4.0.2, Thermo Fisher Scientific) was used for data preprocessing. The 'affy' package (version 1.78.0) implemented the Robust Multi-array Average (RMA) method for normalization.

Principal Component and Clustering Analysis: Principal Component Analysis (PCA), Multidimensional Scaling (MDS), and t-distributed Stochastic Neighbor Embedding (t-SNE) were applied to RMA-normalized gene expression data using the Transcriptomic Analysis Console (TAC). MDS revealed that dimension1 accounted for the greatest variance and clearly separated sepsis patients from healthy controls. Additional components (PC2–PC5) supported sample-specific variance. MDS and t-SNE analyses confirmed the distinct transcriptomic profiles of patient and control groups.

Differential Expression Analysis: DEGs between sepsis patients and healthy controls were identified using linear modeling and empirical Bayes statistics. Genes with |log2 fold change| > 1 and adjusted *p*-value < 0.05 were considered significant. A volcano plot was generated to visualize global transcriptional changes, plotting log2 fold change against -log10-adjusted *p*-value.

Pathway and Functional Enrichment: Enrichment analyses were performed using DAVID and Reactome databases. Gene Ontology (GO) terms and KEGG pathways were used to interpret biological significance.

K-Means Clustering and Functional Module Analysis: To identify gene co-expression modules, unsupervised K-means clustering was applied to the normalized expression matrix. K-means clustering was performed using the 'stats' package (version 4.4.1) with k = 6, selected based on the elbow method to optimize within-cluster sum of squares, ensuring biologically meaningful gene modules. The 'cluster' package (version 2.1.6) was used for silhouette analysis to validate cluster quality. Genes were grouped into six major clusters (A–F), which were then visualized via heatmap. Functional enrichment analysis was performed for each cluster using GO biological processes with adjusted *p*-values.

Bi-clustering Analysis: To identify coherent gene modules regulated across subsets of samples, we performed bi-clustering using the biclust R package. Unlike traditional clustering, which captures patterns across all samples, bi-clustering identifies genes that are co-expressed within specific sample subsets. We applied the BCPlaid algorithm under default parameters, modeling the expression matrix as a sum of additive layers to capture distinct transcriptional patterns. This approach enabled detection of a large co-expression bi-cluster associated with coordinated downregulation of metabolic and translational programs in sepsis patients. Further details are provided in Supplemental Information Table S5.

Co-expression Network Analysis: To identify co-regulated gene modules associated with early-stage sepsis, we implemented Weighted Gene Co-expression Network Analysis (WGCNA) using R. WGCNA was implemented using the 'WGCNA' package (version 1.72-5). A soft-thresholding power of $\beta = 6$ was chosen based on scale-free topology fit ($R^2 > 0.85$), determined using the pickSoftThreshold function. The minimum module size was set to 30 genes, and dynamic tree cutting was performed with a deepSplit of 2 to ensure robust module detection.

A practical clinical scenario for applying these transcriptomic signatures involves the rapid identification of early-stage sepsis in emergency departments. For example, a patient presenting with fever and tachycardia could undergo a blood-based transcriptomic assay targeting OLFM4, S100A12, and HLA-DRA. Elevated OLFM4 and S100A12 combined with suppressed HLA-DRA could confirm sepsis within hours, enabling the prompt initiation of antibiotics and fluids, potentially reducing progression to septic shock. Such an assay, deployable via point-of-care platforms, could integrate with existing electronic health record systems to stratify patients by risk of organ dysfunction (e.g., high SOFA score) and guide immunomodulatory therapies, such as anti-inflammatory agents for hyperinflammatory profiles or immune stimulants for immunosuppressive states [42,45]. This approach addresses the current diagnostic delay and heterogeneity in sepsis management.

Normalized gene expression data were filtered to include genes with sufficient variance across samples. An unsigned adjacency matrix was created using a soft-thresholding power β, selected based on scale-free topology criteria. The topological overlap matrix (TOM) was computed to measure network connectivity. Genes were then hierarchically clustered and grouped into modules using dynamic tree cutting. Module eigengenes (MEs) were calculated to represent the expression profile of each module, and their correlation with clinical traits (sepsis vs. control) was assessed. Modules significantly correlated with sepsis status underwent functional enrichment analysis using GO terms and Reactome pathways.

5. Conclusions

This study provides a comprehensive transcriptomic landscape of early-stage sepsis, illustrating dual-pattern immune dysregulation characterized by innate immune hyperactivation and concurrent suppression of adaptive immunity, translation, and metabolism. Employing an integrative systems biology approach—MDS, differential expression, pathway enrichment, GSEA, K-means clustering, bi-clustering, and WGCNA—we identified multi-scale transcriptional signatures distinguishing sepsis patients from healthy controls.

Upregulated genes and pathways underscored excessive neutrophil activation, inflammatory signaling, and innate immune priming, whereas downregulated programs revealed widespread impairments in antigen presentation, protein synthesis, and energy metabolism. These concurrent opposing shifts highlight the immune paradox of sepsis: simultaneous hyperinflammation and immune paralysis [1,2,42].

Critically, WGCNA delineated distinct co-expression modules, such as the turquoise module enriched in inflammatory mediators and the blue module representing suppressed ribosomal and metabolic functions. These modular patterns validate and extend DEG findings by revealing higher-order transcriptional architecture and potential hub regulators [23,41,42,49].

Identifying these network-based modules advances current sepsis models by providing not only individual biomarkers but also functional gene circuits, informing future diagnostic or therapeutic strategies. Specifically, the suppression of translation-related and metabolic modules presents a promising axis for evaluating immune exhaustion and host resilience [42,44,45].

Collectively, this work deepens our understanding of early sepsis biology, laying the foundation for personalized, network-informed interventions targeting immune and metabolic dysregulation at the transcriptomic level.

By pinpointing actionable gene networks, our findings pave the way for point-of-care diagnostic tools and personalized therapies, potentially transforming sepsis management in critical care settings.

Supplementary Materials: The following supporting information can be downloaded at: https://www.mdpi.com/article/10.3390/ijms26146647/s1.

Author Contributions: Conceptualization, S.T. and K.B.; methodology, M.A., A.S. and N.A.-M.; software, S.T.; validation, S.T., K.B. and M.A.; formal analysis, S.T.; investigation, S.T.; resources, S.T. and K.B.; data curation, S.T. and K.B.; writing—original draft preparation, S.T.; writing—review and editing, S.T.; visualization, S.T.; supervision, S.T. and K.B.; project administration, S.T. and K.B.; funding acquisition, K.B. All authors have read and agreed to the published version of the manuscript.

Funding: This research was funded by the College of Medicine and Health Sciences, Arabian Gulf University, grant number E021-PI-10/17.

Institutional Review Board Statement: Ethical approval obtained from the Research and Ethics Committee of the Arabian Gulf University, reference number E021-PI-10/17, and the Research Technical Support Team of the Ministry of Health, reference number AURS/45/2019. Informed consent was obtained from all participants.

Informed Consent Statement: Informed consent was obtained from all subjects involved in the study.

Data Availability Statement: Data will be available upon request. To clarify, normalized gene expression matrices and de-identified clinical metadata (e.g., age, sex, sepsis status) are available upon reasonable request to the corresponding author, subject to ethics committee approval.

Conflicts of Interest: The authors declare no conflicts of interest. The authors declare that the research was conducted in the absence of any commercial or financial relationships that could be construed as a potential conflict of interest. The funders had no role in the design of the study; in the collection, analyses, or interpretation of data; in the writing of the manuscript; or in the decision to publish the results.

References

1. Singer, M.; Deutschman, C.S.; Seymour, C.W.; Shankar-Hari, M.; Annane, D.; Bauer, M.; Bellomo, R.; Bernard, G.R.; Chiche, J.-D.; Coopersmith, C.M.; et al. The third international consensus definitions for sepsis and septic shock (sepsis-3). *JAMA* **2016**, *315*, 801–810. [CrossRef] [PubMed]
2. Hotchkiss, R.S.; Monneret, G.; Payen, D. Sepsis-induced immunosuppression: From cellular dysfunctions to immunotherapy. *Nat. Rev. Immunol.* **2013**, *13*, 862–874. [CrossRef]
3. Tang, B.M.P.; McLean, A.S.; Huang, S.J.; Dawes, I.W.; Lin, R.C.Y. Gene-expression profiling of peripheral blood mononuclear cells in sepsis. *Crit. Care Med.* **2009**, *37*, 2324. [CrossRef]
4. Sweeney, T.E.; Shidham, A.; Wong, H.R.; Khatri, P. A comprehensive time-course–based multicohort analysis of sepsis and sterile inflammation reveals a robust diagnostic gene set. *Sci. Transl. Med.* **2015**, *7*, 287ra71. [CrossRef] [PubMed]
5. Maslove, D.M.; Wong, H.R. Gene expression profiling in sepsis: Timing, tissue, and translational considerations. *Trends Mol. Med.* **2014**, *20*, 204–213. [CrossRef]
6. Davenport, E.E.; Burnham, K.L.; Radhakrishnan, J.; Humburg, P.; Hutton, P.; Mills, T.C.; Rautanen, A.; Gordon, A.C.; Garrard, C.; Hill, A.V.S.; et al. Genomic landscape of the individual host response and outcomes in sepsis: A prospective cohort study. *Lancet Respir. Med.* **2016**, *4*, 259–271. [CrossRef]
7. Scicluna, B.P.; Klouwenberg, P.M.C.K.; van Vught, L.A.; Wiewel, M.A.; Ong, D.S.Y.; Zwinderman, A.H.; Franitza, M.; Toliat, M.R.; Nürnberg, P.; Hoogendijk, A.J.; et al. A molecular biomarker to diagnose community-acquired pneumonia on intensive care unit admission. *Am. J. Respir. Crit. Care Med.* **2015**, *192*, 826–835. [CrossRef]
8. Pérez-García, F.; Resino, S.; Gómez-Sánchez, E.; Gonzalo-Benito, H.; Fernández-Rodríguez, A.; Lorenzo-López, M.; Heredia-Rodríguez, M.; Gómez-Pesquera, E.; Tamayo, E.; Jiménez-Sousa, M.Á.; et al. *OLFM4* polymorphisms predict septic shock survival after major surgery. *Eur. J. Clin. Investig.* **2020**, *51*, e13416. [CrossRef]
9. Foell, D.; Wittkowski, H.; Vogl, T.; Roth, J. S100 proteins expressed in phagocytes: A novel group of damage-associated molecular pattern molecules. *J. Leukoc. Biol.* **2007**, *81*, 28–37. [CrossRef]
10. Zhang, Y.; Xing, C.-J.; Liu, X.; Li, Y.-H.; Jia, J.; Feng, J.-G.; Yang, C.-J.; Chen, Y.; Zhou, J. Thioredoxin-Interacting Protein (TXNIP) Knockdown Protects against Sepsis-Induced Brain Injury and Cognitive Decline in Mice by Suppressing Oxidative Stress and Neuroinflammation. *Oxidative Med. Cell. Longev.* **2022**, *2022*, 1–23. [CrossRef]
11. Flo, T.H.; Smith, K.D.; Sato, S.; Rodriguez, D.J.; Holmes, M.A.; Strong, R.K.; Akira, S.; Aderem, A. Lipocalin 2 mediates an innate immune response to bacterial infection by sequestrating iron. *Nature* **2004**, *432*, 917–921. [CrossRef]
12. Ramilo, O.; Allman, W.; Chung, W.; Mejias, A.; Ardura, M.; Glaser, C.; Wittkowski, K.M.; Piqueras, B.; Banchereau, J.; Palucka, A.K.; et al. Gene expression patterns in blood leukocytes discriminate patients with acute infections. *Blood* **2006**, *109*, 2066–2077. [CrossRef]
13. Wu, H.-P.; Chuang, L.-P.; Liu, P.-H.; Chu, C.-M.; Yu, C.-C.; Lin, S.-W.; Kao, K.-C.; Li, L.-F.; Chuang, D.-Y. Decreased Monocyte HLA-DR Expression in Patients with Sepsis and Acute Kidney Injury. *Medicina* **2022**, *58*, 1198. [CrossRef]
14. Pankla, R.; Buddhisa, S.; Berry, M.; Blankenship, D.M.; Bancroft, G.J.; Banchereau, J.; Lertmemongkolchai, G.; Chaussabel, D. Genomic transcriptional profiling identifies a candidate blood biomarker signature for the diagnosis of septicemic melioidosis. *Genome Biol.* **2009**, *10*, R127. [CrossRef]
15. Zweigner, J.; Gramm, H.-J.; Singer, O.C.; Wegscheider, K.; Schumann, R.R. High concentrations of lipopolysaccharide-binding protein in serum of patients with severe sepsis or septic shock inhibit the lipopolysaccharide response in human monocytes. *Blood* **2001**, *98*, 3800–3808. [CrossRef]
16. Meisel, C.; Schwab, J.M.; Prass, K.; Meisel, A.; Dirnagl, U. Central nervous system injury-induced immune deficiency syndrome. *Nat. Rev. Neurosci.* **2005**, *6*, 775–786. [CrossRef] [PubMed]
17. Venet, F.; Monneret, G. Advances in the understanding and treatment of sepsis-induced immunosuppression. *Nat. Rev. Nephrol.* **2017**, *14*, 121–137. [CrossRef] [PubMed]
18. Cavaillon, J.-M.; Adib-Conquy, M. Bench-to-bedside review: Endotoxin tolerance as a model of leukocyte reprogramming in sepsis. *Crit. Care* **2006**, *10*, 233. [CrossRef] [PubMed]
19. Medzhitov, R. Origin and physiological roles of inflammation. *Nature* **2008**, *454*, 428–435. [CrossRef]
20. Vandewalle, J.; Libert, C. Sepsis: A failing starvation response. *Trends Endocrinol Metab.* **2022**, *33*, 292–304. [CrossRef]
21. Wong, H.R.; Shanley, T.P.; Sakthivel, B.; Cvijanovich, N.; Lin, R.; Allen, G.L.; Thomas, N.J.; Doctor, A.; Kalyanaraman, M.; Tofil, N.M.; et al. Genome-level expression profiles in pediatric septic shock indicate a role for altered zinc homeostasis in poor outcome. *Physiol. Genom.* **2007**, *30*, 146–155. [CrossRef]
22. Mootha, V.K.; Lindgren, C.M.; Eriksson, K.-F.; Subramanian, A.; Sihag, S.; Lehar, J.; Puigserver, P.; Carlsson, E.; Ridderstråle, M.; Laurila, E.; et al. PGC-1α-responsive genes involved in oxidative phosphorylation are coordinately downregulated in human diabetes. *Nat. Genet.* **2003**, *34*, 267–273. [CrossRef]
23. Blander, J.M.; Sander, L.E. Beyond pattern recognition: Five immune checkpoints for scaling the microbial threat. *Nat. Rev. Immunol.* **2012**, *12*, 215–225. [CrossRef] [PubMed]

24. Gao, Z.; Feng, Y.; Xu, J.; Liang, J. T-cell exhaustion in immune-mediated inflammatory diseases: New implications for immunotherapy. *Front. Immunol.* **2022**, *13*, 977394. [CrossRef] [PubMed]
25. McKinney, E.F.; Smith, K.G. T cell exhaustion and immune-mediated disease—The potential for therapeutic exhaustion. *Curr. Opin. Immunol.* **2016**, *43*, 74–80. [CrossRef]
26. Subramanian, A.; Tamayo, P.; Mootha, V.K.; Mukherjee, S.; Ebert, B.L.; Gillette, M.A.; Paulovich, A.; Pomeroy, S.L.; Golub, T.R.; Lander, E.S.; et al. Gene set enrichment analysis: A knowledge-based approach for interpreting genome-wide expression profiles. *Proc. Natl. Acad. Sci. USA* **2005**, *102*, 15545–15550. [CrossRef]
27. Xu, J.; Li, J.; Xiao, K.; Zou, S.; Yan, P.; Xie, X.; Xie, L. Dynamic changes in human HLA-DRA gene expression and Th cell subsets in sepsis: Indications of immunosuppression and associated outcomes. *Scand. J. Immunol.* **2019**, *91*, e12813. [CrossRef]
28. dela Cruz, C.M.P.; Paner, J.R.O.; Nevado, J.B. Identification of Potential Prognosticators for Sepsis through Expression Analysis of Transcriptomic Data from Sepsis Survivors and Nonsurvivors. *Acta Med. Philipp.* **2023**, *57*, 11–23. [CrossRef] [PubMed]
29. Guo, P.; Wang, R.; Shen, J.; Zhang, L.; Mo, W. Identification of Key Inflammation-related Genes as Potential Diagnostic Biomarkers of Sepsis. *Altern. Ther. Health Med.* **2023**, *29*, 24–31.
30. Wang, T.; Fang, X.; Sheng, X.; Li, M.; Mei, Y.; Mei, Q.; Pan, A. Identification of immune characteristic biomarkers and therapeutic targets in cuproptosis for sepsis by integrated bioinformatics analysis and single-cell RNA sequencing analysis. *Heliyon* **2024**, *10*, e27379. [CrossRef]
31. Schouten, M.; Wiersinga, W.J.; Levi, M.; van der Poll, T. Inflammation, endothelium, and coagulation in sepsis. *J. Leukoc. Biol.* **2008**, *83*, 536–545. [CrossRef] [PubMed]
32. Schüller, S.S.; Kramer, B.W.; Villamor, E.; Spittler, A.; Berger, A.; Levy, O. Immunomodulation to prevent or treat neonatal sepsis: Past, present, and future. *Front. Pediatr.* **2018**, *6*, 199. [CrossRef]
33. Takeda, K.; Akira, S. Toll-like receptors in innate immunity. *Int. Immunol.* **2005**, *17*, 1–14. [CrossRef]
34. Yuk, J.M.; Jo, E.K. Toll-like receptors and innate immunity. *Biochem. Biophys. Res. Commun.* **2009**, *388*, 621–625. [CrossRef]
35. Coornaert, B.; Carpentier, I.; Beyaert, R. A20: Central gatekeeper in inflammation and immunity. *J. Biol. Chem.* **2009**, *284*, 8217–8221. [CrossRef]
36. Mussbacher, M.; Derler, M.; Basílio, J.; Schmid, J.A. NF-κB in monocytes and macrophages—An inflammatory master regulator in multitalented immune cells. *Front. Immunol.* **2023**, *14*, 1134661. [CrossRef]
37. Arina, P.; Singer, M. Pathophysiology of sepsis. *Curr. Opin. Anaesthesiol.* **2021**, *34*, 77–84. [CrossRef] [PubMed]
38. Koutroulis, I.; Batabyal, R.; McNamara, B.; Ledda, M.; Hoptay, C.; Freishtat, R.J. Sepsis Immunometabolism: From Defining Sepsis to Understanding How Energy Production Affects Immune Response. *Crit. Care Explor.* **2019**, *1*, e0061. [CrossRef]
39. Xiao, W.; Oldham, W.M.; Priolo, C.; Pandey, A.K.; Loscalzo, J. Immunometabolic Endothelial Phenotypes: Integrating Inflammation and Glucose Metabolism. *Circ. Res.* **2021**, *129*, 9–29. [CrossRef]
40. Liu, J.; Wang, H.; Xiao, H.; Ji, L.; Yao, Y.; Cao, C.; Liu, Y.; Huang, L. Predicting the prognosis in patients with sepsis by an endoplasmic reticulum stress gene signature. *Aging* **2023**, *15*, 13434–13451. [CrossRef]
41. Honore, P.M.; Jacobs, R.; Hendrickx, I.; Bagshaw, S.M.; Joannes-Boyau, O.; Boer, W.; De Waele, E.; Van Gorp, V.; Spapen, H.D. Prevention and treatment of sepsis-induced acute kidney injury: An update. *Ann. Intensiv. Care* **2015**, *5*, 1–10. [CrossRef] [PubMed]
42. He, J.; Zhao, S.; Duan, M. The Response of Macrophages in Sepsis-Induced Acute Kidney Injury. *J. Clin. Med.* **2023**, *12*, 1101. [CrossRef] [PubMed]
43. Liao, Y.; Pang, S.; Li, W.P.; Shtengel, G.; Choi, H.; Schaefer, K.; Xu, C.S.; Lippincott-Schwartz, J. A Mechanism for ER Exit Site Delivery Into Lysosomes Involving COPII, ALG2 and ESCRTs. *SSRN Electron. J.* **2022**. [CrossRef]
44. Rashid, A.; Brusletto, B.S.; Al-Obeidat, F.; Toufiq, M.; Benakatti, G.; Brierley, J.; Malik, Z.A.; Hussain, Z.; Alkhazaimi, H.; Sharief, J.; et al. A Transcriptomic Appreciation of Childhood Meningococcal and Polymicrobial Sepsis from a Pro-inflammatory and Trajectorial Perspective, a Role for VEGF-A and VEGF-B Modulation? *Shock* **2023**, *60*, 503–516. [CrossRef]
45. Abbas, M.; El-Manzalawy, Y. Machine learning based refined differential gene expression analysis of pediatric sepsis. *BMC Med. Genom.* **2020**, *13*, 1–10. [CrossRef]
46. Kim, J.Y.; Anderson, E.D.; Huynh, W.; Dey, A.; Ozato, K. Proteomic survey of ubiquitin-linked nuclear proteins in interferon-stimulated macrophages. *J. Interf. Cytokine Res.* **2011**, *31*, 619–628. [CrossRef] [PubMed]
47. Gómez, H.; Kellum, J.A.; Ronco, C. Metabolic reprogramming and tolerance during sepsis-induced AKI. *Nat. Rev. Nephrol.* **2017**, *13*, 143–151. [CrossRef]
48. Vanderhaeghen, T.; Vandewalle, J.; Libert, C. Hypoxia-inducible factors in metabolic reprogramming during sepsis. *FEBS J.* **2020**, *287*, 1478–1495. [CrossRef]
49. Liu, W.; Liu, T.; Zheng, Y.; Xia, Z. Metabolic Reprogramming and Its Regulatory Mechanism in Sepsis-Mediated Inflammation. *J. Inflamm. Res.* **2023**, *16*, 1195–1207. [CrossRef]
50. Liu, J.; Zhou, G.; Wang, X.; Liu, D. Metabolic reprogramming consequences of sepsis: Adaptations and contradictions. *Cell. Mol. Life Sci.* **2022**, *79*, 1–15. [CrossRef]

51. Vincent, J.-L.; Sakr, Y. Clinical trial design for unmet clinical needs: A spotlight on sepsis. *Expert Rev. Clin. Pharmacol.* **2019**, *12*, 893–900. [CrossRef] [PubMed]
52. Wen, R.; Liu, Y.P.; Tong, X.X.; Zhang, T.N.; Yang, N. Molecular mechanisms and functions of pyroptosis in sepsis and sepsis-associated organ dysfunction. *Front. Cell Infect. Microbiol.* **2022**, *12*, 962139. [CrossRef] [PubMed]
53. Yang, J.O.; Zinter, M.S.; Pellegrini, M.; Wong, M.Y.; Gala, K.; Markovic, D.; Nadel, B.; Peng, K.; Do, N.; Mangul, S.; et al. Whole blood transcriptomics identifies subclasses of pediatric septic shock. *Crit. Care* **2023**, *27*, 1–13. [CrossRef]
54. Dhillon, B.K.; Kortbeek, S.; Baghela, A.; Brindle, M.; Martin, D.-A.; Jenne, C.N.; Vogel, H.J.; Lee, A.H.Y.; Thompson, G.C.; Hancock, R.E.W. Gene Expression Profiling in Pediatric Appendicitis. *JAMA Pediatr.* **2024**, *178*, 391–400. [CrossRef] [PubMed]

International Journal of *Molecular Sciences*

MDPI

Article

Sex-Specific Differences in LPS-Induced Rapid Myocardial Dysfunction

Brianna I. Harvey [1,†], Arris M. Yoniles [1,†], Andrea Monsivais [1], Jiayue Du [1,2], Lauren Zadorozny [1,2], Qing Yu [1,2] and Meijing Wang [1,2,*]

1 Center for Surgical Sciences, Department of Surgery, Indiana University School of Medicine, Indianapolis, IN 46202, USA; ayoniles@iu.edu (A.M.Y.); qyu@iu.edu (Q.Y.)
2 Division of Cardiothoracic Surgery, Department of Surgery, Indiana University School of Medicine, Indianapolis, IN 46202, USA
* Correspondence: meiwang@iu.edu
† These authors contributed equally to this work.

Abstract: Cardiac dysfunction is a severe complication of sepsis that significantly increases mortality in affected patients. Previous studies have shown better myocardial responses with preserved cardiac function in female animals compared to males following lipopolysaccharide (LPS)-induced sepsis. Our published findings have revealed that females exhibited less cardiac dysfunction than males when exposed to equivalent doses of tumor necrosis factor (TNF)α, which is markedly elevated in both heart tissue and serum following LPS. These raise the question of whether the observed sex differences in LPS-induced myocardial dysfunction are a direct effect of LPS or a secondary consequence mediated by inflammatory cytokines, like TNFα. In this study, we aimed to uncover sex differences in LPS-caused direct effects on cardiac function. To do so, isolated hearts from aged-matched adult male and female mice were subjected to LPS infusion using a Langendorff method. Left ventricular developed pressure (LVDP) was continuously recorded. The female estrous cycle was determined via vaginal smear. The oxidative phosphorylation (OXPHOS) pathway and estrogen receptors (ERs) were determined in heart tissue using Western blot. We found that males exhibited worse LV function than females following the infusion of LPS at 5.0 mg/kg body weight. However, no significant differences in cardiac function and expression of ERs were observed between female groups at different estrous stages. Interestingly, LV function returned to baseline after the initial depression of LVDP during the rapid response to LPS and then depressed again following the 50 min LPS infusion. Protein levels of OXPHOS were altered differently between male and female hearts after 50 min LPS infusion. Our data demonstrate that male hearts exhibit higher sensitivity to LPS-induced rapid cardiac dysfunction compared to females, although estrogen may have a minimal influence on LPS-induced rapid functional depression. Sex differences may exist in myocardial mitochondrial responses to direct LPS insult via the OXPHOS pathway.

Keywords: cardiac dysfunction; endotoxemia; gender difference; OXPHOS

1. Introduction

Lipopolysaccharide (LPS), a component of the outer membrane of Gram-negative bacteria, is a major trigger of endotoxemia. LPS can lead to sepsis—a life-threatening syndrome marked by organ dysfunction due to a dysregulated host response. A serious complication of sepsis is cardiac dysfunction, known as sepsis-induced cardiomyopathy, which significantly contributes to increased mortality in septic patients [1–4]. Understanding the molecular mechanisms driving cardiac dysfunction and damage is critical for developing effective therapeutic approaches to improve patient outcomes.

Accumulating evidence suggests sex-specific differences in the cardiovascular system response to injury. Of note, previous studies have demonstrated that female animals exhibit improved myocardial responses and better cardiac function compared to males following LPS challenge [5,6]. However, it remains unclear whether these sex differences are due to the direct effects of LPS or are mediated by LPS-induced inflammatory cytokines. In fact, our published study, along with others, has shown a significant increase in tumor necrosis factor (TNF)α levels in both heart tissue and serum after LPS challenge [5,7–9]. In addition, females experienced less cardiac dysfunction than males when exposed to an equivalent dose of TNFα [10,11]. This suggests that sex-related disparities in myocardial impairment could be attributable to indirect or secondary effects of LPS-induced inflammatory cytokines, such as TNFα. Therefore, in this study, to simulate endotoxemia and assess myocardial responses without the influence of confounding blood-borne factors, we employed the Langendorff perfusion technique. We aimed to investigate the direct effects of LPS on cardiac function by administering a coronary infusion of LPS to isolated male and female mouse hearts.

2. Results

2.1. LPS Directly Induces Cardiac Functional Depression

The lethal dose (LD50—the dose causing death in 50% of the mice) of LPS is 10 mg/kg body weight for C57BL/6 mice [12]. We first conducted dose-responsive experiments with LPS at 0, 2.5, 5.0, and 7.5 mg/kg body weight in isolated male mouse hearts (the infusion concentrations of LPS were 0, 31.25, 62.5, and 93.75 µg/mL, according to if a mouse had a total blood volume of about 80 mL/kg body weight [13]). Our data demonstrated that myocardial function was impaired by direct LPS infusion (Figure 1B), with a significant depression of left ventricular developed pressure (LVDP), and the maximal positive and negative values of the first derivative of pressure (+dP/dt and −dP/dt) in doses of LPS at 5 and 7.5 mg/kg body weight. However, the infusion of LPS at 2.5 mg/kg body weight did not cause myocardial dysfunction in male hearts. Of note, the 7.5 mg/kg dose of LPS resulted in a comparable level of cardiac functional depression to that observed with the 5 mg/kg LPS infusion (Figure 1B), in line with the previous report showing that both 5 and 10 mg/kg LPS challenges caused a substantial and comparable reduction in cardiac function in vivo [14]. In addition, we found that the myocardium responded to LPS as quickly as 5 min after a 5 mg/kg infusion of LPS (Figure 1A). Collectively, we did not increase the LPS dose further to 10 mg/kg and selected 5 mg/kg to investigate the direct effect of LPS on cardiac dysfunction in male versus female hearts in the experiments.

2.2. Male Hearts Experienced Greater Depression of Myocardial Function Compared to Female Hearts in Response to Infusion of LPS at 5 mg/kg Body Weight

Following exposure to a 5 mg/kg infusion of LPS, male myocardial function significantly decreased by about 50% in LVDP and −dP/dt and by 40% in dP/dt (Figure 2A), while female hearts exhibited a decrease of approximately 30% in LVDP and 20% in dP/dt and −dP/dt, highlighting a sex difference in LPS-induced acute myocardial functional depression. Additionally, LPS triggered a significantly faster cardiac response in male hearts (6.15 $\pm$ 1.22 min) compared to female myocardium (13.09 $\pm$ 1.92 min) (Figure 2B).

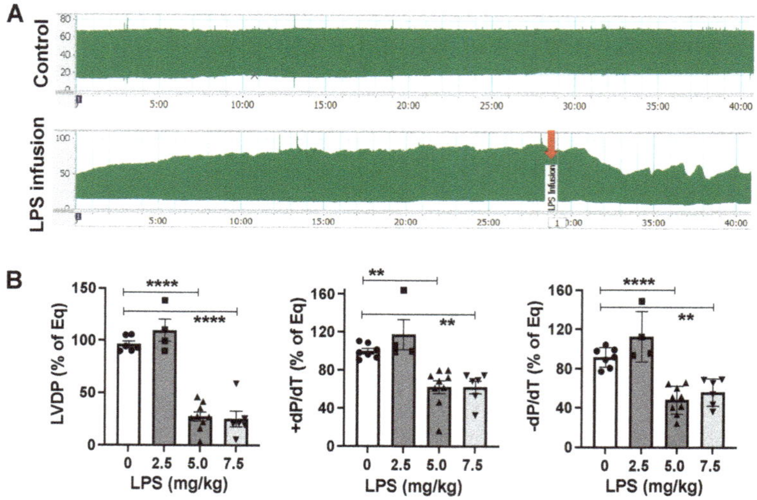

Figure 1. (**A**) LVDP (left ventricular developed pressure) trace in male hearts without (control) or with LPS infusion (5.0 mg/kg). (**B**) Dose–response study of LPS infusion in isolated male mouse hearts using Langendorff technique. Dots represent individual mouse heart function. Mean +/− SEM, ** $p < 0.01$, **** $p < 0.0001$.

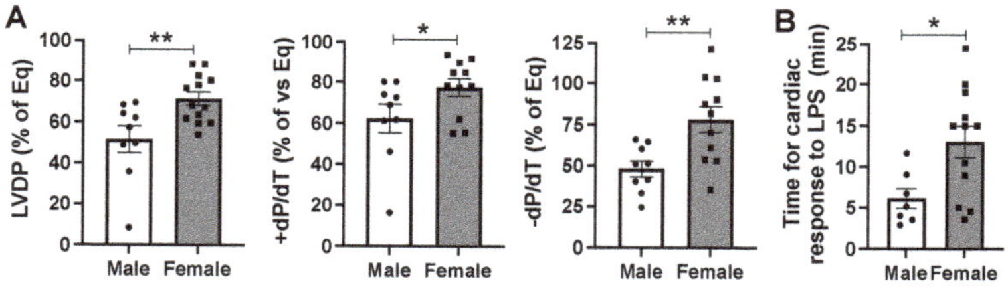

Figure 2. (**A**) Heart function in male and female hearts after infusion of 5.0 mg/kg LPS at rapid response/initial depression of LV function. (**B**) Time required for rapid response/initial depression of LV function in male and female hearts after infusion of 5.0 mg/kg LPS. Dots represent individual mouse heart values. Mean +/− SEM, * $p < 0.05$, ** $p < 0.01$.

2.3. Effects of Estrous Cycle on LPS Caused Myocardial Dysfunction in Females and LPS' Role in Modulating Expression of Estrogen Receptors in Male and Female Hearts

Estrogen, a sex hormone, plays a role in influencing cardiac function during injury. Female animals at different estrous stages have varying estrogen levels, which may impact myocardial responses to LPS. To explore this, we divided the female mice into two groups based on vaginal smear results (Figure 3A) as follows: proestrus/estrus females with high estrogen levels and metestrus/diestrus females with low estrogen levels. Interestingly, there was no significant difference in myocardial function between proestrus/estrus and metestrus/diestrus females following a 5 mg/kg infusion of LPS (Figure 3B). Additionally, considering that estrogen exerts its biological function through binding to estrogen receptors (ERs), we investigated whether the differential expression of the classical receptors ERα and ERβ occurs in the heart following LPS infusion. We found that there were no sex differences in the myocardial expression of ERα and ERβ without LPS stress (Figure 3(C1,C2,D1,D2)). In addition, LPS did not change the levels of ERα and ERβ in male hearts (Figure 3(C2,D2)). However, significantly reduced ERα and ERβ expression was observed in female hearts following LPS infusion (Figure 3(C2,D2)). Furthermore, the estrus cycle did not alter LPS-decreased levels of ERα and ERβ in female hearts (Figure 3(C3,D3)).

These data suggest that estrogen and/or estrogen signaling may not influence the direct effects of LPS on myocardial function.

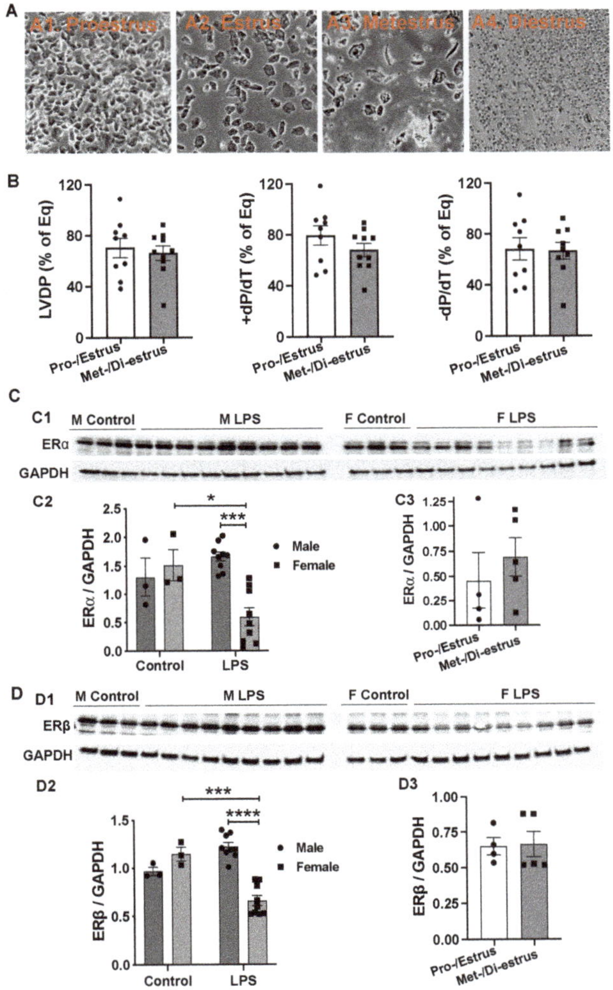

Figure 3. (**A**) Estrus cycle in female mice by vaginal smear. High-estrogen stages: (**A1**) proestrus with clusters of well-formed nucleated epithelial cells; (**A2**) estrus with clusters of cornified squamous epithelial cells. Low-estrogen stages: (**A3**) metestrus shows fragmented cornified squamous epithelial cells accompanied by small leukocytes; (**A4**) diestrus dominated by small leukocytes with few cornified squamous epithelial cells. (**B**) Cardiac function in female mouse hearts during proestrus/estrus (high estrogen) versus metestrus/diestrus (low estrogen) phases following LPS infusion. (**C**) ERα expression in male and female hearts without LPS infusion. (**C1**) Western blot images of ERα and GAPDH across groups; (**C2**) quantification of ERα band intensity normalized to GAPDH; (**C3**) comparison of relative ERα levels (normalized to GAPDH) between high-estrogen (proestrus/estrus) and low-estrogen (metestrus/diestrus) female hearts following LPS infusion. (**D**) ERβ expression in male and female hearts +/− LPS infusion. (**D1**) Western blot images of ERβ and GAPDH among groups; (**D2**) quantification of ERβ band intensity normalized to GAPDH; (**D3**) comparison of relative ERβ levels (normalized to GAPDH) between high-estrogen (proestrus/estrus) and low-estrogen (metestrus/diestrus) female hearts after LPS infusion. Dots represent individual mouse heart functions. Mean +/− SEM; two-way ANOVA in C2 and D2, *t*-test in others; * $p < 0.05$, *** $p < 0.001$, **** $p < 0.0001$.

2.4. Effects of Longer LPS Infusion on Isolated Male and Female Heart Function and on Myocardial Expression of Toll-like Receptor 4

Notably, when the duration of the LPS infusion (5 mg/kg body weight) was extended to 50 min (50′), we observed that LV function returned to normal after the initial rapid depression/first response to the LPS (<20′ infusion). However, LV function significantly decreased again in male hearts following the 50′-LPS infusion (Figure 4A,B). In contrast, although female hearts showed a similar trend, no statistically significant difference was observed during the 50′-LPS infusion (Figure 4C). This suggests that the female myocardium may be more tolerant to direct LPS-induced injury.

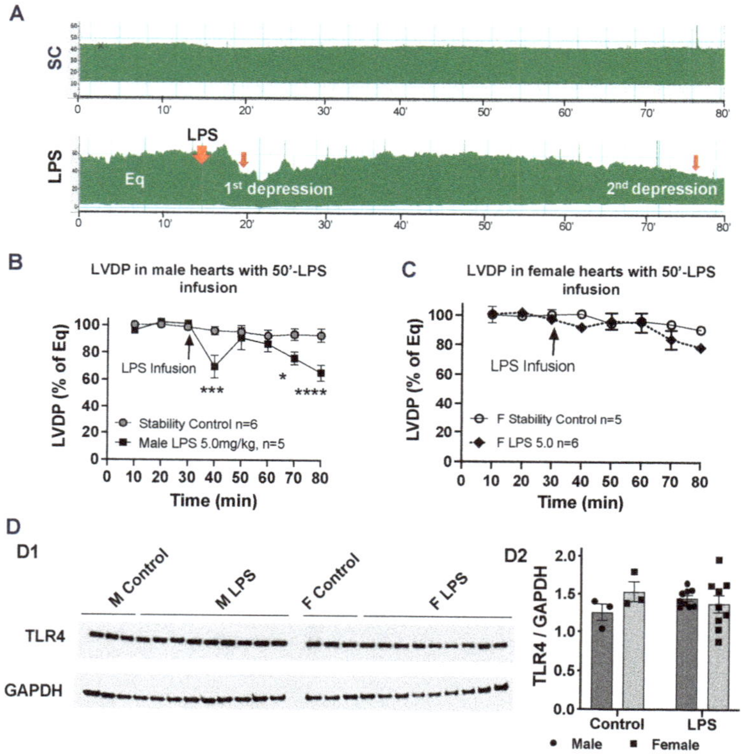

Figure 4. (**A**) Representative LVDP trace of male stability control (SC) with 80 min of perfusate perfusion and male heart with 50 min of LPS infusion (5.0 mg/kg). Changes in LVDP in SC and LPS-infused male hearts (**B**) and female hearts (**C**). (**D**) TLR4 expression in LPS-infused male and female hearts compared to their untreated counterparts. (**D1**) Western blot images of TLR4 and GAPDH across groups; (**D2**) quantification of TLR4 band intensity normalized to GAPDH. Mean +/− SEM; two-way ANOVA; * $p < 0.05$, *** $p < 0.001$, **** $p < 0.0001$.

LPS binds to Toll-like receptor 4 (TLR4), initiating the LPS/TLR4 signaling pathway to exert its biological effects. Therefore, we assessed myocardial TLR4 expression in male and female hearts in response to LPS infusion. We found that LPS infusion did not change TLR4 levels in either male or female hearts (Figure 4D).

2.5. Direct Effects of LPS on Myocardial Mitochondrial OXPHOS Between Male and Female Hearts

LPS has been shown to impair mitochondrial metabolism in vivo via the OXPHOS pathway in the heart [15]. To dissect the molecular mechanisms underlying the sex differences in LPS-induced cardiac dysfunction, we examined the myocardial protein levels of mitochondrial OXPHOS. Increased levels of ATP5A, UQCRC2, and NDUF8 were observed in male hearts following 50′-LPS infusion (Figure 5A,B), whereas 50′-LPS infusion significantly reduced UQCRC2 and MTCO1 levels in female hearts (Figure 5A,B), indicating sex-specific differences in myocardial mitochondrial responses to direct LPS insult.

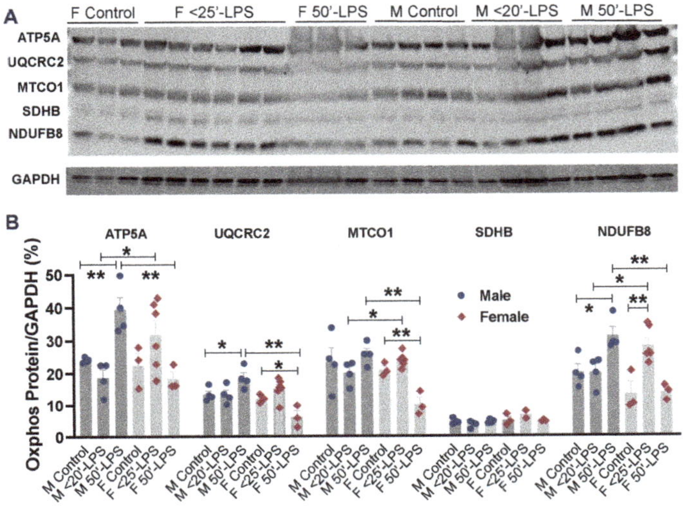

Figure 5. (**A**) Immunoblots of five OXPHOS protein levels in female (F) and male (M) hearts with +/− <25 min or 50 min LPS infusion. (**B**) Quantification of immunoblotting band intensity of ATP5A-complex V, UQCRC2-complex III, MTCO1-complex IV, SDHB-complex II, and NDUFB8-complex I compared to GAPDH, respectively. Mean +/− SEM; * $p < 0.05$, ** $p < 0.01$. One-way ANOVA with multiple comparisons within the same sex group and a *t*-test between M and F at the same dose of LPS infusion.

3. Discussion

Sex differences in myocardial responses have been reported following LPS challenge in vivo [5,6]. However, our published studies and others have indicated that inflammatory cytokines, including TNFα, substantially increased following LPS injection [5,7–9]. Additionally, male hearts had more severe cardiac contractile depression than female hearts when exposed to TNFα [10,11], raising the question as to whether sex differences in the myocardial response to LPS in vivo are due to LPS-increased inflammatory cytokines in the circulation, particularly TNFα. In this study, we investigated the direct effects of LPS on myocardial function between male and female hearts using the Langendorff approach, which eliminates the influence of confounding blood-borne factors. Our results showed that when exposed to the same dose of LPS (1) male hearts experienced greater myocardial functional depression compared to female hearts; (2) no significant differences in cardiac dysfunction and myocardial ER expression were observed between proestrus/estrus and metestrus/diestrus females; and (3) distinct differences in OXPHOS responses were noticed between male and female hearts.

LPS is a pathogen-associated molecule and functions as TLR4 agonists to initiate the LPS/TLR4 signaling pathway. All cardiac cell types including cardiomyocytes express TLR4 [16]. However, most studies focus on evaluating LPS/TLR4 signaling in inflammatory responses and reactive oxygen species (ROS) production [17,18], thus subsequently regulating myocardial function during endotoxemia. In fact, LPS decreased the sarcoplasmic reticulum Ca^{2+} content, the systolic Ca^{2+} transient, and cardiomyocyte contraction, all of which were reversed by using the TLR4-specific inhibitor or deletion of TLR4 [19]. While LPS-induced cardiomyocyte impairment requires TLR4 on immune cells not on cardiomyocytes, as LPS does not cause myocyte shortening in mice with TLR4-deficient leukocytes [20], other studies have challenged this view by demonstrating that LPS-depressed cardiac function was not observed in mice with TLR4KO in cardiomyocytes [21]. Such a discrepancy may be due to the in vivo LPS treatment, which induces systematic responses and changes in blood-borne factors to complicate outcomes. In the current study, we explored the direct effects of LPS on impairing myocardial function in isolated mouse hearts, excluding other confounding variables. Our previous work has also shown that the direct infusion of LPS into isolated rat hearts via coronary delivery led to a progressive depression of LV contractile function [22]. Interestingly, in this study, we found that the myocardial responses to LPS appeared time-dependent, with a cycle of rapid depression, returning to normal, and decreasing in LV function again along with continuing LPS infusion. This result suggests that a low dose/amount of LPS (the first depression) likely induces the defense mechanisms to prevent the heart from further injury, leading to LV function returning to normal. Our finding confirmed the possibility to use LPS for eliciting the preconditioning mechanism in the heart, aligning with the previous studies in which LPS induced preconditioning to improve postischemic cardiac function and reduce infarct size against myocardial infarction [23–25].

Of note, sex differences have been observed in the prognosis of sepsis. Clinically, epidemiological studies consistently indicate that severe sepsis with developed organ dysfunction/failure, including cardiac dysfunction, often occur in male patients [26–29]. In line with this, myocardial functional depression was significantly less noticeable in female mice compared to males following LPS (3 mg/kg) injection [5]. Additionally, endotoxic shock remained in male rats with depressed LV function and decreased stork work 24 h after LPS challenge, whereas cardiac function was significantly improved in 24 h LPS-treated female rats [6]. In our study, by excluding the confounding systematic and blood-borne influences, sex differences in cardiac dysfunction were further noticed following the direct infusion of LPS, with female mouse hearts more resistant to an equal amount of LPS compared to male hearts. Accumulated evidence has reported that the sex differences in cardiac function and inflammatory responses appears attributable to sex hormones—estrogen and its downstream signals during endotoxemia [8]. Using estrogen or selective agonists of ERs protected male rats against LPS-induced damage, while the depletion of estrogen by ovariectomy worsened the detrimental effects of LPS on female rats [8,30]. To this end, we investigated whether estrogen played a role in LPS-induced rapid LV dysfunction in female mice with various estrogen levels in the present study. However, we did not see significant differences in the LPS-depressed cardiac function between the proestrus/estrus and metestrus/diestrus female hearts, implying that fluctuations in estrogen may have little influence on the acute myocardial response to LPS. Notably, LPS significantly reduced the myocardial expression of ERα and ERβ in female hearts but not in male hearts. Interestingly, endogenous estrogen levels did not appear to impact the levels of ERs. These findings suggest potentially changed estrogen signaling in female hearts compared to the male myocardium during endotoxemia, warranting further investigation.

Next, we asked a question as to how differences in myocardial dysfunction following the direct infusion of LPS exist between male and female mouse hearts. Indeed, accumulating evidence has shown sex differences in sarcomeric protein composition and calcium-handling function, contributing to stronger and faster contractions in male cardiomyocytes compared to female cells [31,32]. These sex-specific differences in cardiac structure and function may influence the heart's response to LPS infusion. However, we did not observe differences in TLR4 levels between male and female hearts in response to LPS, suggesting that the observed sex disparities in cardiac function are not due to differential TLR4 signaling following LPS infusion. Nevertheless, the Four Core Genotypes mouse model can be employed in future studies to investigate the relative contributions of sex chromosomes and gonadal sex to the molecular mechanisms underlying sex differences during sepsis.

On the other hand, compelling evidence has suggested a key role of mitochondrial dysfunction and metabolic shutdown in the pathogenesis of sepsis-induced organ dysfunction/failure [33,34]. Notably, emerging studies raise the possibility that cardiac mitochondria are more vulnerable to sepsis-induced impairment than those from kidneys, the liver, and skeletal muscles [35–37]. In fact, sex differences in mitochondrial function have been reported, with less mitochondrial ROS production and oxidative damage in female hearts [38–40]. Our previous study has also shown better mitochondrial metabolic function in cardiomyocytes from female mice compared to those from males when exposed to inflammatory mediators—TNFα or oxidative stress—H_2O_2 [41]. In the present study, we observed a significant increase in mitochondrial respiratory chain proteins complex I-NDUFB8, complex III-UQCRC2, and complex V-ATP5A in male mouse hearts subjected to LPS, while there was a marked decrease in complex III-UQCRC2 and complex IV-MTCO1 in the LPS-infused female mouse hearts. The activity of mitochondrial complex I determines the overall electron flux through the respiratory chain (complexes I-IV), significantly contributing to ROS production. Elevated levels of complex I have been observed in the male brain [42,43], which may help explain the higher oxidative stress reported in males [44]. Our findings of increased complex I content are consistent with these observations, suggesting that sex differences likely exist in mitochondrial respiratory function, with female hearts experiencing less oxidative stress than male hearts following 50 min of LPS infusion. In addition, our results on sex differences in OXPHOS enzyme content may also suggest differing adaptive capacities to altered metabolic conditions between male and female hearts. Indeed, stressed females exhibited a more protective and resilient phenotype of major mitochondrial respiratory complexes compared to males [45]. Furthermore, enhanced metabolic adaptability has been reported in female skeletal muscle under changed energy conditions [46].

Limitations: In this study, we utilized a dose of LPS at 5 mg/kg body weight to investigate sex differences in cardiac dysfunction. It is unknown whether these sex disparities persist with higher doses of LPS. Additionally, the longest duration of LPS infusion in the current study was 50 min, and it remains unclear what effects might occur with an infusion lasting longer than 50 min. While vaginal smear can serve as a useful tool for training medical students in basic techniques in the current study, measuring estradiol levels in serum provides more accurate results for determining estrogen level in circulation and should be used in future research. Furthermore, future studies incorporating exogenous estrogen or ER modulators (both agonists and antagonists) into the perfusate should be undertaken to investigate the role of exogenous estrogen and membrane-associated ERs in acute/rapid cardioprotection during LPS infusion.

4. Materials and Methods

4.1. Animals

Male and female C57BL/6J mice (9–12 weeks) were purchased from Jackson Laboratories (Bar Harbor, ME, USA). All mice were acclimated for >5 days with a standard diet feeding prior to the experiments. Age-matched male and female mice at 12–16 weeks old were used for the experiments. The animal protocol was reviewed and approved by the Institutional Animal Care and Use Committee of Indiana University. All animals received humane care in compliance with the Guide for the Care and Use of Laboratory Animals (NIH Pub. No. 85-23, revised 1996).

4.2. Assessment of Cardiac Function Using Langendorff Method

A modified isovolumetric Langendorff technique was employed to evaluate intrinsic cardiac contractility without or with LPS infusion. Isolated mouse hearts were subjected to the Langendorff technique, as previously described [10,11,22,47,48]. Briefly, mice were anesthetized with isoflurane and heparinized (100 IU i.p.). Hearts were then rapidly excised into ice-cold Krebs–Henseleit (K-H) buffer. The aorta was annulated under a dissection microscope and the heart was perfused in the isovolumetric Langendorff mode (70 mmHg) with oxygenated (95% O_2-5% CO_2) K-H solution (37 °C). The hearts were paced at 420–460 bpm/min during the whole experimental time. Data were continuously recorded using a PowerLab 8 preamplifier/digitizer (ADInstruments Inc., Colorado Springs, CO, USA). The LVDP was measured, +dP/dt and −dP/dt) were calculated using PowerLab software (LabChart 8).

4.3. Experimental Protocols

A dose–response study was performed in isolated adult male mouse hearts with LPS (from *Escherichia coli* O127:B8, L3129, MilliporeSigma, Burlington, MA, USA) at 0, 2.5, 5.0, and 7.5 mg/kg body weight. The infusion concentrations of LPS were 0, 31.25, 62.5, and 93.75 μg/mL, based on the fact that the total blood volume of a mouse is approximately 80 mL/kg [13]. Isolated mouse hearts were subjected to an infusion protocol consisting of a minimum 20 min equilibration period, followed by LPS infusion through the aortic root. The experimental workflow is shown in Figure 6. The concentration was determined with 5 mg/kg body weight (62.5 μg/mL) for all experiments in female hearts and the study in male hearts with a 50 min infusion period. The hearts were harvested at the time point when a significant depression of LVDP occurred, with a >20% drop following LPS infusion in male hearts and a >10% drop in female hearts and after a 50 min infusion period. Heart tissue was snap-frozen in liquid nitrogen and stored at −80 °C.

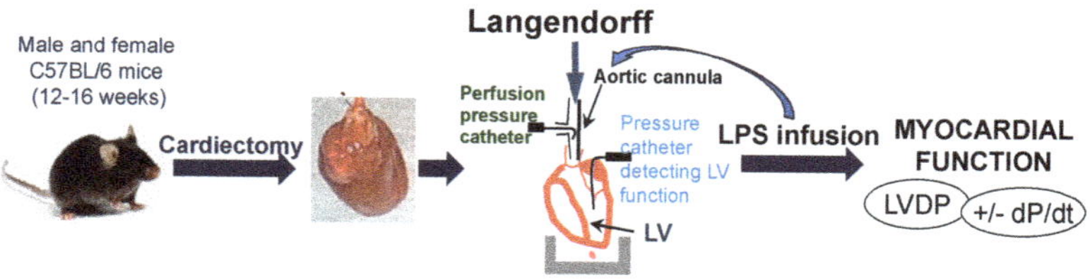

Figure 6. The scheme shows the experimental workflow.

4.4. Vaginal Smear

After the heart was removed, 50 μL of sterile PBS was gently introduced into the vaginal canal of female mice using a pipette. The pipette was aspirated and dispensed several times to wash the vaginal canal and collect an adequate number of cells for a single sample. The fluid was then placed on a glass slide. After allowing the smear to air dry for 10 min, it was examined under light microscopy, and photomicrographs were taken. The images were analyzed by at least three researchers to determine the cell type present. Based on vaginal cytology, four estrus stages were identified [49], namely proestrus, characterized by clusters of well-formed nucleated epithelial cells; estrus, marked by clusters of cornified squamous epithelial cells; metestrus, showing fragmented cornified squamous epithelial cells with small leukocytes; and diestrus, dominated by small leukocytes with a few cornified squamous epithelial cells.

4.5. Western Blotting

The heart tissues were lysed in cold RIPA buffer containing Halt protease and phosphatase inhibitor cocktail (ThermoFisher Scientific, Waltham, MA, USA). The protein extracts (10–20 μg) from heart tissue were subjected to electrophoresis on a 4–15% Criterion TGX Precast midi protein gel (Bio-Rad, Hercules, CA, USA) and transferred to a nitrocellulose membrane. The membranes were incubated with the following primary antibodies, respectively: OXPHOS antibody cocktail (complex I-NDUFB8, complex II-SDHB, complex IV-MTCO1, complex III-UQCRC2, and complex V-ATP5A) (ThermoFisher Scientific), ERα (SC-543), ERβ (SC-8974), TLR4 (SC-293072) (Santa Cruz, Dallas, TX, USA), and GAPDH (#5174) (Cell Signaling Technology, Beverly, MA, USA), followed by a HRP-conjugated secondary antibody. The images were detected by a ChemiDoc system (Bio-Rad). Image J software (Version 1.51, NIH) was utilized for immunoblotting band density measurement.

4.6. Statistical Analysis

All reported results were means ± SEM, and each dot was an individual heart measurement. Data were checked for variables using the Shapiro–Wilk normality test and then evaluated using an unpaired t-test or analysis of variance (ANOVA) followed by a multiple comparisons test. Differences were considered statistically significant when $p < 0.05$. All statistical analyses were performed using GraphPad Prism (Version 10.5.0, GraphPad, La Jolla, CA, USA).

5. Conclusions

In summary, the present study clearly demonstrates that sex differences exist in cardiac dysfunction following the direct infusion of LPS, with significantly depressed LV contractile function in male hearts compared to female hearts. Given the comparable levels of LPS-induced cardiac dysfunction between the proestrus/estrus and metestrus/diestrus groups, estrogen itself may have little effect on female hearts in response to direct LPS infusion. However, the current findings cannot fully rule out estrogen's role in regulating the female myocardial response to LPS infusion for the two following reasons: (1) it remains unclear whether estrogen levels varied in the hearts of female mice at different estrus stages and (2) the isolated hearts were perfused with the same buffer without estrogen. Further research is needed to explore the mechanisms behind sex-mediated LPS-induced cardiac dysfunction, particularly the mitochondrial factors driving differences in the myocardium. Understanding these important unknowns could pave the way for the development of novel therapies for septic cardiomyopathy.

Author Contributions: Conceptualization, M.W.; methodology, B.I.H., A.M.Y., A.M., J.D., Q.Y., and M.W.; formal analysis, A.M.Y., J.D., L.Z., and M.W.; investigation, B.I.H., A.M.Y., A.M., and L.Z.; resources, M.W.; data curation, Q.Y. and M.W.; writing—original draft preparation, B.I.H. and M.W.; writing—review and editing, B.I.H., A.M.Y., A.M., J.D., L.Z., Q.Y., and M.W.; supervision, M.W.; funding acquisition, M.W. All authors have read and agreed to the published version of the manuscript.

Funding: This research was funded by the National Institutes of Health-National Heart, Lung, and Blood Institute (NIH-NHLBI) R01 HL155957 (to M. Wang) and the Indiana University School of Medicine Strategic Research Initiative. We also acknowledge the Indiana University Medical Student Program for Research and Scholarship (IMPRS) for supporting the medical students working on this project during the summer. The content is solely the responsibility of the authors and does not necessarily represent the official views of the funding agencies.

Institutional Review Board Statement: The animal study protocol was approved by the Institutional Animal Care and Use Committee of Indiana University (protocol #23000 and date of approval 31

March 2023). All animals received humane care in compliance with the Guide for the Care and Use of Laboratory Animals (NIH Pub. No. 85-23, revised 1996).

Informed Consent Statement: Not applicable.

Data Availability Statement: Data is contained within the article.

Conflicts of Interest: The authors declare no conflicts of interest.

Abbreviations

LPS	lipopolysaccharide
LVDP	left ventricular developed pressure
OXPHOS	oxidative phosphorylation
+/− dP/dt	positive and negative values of the first derivative of pressure
ROS	reactive oxygen species
TLR4	Toll-like receptor 4
TNFα	tumor necrosis factor α

References

1. Martin, G.S.; Mannino, D.M.; Eaton, S.; Moss, M. The epidemiology of sepsis in the United States from 1979 through 2000. *N. Engl. J. Med.* **2003**, *348*, 1546–1554. [CrossRef]
2. Paoli, C.J.; Reynolds, M.A.; Sinha, M.; Gitlin, M.; Crouser, E. Epidemiology and Costs of Sepsis in the United States-An Analysis Based on Timing of Diagnosis and Severity Level. *Crit. Care Med.* **2018**, *46*, 1889–1897. [CrossRef] [PubMed]
3. Landesberg, G.; Gilon, D.; Meroz, Y.; Georgieva, M.; Levin, P.D.; Goodman, S.; Avidan, A.; Beeri, R.; Weissman, C.; Jaffe, A.S.; et al. Diastolic dysfunction and mortality in severe sepsis and septic shock. *Eur. Heart J.* **2012**, *33*, 895–903. [CrossRef]
4. Sanfilippo, F.; Corredor, C.; Fletcher, N.; Landesberg, G.; Benedetto, U.; Foex, P.; Cecconi, M. Diastolic dysfunction and mortality in septic patients: A systematic review and meta-analysis. *Intensive Care Med.* **2015**, *41*, 1004–1013. [CrossRef] [PubMed]
5. Chen, J.; Chiazza, F.; Collino, M.; Patel, N.S.; Coldewey, S.M.; Thiemermann, C. Gender dimorphism of the cardiac dysfunction in murine sepsis: Signalling mechanisms and age-dependency. *PLoS ONE* **2014**, *9*, e100631. [CrossRef] [PubMed]
6. Goncalves, R.P.; Guarido, K.L.; Assreuy, J.; da Silva-Santos, J.E. Gender-specific differences in the in situ cardiac function of endotoxemic rats detected by pressure-volume catheter. *Shock* **2014**, *42*, 415–423. [CrossRef]
7. Wang, M.; Meng, X.; Tsai, B.; Wang, J.F.; Turrentine, M.; Brown, J.W.; Meldrum, D.R. Preconditioning up-regulates the soluble TNF receptor I response to endotoxin. *J. Surg. Res.* **2004**, *121*, 20–24. [CrossRef]
8. El-Lakany, M.A.; Fouda, M.A.; El-Gowelli, H.M.; El-Gowilly, S.M.; El-Mas, M.M. Gonadal hormone receptors underlie the resistance of female rats to inflammatory and cardiovascular complications of endotoxemia. *Eur. J. Pharmacol.* **2018**, *823*, 41–48. [CrossRef]
9. Zhu, H.; Shan, L.; Peng, T. Rac1 mediates sex difference in cardiac tumor necrosis factor-alpha expression via NADPH oxidase-ERK1/2/p38 MAPK pathway in endotoxemia. *J. Mol. Cell. Cardiol.* **2009**, *47*, 264–274. [CrossRef]
10. Wang, M.; Tsai, B.M.; Crisostomo, P.R.; Meldrum, D.R. Tumor necrosis factor receptor 1 signaling resistance in the female myocardium during ischemia. *Circulation* **2006**, *114*, I282–I289. [CrossRef]
11. Sando, I.C.; Wang, Y.; Crisostomo, P.R.; Markel, T.A.; Sharma, R.; Erwin, G.S.; Guzman, M.J.; Meldrum, D.R.; Wang, M. Females exhibit relative resistance to depressive effects of tumor necrosis factor-alpha on the myocardium. *J. Surg. Res.* **2008**, *150*, 92–99. [CrossRef]
12. Fink, M.P. Animal models of sepsis. *Virulence* **2014**, *5*, 143–153. [CrossRef] [PubMed]
13. Harkness, J.E.; Wagner, J.E. *The Biology and Medicine of Rabbits and Rodents*, 3rd ed.; Lea & Febiger: Philadelphia, PA, USA, 1989; p. 230.
14. Sun, Y.; Yao, X.; Zhang, Q.J.; Zhu, M.; Liu, Z.P.; Ci, B.; Xie, Y.; Carlson, D.; Rothermel, B.A.; Sun, Y.; et al. Beclin-1-Dependent Autophagy Protects the Heart During Sepsis. *Circulation* **2018**, *138*, 2247–2262. [CrossRef]
15. Zang, Q.S.; Martinez, B.; Yao, X.; Maass, D.L.; Ma, L.; Wolf, S.E.; Minei, J.P. Sepsis-induced cardiac mitochondrial dysfunction involves altered mitochondrial-localization of tyrosine kinase Src and tyrosine phosphatase SHP2. *PLoS ONE* **2012**, *7*, e43424. [CrossRef]
16. Frantz, S.; Kobzik, L.; Kim, Y.D.; Fukazawa, R.; Medzhitov, R.; Lee, R.T.; Kelly, R.A. Toll4 (TLR4) expression in cardiac myocytes in normal and failing myocardium. *J. Clin. Investig.* **1999**, *104*, 271–280. [CrossRef]
17. Avlas, O.; Fallach, R.; Shainberg, A.; Porat, E.; Hochhauser, E. Toll-like receptor 4 stimulation initiates an inflammatory response that decreases cardiomyocyte contractility. *Antioxid. Redox Signal.* **2011**, *15*, 1895–1909. [CrossRef] [PubMed]

18. Zhao, H.; Zhang, M.; Zhou, F.; Cao, W.; Bi, L.; Xie, Y.; Yang, Q.; Wang, S. Cinnamaldehyde ameliorates LPS-induced cardiac dysfunction via TLR4-NOX4 pathway: The regulation of autophagy and ROS production. *J. Mol. Cell. Cardiol.* **2016**, *101*, 11–24. [CrossRef]
19. Yang, J.; Zhang, R.; Jiang, X.; Lv, J.; Li, Y.; Ye, H.; Liu, W.; Wang, G.; Zhang, C.; Zheng, N.; et al. Toll-like receptor 4-induced ryanodine receptor 2 oxidation and sarcoplasmic reticulum Ca^{2+} leakage promote cardiac contractile dysfunction in sepsis. *J. Biol. Chem.* **2018**, *293*, 794–807. [CrossRef] [PubMed]
20. Tavener, S.A.; Long, E.M.; Robbins, S.M.; McRae, K.M.; Van Remmen, H.; Kubes, P. Immune cell Toll-like receptor 4 is required for cardiac myocyte impairment during endotoxemia. *Circ. Res.* **2004**, *95*, 700–707. [CrossRef]
21. Fallach, R.; Shainberg, A.; Avlas, O.; Fainblut, M.; Chepurko, Y.; Porat, E.; Hochhauser, E. Cardiomyocyte Toll-like receptor 4 is involved in heart dysfunction following septic shock or myocardial ischemia. *J. Mol. Cell. Cardiol.* **2010**, *48*, 1236–1244. [CrossRef]
22. Wang, M.; Sankula, R.; Tsai, B.M.; Meldrum, K.K.; Turrentine, M.; March, K.L.; Brown, J.W.; Dinarello, C.A.; Meldrum, D.R. P38 MAPK mediates myocardial proinflammatory cytokine production and endotoxin-induced contractile suppression. *Shock* **2004**, *21*, 170–174. [CrossRef] [PubMed]
23. Meng, X.; Brown, J.M.; Ao, L.; Shames, B.D.; Banerjee, A.; Harken, A.H. Reduction of infarct size in the rat heart by LPS preconditioning is associated with expression of angiogenic growth factors and increased capillary density. *Shock* **1999**, *12*, 25–31. [CrossRef] [PubMed]
24. Wang, Y.P.; Sato, C.; Mizoguchi, K.; Yamashita, Y.; Oe, M.; Maeta, H. Lipopolysaccharide triggers late preconditioning against myocardial infarction via inducible nitric oxide synthase. *Cardiovasc. Res.* **2002**, *56*, 33–42. [CrossRef]
25. Fan, M.H.; Wong, K.L.; Wu, S.; Leung, W.K.; Yam, W.C.; Wong, T.M. Preconditioning with Porphyromonas gingivalis lipopolysaccharide may confer cardioprotection and improve recovery of the electrically induced intracellular calcium transient during ischemia and reperfusion. *J. Periodontal Res.* **2010**, *45*, 100–108. [CrossRef]
26. Angus, D.C.; Linde-Zwirble, W.T.; Lidicker, J.; Clermont, G.; Carcillo, J.; Pinsky, M.R. Epidemiology of severe sepsis in the United States: Analysis of incidence, outcome, and associated costs of care. *Crit. Care Med.* **2001**, *29*, 1303–1310. [CrossRef]
27. Dombrovskiy, V.Y.; Martin, A.A.; Sunderram, J.; Paz, H.L. Rapid increase in hospitalization and mortality rates for severe sepsis in the United States: A trend analysis from 1993 to 2003. *Crit. Care Med.* **2007**, *35*, 1244–1250. [CrossRef] [PubMed]
28. Sakr, Y.; Elia, C.; Mascia, L.; Barberis, B.; Cardellino, S.; Livigni, S.; Fiore, G.; Filippini, C.; Ranieri, V.M. The influence of gender on the epidemiology of and outcome from severe sepsis. *Crit. Care* **2013**, *17*, R50. [CrossRef]
29. Mayr, F.B.; Yende, S.; Angus, D.C. Epidemiology of severe sepsis. *Virulence* **2014**, *5*, 4–11. [CrossRef]
30. El-Lakany, M.A.; Fouda, M.A.; El-Gowelli, H.M.; El-Mas, M.M. Ovariectomy provokes inflammatory and cardiovascular effects of endotoxemia in rats: Dissimilar benefits of hormonal supplements. *Toxicol. Appl. Pharmacol.* **2020**, *393*, 114928. [CrossRef]
31. Farrell, S.R.; Ross, J.L.; Howlett, S.E. Sex differences in mechanisms of cardiac excitation-contraction coupling in rat ventricular myocytes. *Am. J. Physiol.-Heart Circ. Physiol.* **2010**, *299*, H36–H45. [CrossRef]
32. Trexler, C.L.; Odell, A.T.; Jeong, M.Y.; Dowell, R.D.; Leinwand, L.A. Transcriptome and Functional Profile of Cardiac Myocytes Is Influenced by Biological Sex. *Circ. Cardiovasc. Genet.* **2017**, *10*, e001770. [CrossRef] [PubMed]
33. Singer, M. The role of mitochondrial dysfunction in sepsis-induced multi-organ failure. *Virulence* **2014**, *5*, 66–72. [CrossRef] [PubMed]
34. Stanzani, G.; Duchen, M.R.; Singer, M. The role of mitochondria in sepsis-induced cardiomyopathy. *Biochim. Biophys. Acta Mol. Basis Dis.* **2019**, *1865*, 759–773. [CrossRef]
35. Fukumoto, K.; Pierro, A.; Spitz, L.; Eaton, S. Cardiac and renal mitochondria respond differently to hydrogen peroxide in suckling rats. *J. Surg. Res.* **2003**, *113*, 146–150. [CrossRef]
36. Kozlov, A.V.; Staniek, K.; Haindl, S.; Piskernik, C.; Ohlinger, W.; Gille, L.; Nohl, H.; Bahrami, S.; Redl, H. Different effects of endotoxic shock on the respiratory function of liver and heart mitochondria in rats. *Am. J. Physiol.-Gastrointest. Liver Physiol.* **2006**, *290*, G543–G549. [CrossRef]
37. Trumbeckaite, S.; Opalka, J.R.; Neuhof, C.; Zierz, S.; Gellerich, F.N. Different sensitivity of rabbit heart and skeletal muscle to endotoxin-induced impairment of mitochondrial function. *Eur. J. Biochem.* **2001**, *268*, 1422–1429. [CrossRef] [PubMed]
38. Lagranha, C.J.; Deschamps, A.; Aponte, A.; Steenbergen, C.; Murphy, E. Sex differences in the phosphorylation of mitochondrial proteins result in reduced production of reactive oxygen species and cardioprotection in females. *Circ. Res.* **2010**, *106*, 1681–1691. [CrossRef]
39. Colom, B.; Oliver, J.; Roca, P.; Garcia-Palmer, F.J. Caloric restriction and gender modulate cardiac muscle mitochondrial H_2O_2 production and oxidative damage. *Cardiovasc. Res.* **2007**, *74*, 456–465. [CrossRef]
40. Khalifa, A.R.; Abdel-Rahman, E.A.; Mahmoud, A.M.; Ali, M.H.; Noureldin, M.; Saber, S.H.; Mohsen, M.; Ali, S.S. Sex-specific differences in mitochondria biogenesis, morphology, respiratory function, and ROS homeostasis in young mouse heart and brain. *Physiol. Rep.* **2017**, *5*, e13125. [CrossRef]
41. Scott, S.R.; Singh, K.; Yu, Q.; Sen, C.K.; Wang, M. Sex as Biological Variable in Cardiac Mitochondrial Bioenergetic Responses to Acute Stress. *Int. J. Mol. Sci.* **2022**, *23*, 9312. [CrossRef]

42. Arias-Reyes, C.; Losantos-Ramos, K.; Gonzales, M.; Furrer, D.; Soliz, J. NADH-linked mitochondrial respiration in the developing mouse brain is sex-, age- and tissue-dependent. *Respir. Physiol. Neurobiol.* **2019**, *266*, 156–162. [CrossRef] [PubMed]
43. Guerrero, I.; Yoval-Sanchez, B.; Konrad, C.; Manfredi, G.; Wittig, I.; Galkin, A. Sex-dependent differences in macaque brain mitochondria. *Biochim. Biophys. Acta Bioenerg.* **2024**, *1865*, 149494. [CrossRef] [PubMed]
44. Guevara, R.; Santandreu, F.M.; Valle, A.; Gianotti, M.; Oliver, J.; Roca, P. Sex-dependent differences in aged rat brain mitochondrial function and oxidative stress. *Free. Radic. Biol. Med.* **2009**, *46*, 169–175. [CrossRef]
45. Odendaal-Gambrell, C.P.; O'Brien, C.; Cairns, M.; Maarman, G.J.; Joseph, D.E.; Smith, C.; Rautenbach, F.; Marnewick, J.L.; Essop, M.F. Chronic stress elicits sex-specific mitochondrial respiratory functional changes in the rat heart. *Physiol. Rep.* **2025**, *13*, e70371. [CrossRef]
46. Colom, B.; Alcolea, M.P.; Valle, A.; Oliver, J.; Roca, P.; Garcia-Palmer, F.J. Skeletal muscle of female rats exhibit higher mitochondrial mass and oxidative-phosphorylative capacities compared to males. *Cell. Physiol. Biochem.* **2007**, *19*, 205–212. [CrossRef]
47. Wang, L.; Gu, H.; Turrentine, M.; Wang, M. Estradiol treatment promotes cardiac stem cell (CSC)-derived growth factors, thus improving CSC-mediated cardioprotection after acute ischemia/reperfusion. *Surgery* **2014**, *156*, 243–252. [CrossRef] [PubMed]
48. Wang, M.; Smith, K.; Yu, Q.; Miller, C.; Singh, K.; Sen, C.K. Mitochondrial connexin 43 in sex-dependent myocardial responses and estrogen-mediated cardiac protection following acute ischemia/reperfusion injury. *Basic Res. Cardiol.* **2019**, *115*, 1. [CrossRef]
49. Byers, S.L.; Wiles, M.V.; Dunn, S.L.; Taft, R.A. Mouse estrous cycle identification tool and images. *PLoS ONE* **2012**, *7*, e35538. [CrossRef]

International Journal of
Molecular Sciences

MDPI

Article

Profiling of miRNAs Contained in Circulating Extracellular Vesicles and Associated with Sepsis Development in Burn Patients: A Proof-of-Concept Study

Martina Schiavello [1], Ornella Bosco [1,†], Barbara Vizio [1,†], Alberto Sciarrillo [2], Anna Pensa [2], Emanuele Pivetta [1], Fulvio Morello [1], Daniela Risso [2], Giuseppe Montrucchio [1,*], Filippo Mariano [1,3,‡] and Enrico Lupia [1,‡]

[1] Department of Medical Science, University of Turin, 10126 Turin, Italy; martina.schiavello@unito.it (M.S.); ornella.bosco@unito.it (O.B.); barbara.vizio@unito.it (B.V.); emanuele.pivetta@unito.it (E.P.); fulvio.morello@unito.it (F.M.); filippo.mariano@unito.it (F.M.); enrico.lupia@unito.it (E.L.)

[2] Plastic Surgery and Burn Center, Department of General and Specialized Surgery, City of Health and Science, CTO Hospital, 10126 Turin, Italy; albertosciarrillo@gmail.com (A.S.); anna.pensa@unito.it (A.P.); drisso@cittadellasalute.to.it (D.R.)

[3] Nephrology, Dialysis and Transplantation Unit, City of Health and Science, CTO Hospital, 10126 Turin, Italy

* Correspondence: giuseppe.montrucchio@unito.it

† These authors contributed equally to this work.

‡ These authors contributed equally to this work.

Abstract: Sepsis is the leading cause of mortality in patients with burn injuries and it may represent, in these patients, a real diagnostic challenge. Here we studied the profile of miRNAs contained in extracellular vesicles (EVs) (EV-miRNAs) isolated from plasma from burn patients complicated by sepsis at admission and 7 days later. We enrolled 28 burn patients, 18 with (Burn Septic Patients—BSPs) and 10 without (Burn non-Septic Patients—BnSPs) sepsis. Ten healthy subjects (HSs) were used as additional controls. After EV isolation by charge precipitation and miRNA extraction, we proceeded with a two-phase approach. Through a first screening phase, we identified 178 miRNAs differentially expressed in BSPs compared to HSs. Among these, by a validation phase based on qRT-PCR, we found that miR-483-5p, miR-193a-5p, and miR-188-3p were increased in the BSPs compared to the BnSPs and HSs. Upon ROC analysis, all three miRNAs showed a good accuracy in differentiating BSPs from BnSPs, especially miR-483-5p (AUC = 0.955, p-value = 0.001). Moreover, we found 173 miRNAs differentially expressed in BSPs after 7 days from enrollment compared to T0, among whose miR-1-3p, miR-34a-3p, and miR-193a-5p decreased in BSPs after 7 days, in parallel with a decrease in SOFA scores. Finally, the other two miRNAs, miR-34a-3p and miR-193a-5p, positively correlated with the SOFA score. In conclusion, we identified several miRNAs—namely miR-483-5p, miR-193a-5p, and miR-188-3p—with potential clinical utility as diagnostic biomarkers in a heterogeneous population of burn patients at high risk of developing sepsis. Moreover, we found some miRNAs (miR-1-3p, miR-34a-3p, and miR-193a-5p) that vary according to the course of sepsis and others (miR-34a-3p and miR-193a-5p) that are associated with its clinical severity.

Keywords: extracellular vesicles; miRNAs; sepsis; burn patients

1. Introduction

In patients with burn injuries caused by serious thermodynamic damage the incidence of sepsis is extremely high [1]. The prognosis for burn patients with sepsis is poor, with estimates of a >60% mortality rate in burn patients resulting from infectious complications [2]. These patients have a higher susceptibility to bacterial invasion and sepsis due to the compromised skin barrier and to the systemic dysregulation and immunosuppression brought about in response to burn injury. For these reasons, an early diagnosis of sepsis is crucial for the management and outcome of critically burned patients.

Several clinical scores have been proposed to help in diagnosing sepsis [3,4]; however, some of these are not appropriate for burn patients [5–7]. Moreover, although many biomarkers have been proposed, there is still a lack of reliable indicators that are useful for diagnosis and disease assessment, whereas, due to the complexity of burn patients, it seems wise to find a combination of biomarkers, instead of a single biomarker, that are potentially applicable in these patients [8–10].

Extracellular vesicles (EVs) are functional vesicles released by all human cells and found in various body fluids [11]. They act as pivotal vehicles for intercellular communication [12]. EVs are composed of lipid bilayers and carry various cargos, such as lipids, proteins, and miRNAs, to target cells or organs via systemic circulation [11]. The contents of EV cargoes differ significantly depending on the origin and the state of cells [12]. In recent years, the study of EVs has deeply evolved as a consequence of the availability of more sophisticated isolation methods, and EVs have been widely investigated as markers for diseases, including chronic and critical illnesses [13–16].

miRNAs are small non-coding 18–25 nucleotide RNAs that interfere with the expression of up to 30% of protein-coding genes in mammalian cells [17]. The clinical relevance of miRNAs in sepsis has been previously reported [18,19]. For instance, miR-150 has been shown to be a predictor for survival in patients with critical illness and sepsis [20]. Increased levels of serum miR-133a has also been demonstrated to be an independent predictor for mortality in sepsis patients [21]. Moreover, plasma miR-15 and miR-27a levels were significantly reduced while levels of miR-34a were increased in patients with septic shock [22]. Despite a long road travelled in the study of EVs in several diseases, the nature and function of miRNAs contained in EVs (EV-miRNAs) isolated from plasma from patients with sepsis-associated burn injuries are still unknown.

Here, we conducted a proof-of-concept study aimed at evaluating the utility of EV-miRNAs isolated from plasma from burn patients complicated by sepsis as diagnostic biomarkers for the rapid detection of sepsis. Aiming to establish a comprehensive workflow to evaluate miRNA expression in EVs from plasma from burn patients, the following two-phase approach was used: (i) a preliminary screening phase of EV-miRNAs followed by (ii) a validation phase.

2. Results

2.1. Patient Characteristics

A total of 28 burn patients were included in this study. Among these, sepsis was present in 18 cases. A total of 10 healthy subjects (HSs) were also enrolled and used as additional controls. The study groups (Burn non-Septic Patients—BnSPs vs. Burn-Septic Patients—BSPs) did not differ in age or gender distribution, as well as in average % total body surface area (TBSA). At 1 month of hospitalization, all 28 patients were alive. Blood cultures were positive in all BSPs. Detailed information on the demographic and clinical characteristics of the patients and controls is summarized in Table 1.

Table 1. Demographic and clinical characteristics of patients with burn injuries and healthy subjects.

Characteristics	Healthy Subjects (HSs) (n = 10)	Burn Non-Septic Patients (BnSPs) (n = 10)	Burn-Septic Patients (BSPs) (n = 18)	p-Value
Age, year, mean ± SD	57.60 (±13.28)	52.43 (±18.43)	58.07 (±16.41)	0.659
Gender ratio (M/F)	5/5	6/4	11/7	0.317
Comorbidities				
Diabetes Mellitus, n (%)	0	0	2	0.117
Hypertension, n (%)	0	0	8	<0.0001
% TBSA	-	20.00 (10.00–35.00)	30.00 (19.00–41.50)	0.121
MAP	-	80.00 (43.00–83.00)	81.50 (33.00–100.00)	0.329
SOFA score	-	0	10.39 (±2.35)	<0.0001
Laboratory findings				
White Blood Cell $10^9/L$	4.60 (4.35–5.28)	6.99 (5.73–12.24)	12.24 (11.00–17.78) ****°	<0.0001
Hemoglobin g/dL	13.55 (13.28–13.85)	12.90 (11.93–14.25)	8.85 (8.57–9.57) ****°°	<0.0001
Platelets $10^9/L$	261.0 (±26.44)	218.6 (±45.10)	136.3 (±62.00) ****°°°	<0.0001
Creatinine mg/dL	0.933 (±0.06)	1.14 (±0.81)	1.67 (±0.99)	0.221
Procalcitonin ng/mL	-	0.39 (0.35–0.88)	2.52 (0.15–19.68)	0.021
Lactate mmol/L	-	0.80 (0.50–1.20)	1.40 (1.10–1.80)	0.018
Bilirubin mg/dL	-	0.80 (0.55–1.35)	1.20 (0.60–1.70)	0.368
NT-pro-BNP ng/L	-	157.00 (27.00–500.00)	1528 (143.00–44,552)	0.003
Troponin I ng/L	-	4.50 (±1.80)	28.00 (6.00–303.00)	0.005
Myoglobin µg/L	-	79.00 (±50.76)	128.00 (41.00–14,265)	0.227

% TBSA, Total Body Surface Area; MAP, mean arterial pressure; SOFA, Sequential Organ Failure Assessment; mean (±SD) or median (IQR) as appropriate. **** vs. HSs, $p < 0.0001$; ° vs. BnSPs, $p < 0.05$; °° vs. BnSPs, $p < 0.01$; °°° vs. BnSPs, $p < 0.001$.

2.2. Characterization of EVs Isolated from Plasma from Burn Patients and Healthy Subjects

EVs were isolated via a charge-based precipitation method from plasma samples of 18 BSPs, 10 BnSPs, and 10 HSs. We used Nanoparticle Tracking Analysis (NTA) to determine the size and the concentration of the particles isolated from plasma samples. The diameter of the particles prepared was in the ranges of 100–400 nm in the three study groups (Figure S1), whereas the concentration of particles was 2.12×10^{10} in HSs, 5.17×10^{10} in BnSPs, and 8.20×10^{10} in BSPs. We used flow cytometric analysis to verify the expression of specific EV surface markers, showing that CD9 and CD63, considered specific EV markers, were expressed in particles isolated from plasma samples of the HSs, BnSPs, and BSPs (Figure S2). Therefore, EVs were successfully isolated from plasma from both burn patients and healthy subjects.

2.3. Sepsis Significantly Alters the Profile of miRNAs Contained in EVs (EV-miRNAs) Isolated from Plasma from Patients with Burn Injuries

Among 754 miRNAs screened, 178 miRNAs were differentially expressed in the BSPs compared to the HSs. Moreover, 16 miRNAs were exclusively detected in EVs isolated from the BSPs, while 32 miRNAs were specific only to EVs isolated from the HSs (Table S1). Finally, the expression of 528 miRNAs was not detected.

2.4. Validation of Differentially Expressed EV-miRNAs in Patients with Burn Injuries Complicated or Not with Sepsis

To validate the results obtained in the preliminary discovery analysis, we enrolled an additional control group represented by patients with burn injuries with no deterioration in SOFA scores > 2 and no blood culture positivity at the enrollment and during the following 72 h of hospitalization (Burn non-Septic Patients—BnSPs).

In this validation phase conducted via qRT-PCR, we considered the nine more abundantly expressed EV-miRNAs. Of these, we chose the eight EV-derived miRNAs with the highest levels of expression in the BSPs compared to the HSs: miR-452-3p, miR-27a-5p, miR-302d-3p, miR-483-5p, miR-1-3p, miR-193a-5p, miR-34a-3p, and miR-1255a (Table S1). Moreover, we chose one miRNA expressed only in EVs prepared from BSPs: miR-188-3p (Table S1). The validation analysis of the more abundantly expressed EV-miRNAs found during the screening phase confirmed that several miRNAs—namely miR-452-3p, miR-302d-3p, miR-27a-5p, miR-34a-3p, miR-1-3p, miR-483-5p, and miR-193a-5p—were significantly more expressed in the BSPs compared to the HSs (Figure 1a–g). Moreover, the qRT-PCR validation showed that miR-188-3p was increased in the BSPs, confirming the results obtained in the screening phase, but was detectable in the HSs at low expression levels, at variance from what was observed in the array screening, where no expression was observed (Figure 1h, Table S1). miR-1255a showed no statistically significant trend of upregulation in the BSPs. Of note, miR-452-3p and miR-302d-3p were found to have increased in the BnSPs compared to the HSs, while miR-483-5p, miR-193a-5p, and miR-188-3p were increased in the BSPs compared to the BnSPs.

2.5. Accuracy of Plasma EV-miRNAs in Patients with Burn Injuries for Sepsis Diagnosis

The diagnostic performance of those EV-miRNAs we found increased in the BSPs compared to the BnSPs (miR-483-5p, miR-193a-5p, and miR-188-3p). Distinguishing features between these two patients groups was evaluated by ROC curve analysis (Figure 2a,b). miR-483-5p showed the best AUC (0.955, p-value = 0.001), but miR-193a-5p (0.917, p-value 0.007) also showed a good accuracy, whereas miR-188-3p was close to reaching a statistical significance (0.822, p-value 0.053). These AUCs were superior to that of procalcitonin (0.798, p-value 0.016), a well-established marker for the diagnosis of sepsis [9,10].

2.6. Temporal Dynamics of Plasma EV-miRNAs During the Course of Sepsis

In order to characterize the temporal trends of miRNAs-derived from EVs isolated from BSPs, we performed a miRNA screening on EVs isolated from plasma from 5 BSPs at the time of enrollment (T0) and after 7 days (T1).

In these patients, we observed a significant decrease in SOFA scores at T1 compared to T0 (p = 0.0004). The clinical characteristics of these BSPs at the different time points are summarized in Table 2.

Table 2. Patients Characteristics.

Characteristics	Burn-Septic Patients BSP T0 (n = 18)	Burn-Septic Patients BSP T1 (n = 18)	p-Value
MAP	81.50 (33.00–100.00)	78.00 (60.00–98.00)	0.170
P/F	286.3 (±106.9)	277.3 (±81.81)	0.948
SOFA score	10.39 (±2.35)	7.33 (±3.51)	<0.001
Laboratory findings			
White Blood Cell 10^9/L	12.24 (11.00–17.78)	12.71 (6.39–35.53)	0.502
Hemoglobin g/dL	8.85 (8.57–9.57)	9.05 (7.70–11.20)	0.412
Platelets 10^9/L	136.3 (±62.00)	344.00 (±127.5)	<0.001
Creatinine mg/dL	1.53 (0.86–3.80)	0.77 (0.30–2.35)	0.003
Procalcitonin ng/mL	2.52 (0.15–99.67)	0.56 (0.16–5.86)	<0.001
Lactate mmol/L	1.40 (0.10–1.80)	1.05 (0.40–2.00)	0.017
Bilirubin mg/dL	1.20 (0.60–1.70)	0.85 (0.30–8.70)	0.734
NT-pro-BNP ng/L	1528 (143.00–44,552)	686.00 (37.00–9622)	0.065
Copeptin pmol/L	42.80 (3.00–167.3)	28.90 (6.40–493.00)	0.464
Troponin I ng/L	28.00 (6.00–303.00)	27.00 (5.00–520.00)	0.452
Myoglobin µg/L	128.00 (41.00–14,265)	63.00 (34.00–503.00)	0.006

SOFA, Sequential Organ Failure Assessment; MAP, mean arterial pressure; P/F, PaO_2/FiO_2; mean (±SD) or median (IQR) as appropriate.

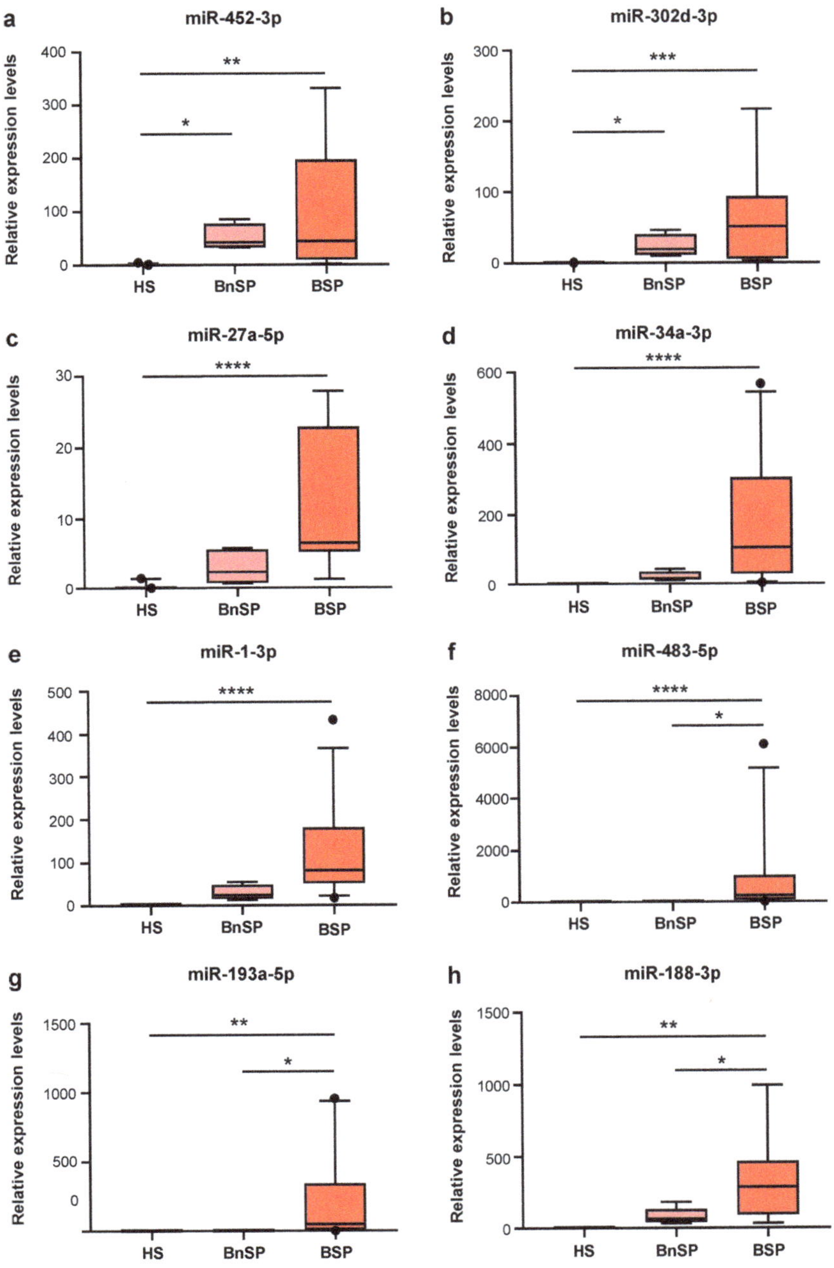

Figure 1. Validation by qRT-PCR of candidate miRNAs contained in plasma EVs. Relative expression levels of miR-452-3p panel (**a**), miR-302d-3p panel (**b**), miR-27a-5p panel (**c**), miR-34a-3p panel (**d**); miR-1-3p panel (**e**); miR-483-5p panel (**f**); miR-193a-5p panel (**g**); miR-188-3p panel (**h**) in EVs isolated from plasma from HSs ($n = 10$), BnSPs ($n = 10$), and BSPs ($n = 18$). Data are presented as median (IQR), normalized with a reference exogenous control (Cel-miR-39). * $p < 0.05$, ** $p < 0.01$, *** $p < 0.001$, **** $p < 0.0001$.

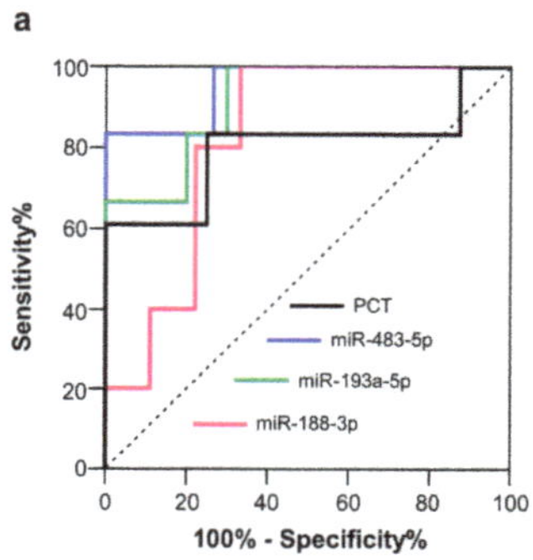

b

	Area	95% confidence interval	P-value
PCT	0.798	0.626-0.971	0.016
miR-483-5p	0.955	0.861-1.000	0.001
miR-193a-5p	0.917	0.778-1.000	0.007
miR-188-3p	0.822	0.598-1.000	0.053

Figure 2. Receiver operating characteristic (ROC) curves of the candidate EV-miRNAs and procalcitonin (PCT) for distinguishing between BSPs and BnSPs. panel (**a**) Area Under the Curve (AUC); panel (**b**) Discriminatory performance of each EV-miRNA examined.

Among 754 miRNAs screened, 173 miRNAs were differentially expressed in the BSPs at T1 compared to T0. Moreover, 31 miRNAs were exclusively detected in the BSPs at T1, while 6 miRNAs were specific only to BSPs at T0 (Table S2). Finally, the expression of 544 miRNAs was not detected.

The validation analysis carried out via qRT-PCR of the more abundantly expressed EV-derived miRNAs showed that miR-1-3p, miR-34a-3p, miR-188-3p, and miR-193a-5p were more expressed in the BSPs at T0 compared to T1 (Figure 3a–d). miR-483-5p showed a trend of increased expression in the BSPs at T0 compared to T1, but was not statistically significant (Figure S3a). On the contrary, miR-452-3p, miR-302d-3p, and miR-27a-5p did not show any difference in the expression levels at T0 compared to T1.

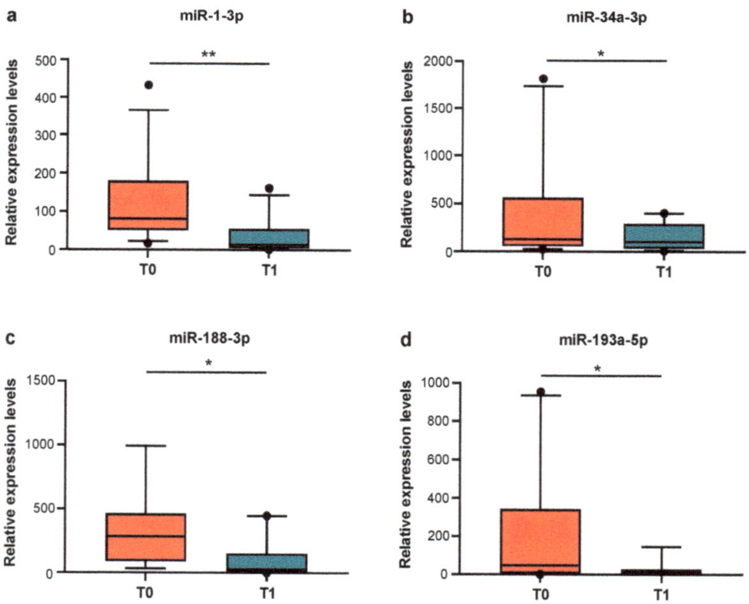

Figure 3. Validation via qRT-PCR of candidate miRNAs contained in EVs isolated from BSPs at T0 and at T1. Relative expression levels of miR-1-3p panel (**a**), miR-34a-3p panel (**b**), miR-188-3p panel (**c**), and miR-193a-5p panel (**d**) in EVs isolated from plasma from BSPs at T0 and at T1. Data are presented as median (IQR), normalized with a reference exogenous control (Cel-miR-39). * $p < 0.05$, ** $p < 0.01$.

We also analyzed the correlation between the SOFA scores, commonly used for the evaluation of the clinical severity of critically ill patients, and selected EV-miRNAs in the BSPs. We found a positive correlation between the highest SOFA score and an increase in miR-34a-3p (r = 0.200, p = 0.028), miR-193a-5p (r = 0.624, p = 0.002), and miR-483-5p (r = 0.509, p = 0.003) expression both at T0 and T1 (Figure 4a,b and S3b). On the contrary, miR-452-3p, miR-302d-3p, and miR-27a-5p were not correlated with SOFA scores.

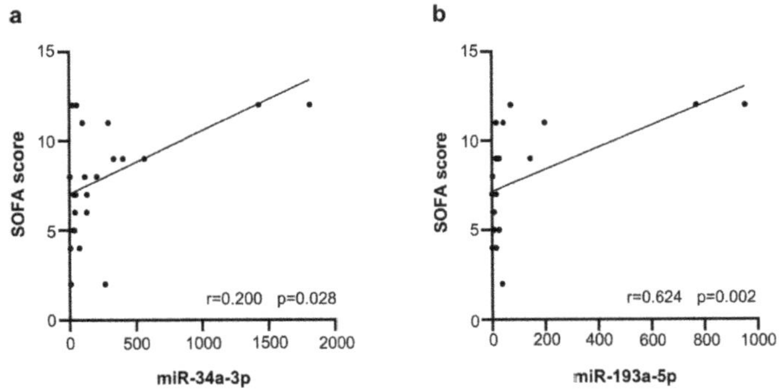

Figure 4. Correlation between EV-miRNA expression levels and SOFA scores in BSPs: panel (**a**) miR-34a-3p; panel (**b**) miR-193a-5p.

3. Discussion

After a severe burn injury, the body enters a pathological condition of excessive inflammation, hypermetabolism, and acute immune response [23]. Understanding early which patients with burn injuries may develop sepsis could be a major milestone in terms of diagnosis and personalized decision therapies.

Sepsis is the most common complication in severe burn patients and tends to be aggressive, rapid, and fatal [24]. Therefore, the prognosis of sepsis in burn patients depends on accurate diagnosis and timely management [25]. The search for sepsis biomarkers is an exciting and never-ending story [26–28]. Recently, the rapid development of multi-level omics biological technologies and computer analytic tools has provided a strong technical foundation for the early warning identification and treatment of the disease [29,30].

In addition to their role in regulating gene expression, circulating miRNAs were proposed as next-generation biomarkers in manifold diseases [31,32]. The diagnostic potential of miRNAs is based on their extraordinary stability and resistance to storage handling [33]. This stability at least partly relies on the inclusion of miRNAs in extracellular vesicles (EVs), where they are protected against degradation or destruction [34].

In our proof-of-concept study, aimed to test the hypothesis that sepsis alters the profile of miRNAs contained in EVs (EV-miRNAs) in burn patients, we used a two-phase approach. In a first set of experiments, we examined circulating EV-miRNA profiles by array technology in patients with burn injury complicated by sepsis (BSPs) in comparison with healthy subjects (HSs). We found that, among 754 miRNAs screened, 178 miRNAs were differentially expressed in the BSPs compared to the HSs. Moreover, 16 miRNAs were exclusively detected in EVs isolated from the BSPs, while 32 miRNAs were specific only to EVs isolated from the HSs. The number of samples in the screening analysis was limited to a pool of five patients, but we further verified the results of the array investigation via qRT-PCR analysis, which was performed on all the patients enrolled in the study. In this set of validation experiments, we performed the analysis in the BSPs, the HSs, and, additionally, in a population of patients with burn injury without evidence of infection (BnSPs). Thus, we identified a pool of miRNAs potentially useful for the diagnosis of sepsis in a heterogeneous population at high risk of developing sepsis like burn patients. We found that eight miRNAs (miR-452-3p, miR-302d-3p, miR-27a-5p, miR-34a-3p, miR-1-3p, miR-483-5p, miR-193a-5p, and miR-188-3p) were more expressed in the BSPs compared to the HSs. Furthermore, two miRNAs (miR-452-3p, miR-302d-3p) were more expressed in the BnSPs compared to the HSs, suggesting a potential association of these miRNAs with burn injuries. Of note, three miRNAs (miR-483-5p, miR-193a-5p, and miR-188-3p) were found to have had a higher expression in BSPs compared to BnSPs, suggesting their potential value for the diagnosis of sepsis in burn patients. All three of these miRNAs showed a good accuracy in discriminating BSPs from BnSPs. This suggests that implementing the use of miRNAs together with the currently used markers, such as procalcitonin (PCT), may be better than the use of a single marker, as has already been established in other diseases [35,36].

Increased expression of selected miRNAs has also been observed in various cancers [37], cardiovascular diseases [38], and in sepsis [18]. In particular, miR-483-5p levels were found to be upregulated in the lung tissues of sepsis-induced acute lung injury (ALI) murine models as compared to the corresponding control groups [39]. The study authors demonstrated that pro-inflammatory cytokines, namely IL-1b and IL-6, were downregulated in mice with sepsis-induced ALI by miR-483-5p knockdown. Similarly, serum miR-483-5p has been proven to be a potential prognostic marker in septic patients in a prospective observational study [40], which is consistent with our results.

Previous research has shown that exosomal miR-193a-5p, together with other miRNAs, predicts the survival of septic patients with high confidence [41].

miR-188-3p is an independent prognostic factor in colorectal cancer [42] and is expressed in atherosclerosis [43]. To the best of our knowledge, no data referring to miR-188-3p are reported to be associated with sepsis and therefore it could be proposed as a novel early warning marker of burns-associated sepsis in the future.

When we look at miRNA expression in a later phase of the disease, when the clinical conditions of BSPs were improving (BSP T1) compared to the time of enrollment (BSP T0), we found that, among the 754 miRNAs screened, 173 were differentially expressed. Moreover, 31 miRNAs were exclusively detected in BSPs at T1, while 6 were specific only to BSPs at T0. In addition, we validated the levels of the most expressed miRNAs and we found that the levels of four miRNAs (miR-1-3p, miR-34a-3p, miR-188-3p, and miR-193a-5p) decreased after 7 days (BSP T1), paralleling the decrease in SOFA scores and the improved clinical conditions of these patients. Interestingly, miR-34a-3p and miR-193a-5p showed a positive correlation with SOFA scores, suggesting that these miRNAs may be proposed as potential markers for assessing disease severity and that combining SOFA scores with specific miRNAs can increase sensitivity when prognosticating the outcome of sepsis.

In a previous study by Chen et al., miR-34a expression was shown to increase in rats with LPS-induced sepsis [44]. In contrast, other authors revealed that the serum expression level of miR-34a-5p was significantly decreased in patients with neonatal sepsis compared with healthy neonates [45]. This discrepancy in the increased and decreased expression of miR-34a in sepsis might be due to the -3p and -5p strands that define the fate of cellular processes as observed in cell proliferation, migration, and invasion in chronic diseases like cervical cancer [46].

Our study presents some advantages compared to others available in the literature. For instance, at variance from other studies that enrolled only healthy controls, our study included an additional control group comprising patients with burn injuries but no evidence of infection or sepsis. In addition, there was no significant difference in %TBSA between the BSPs and BnSPs, making the two groups similar for this important variable. Distinguishing sepsis patients from healthy subjects is easier than distinguishing patients with burn injuries who develop sepsis from those who did not. Therefore, the results from our study are more convincing than those of other studies that exclusively enrolled normal healthy controls.

On the other hand, our study has several limitations. First, the sample size was relatively small, and thus additional multi-center studies are required to confirm our findings. Moreover, we evaluated BSPs only at two different time points, whereas a better evaluation conducted at several time-points would have been useful to improve the evaluation of the proposed EV-miRNAs. Third, it would be of interest to evaluate the same miRNAs in a population of septic patients with different etiology to establish the universal potential value of selected miRNAs for the diagnosis and prognostic stratification of patients with sepsis. Finally, in our study, we did not explore whether and how the EV-miRNAs we identified as differentially expressed may act in terms of mediators of the pathological mechanisms involved in sepsis development and/or progression in burn patients. Further studies will be needed in order to provide mechanistic information on these topics.

Despite these limitations, our results suggest that circulating EV-miRNAs may be proposed as reliable biomarkers in burn patients to differentiate those with sepsis from those without infection. Moreover, EV-miRNAs seem to have a prominent association with the course of sepsis in burn patients. Future developments will include the study of the functional role of EV-miRNAs here identified, with the perspective of proposing future innovative therapeutic approaches useful for the treatment of burn patients complicated by sepsis.

4. Materials and Methods

4.1. Patients and Sample Collection

In this prospective observational study, we recruited 40 patients with Total Body Surface Areas (TBSAs) comprised between 10% and 50%. Of these, 18 burn-septic patients (BSPs) and 10 burn non-septic patients (BnSPs) were considered eligible and enrolled in the study. Patient enrollment was conducted at the Burn Center of the "Città della Salute e della Scienza di Torino" University Hospital—CTO Site from November 2022 to January 2024. A total of 12 patients were excluded and considered non-eligible because they did not fit with the inclusion and exclusion criteria as follows.

The inclusion criteria for burn patients were the following: $\geq$18 years of age, a TBSA >10% and <50%, and informed consent for participation in the study. The exclusion criteria included the following: age < 18 years, a TBSA < 10% and >50%, cancer (active or recent history), autoimmune or chronic inflammatory disease, and HBV/HCV/HIV/SARS-CoV-2 infection. Burn patients admitted to the Burn Center were regularly screened for the insurgence of sepsis, which was diagnosed according to the criteria defined by the Sepsis-3 guidelines [3], modified as follows: an increase in the Sequential Organ Failure Assessment (SOFA) score of $\geq$2 points plus blood culture positivity. The severity of organ dysfunction was estimated using the SOFA score [47]. Patients with burn injuries with no deterioration in SOFA score > 2 and no blood culture positivity at the enrollment and during the following 72 h of hospitalization were classified as Burn non-Septic Patients (BnSPs) and used as controls.

A total of 10 healthy subjects (HS) without comorbidities and paired for sex and age were also enrolled and used to constitute an additional control group.

Written informed consent was acquired from all enrolled patients and healthy volunteers.

We collected the following data concerning the demographic and clinical characteristics of the study patients: age, gender, comorbidities, total body surface burned area (%TBSA), mean arterial pressure (MAP), Sequential Organ Failure Assessments (SOFA) score, and laboratory findings.

The study was approved by the Institutional Ethics and Review Board of the "Citta della Salute e della Scienza di Torino" University Hospital, Turin, Italy (n. CS2/815) and conducted according to the ethical standards set out by the Declaration of Helsinki and its later amendments.

For patients and healthy subjects, whole blood was collected from a central venous catheter or from a peripheral vein via clean venipuncture using a 21-gauge infusion set, respectively, in EDTA tubes (BD Vacutainer, Reading, UK), and processed within 1 h. The blood samples were first centrifuged at 1600× g for 10 min at 4 °C, then the plasma was collected and stored at −80 °C until EV isolation and subsequent analyses were carried out.

4.2. Study Design

This study was designed in two phases (Figure 5): (i) the screening phase and (ii) the validation phase.

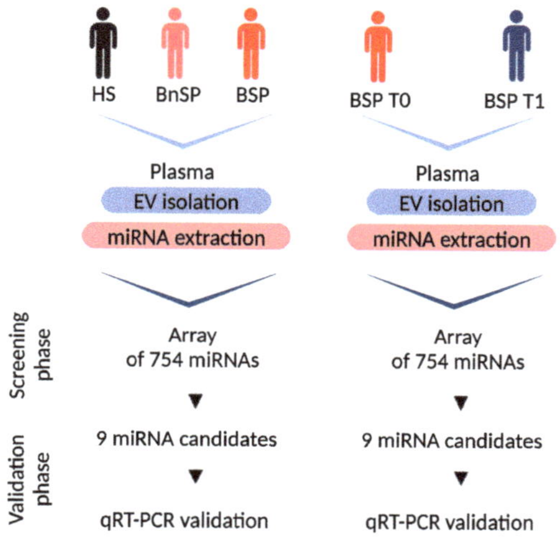

Figure 5. Study design. Created with http://biorender.com/, accessed on 30 December 2024.

For the screening phase, two pooled samples of miRNAs derived from EVs isolated from plasma (EV-miRNAs) prepared from HSs (n = 5) and BSPs (n = 5) were screened using a miRNA array card. Each group was composed of a mix of EV-miRNAs from five individuals paired for sex and age. For all samples, EV isolation and miRNA extraction from EVs were performed separately and mixed only after EV-miRNA extraction.

For the validation phase, EV-miRNAs from individual samples of HSs (n = 10), BnSPs (n = 10), BSPs (n = 18) were analyzed via qRT-PCR for the expression of the nine more abundantly expressed EV-derived miRNAs identified during the screening phase.

Moreover, we studied the temporal trend of expression of selected EV-miRNAs by two additional phases: (i) screening by miRNA array card of two pooled samples composed of EV-miRNAs prepared from five BSPs at the time of enrollment (T0, n = 5) and after 7 days (T1, n = 5); (ii) validation phase: analysis via qRT-PCR of the EV-miRNAs from individual samples prepared from BSPs at T0 (n = 18) and at T1 (n = 18) for the expression of the nine more abundantly expressed EV-derived miRNAs identified during the screening phase.

4.3. Isolation of EVs from Plasma via the Charge-Based Precipitation Method

EVs were isolated using the charge-based precipitation method from plasma samples of 18 BSPs, 10 BnSPs, and 10 HSs.

An amount of 1 mL of plasma samples from patients and healthy subjects, stored at −80 °C, were centrifugated at 5000× *g* at 4 °C for 30 min to remove cellular debris and platelet contamination. EVs were isolated via the charge-based precipitation method, as previously described [48]. Briefly, a protamine (P) (Sigma, St. Louis, MO, USA)/Polyethylene glycol (PEG 35,000; Merck KGaA, Darmstadt, Germany) precipitation solution (P/PEG; Sigma, St. Louis, MO, USA) (0.2 g PEG 35,000 and 1 mg protamine chloride/mL; 1:4) was added to the plasma samples. After overnight incubation at 4 °C, the mixture was centrifugated at 1500× *g* for 30 min at 4 °C, and then a second centrifugation was performed at 1500× *g* for 10 min at 4 °C. Finally, the pellet was re-suspended in 150 μL of PBS-free particles and stored at −80° C for subsequent RNA extraction.

4.4. EV Characterization

4.4.1. Nanoparticle Tracking Analysis (NTA)

The particles isolated as described above were characterized following the recommendations set out in "Minimal Information for Studies of Extracellular Vesicles" (MISEV) 2023 [49]. To characterize particles isolated from plasma in terms of quantity and size distribution, we used Nanoparticle Tracking Analysis (NTA) using a NanoSight LM10 instrument equipped with 405 nm laser and a Nanosight Tracking Analyses 2.3 Analytical Software (Malvern Panalytical Ltd., Malvern, UK). Briefly, EVs were diluted in particle-free PBS before our analysis was carried out (1:1000). Three consequent 30-s records per sample were acquired. The minimum expected particle size, minimum track length, and biomedical light unit setting were set to automatic, and the detection threshold was set to 4 to reveal all the particles.

4.4.2. Flow Cytometry

In order to investigate the EV expression of specific surface markers by flow cytometry, 20 μL of EVs were labelled with either a phycoerythrin (PE; Invitrogen, ThermoFisher Scientific, Carlsbad, CA, USA)-conjugated mouse anti-human IgG1 monoclonal antibody against the tetraspanins CD9 (clone eBioSN4, C3-3A2) or PE-Cyanine7 (Invitrogen, ThermoFisher Scientific)-conjugated mouse anti-human IgG1 monoclonal antibody against the tetraspanins CD63 (clone H5C6) at a volume of 5 μL/test in a final volume of 100 μL of diluted particle-free PBS, for 1 h at room temperature in the dark. Mouse IgG1 kappa isotype control monoclonal antibodies lacking specificity for CD9 or CD63 (P3.6.2.8.1, PE or PE-Cyanine7, Invitrogen, ThermoFisher Scientific) were used to measure the signal from non-specific flow cytometry interactions. The Attune NxT Small Particle Side-Scatter Filter (488/10) (Invitrogen, ThermoFisher Scientific) was installed to enable SSC resolution at the scale required to visualize nanoparticles in the Attune NxT Acoustic Focusing Flow Cytometer system (ThermoFisher Scientific).

For fluorochrome-conjugated antibody compensation, the AbC Total Antibody Compensation Bead Kit (Life Technologies, ThermoFisher Scientific) was used. For the established gating strategies of EV samples, we used Flow Cytometry Sub-Micron Particle Size Reference Kit (Life Technologies, ThermoFisher Scientific), which provides a set of green fluorescent microsphere suspensions (with a nominal diameter of 0.1, 0.2, 0.5, and 1.0 μm) to serve as reliable size references for flow cytometry, according to the minimal information for the standardized reporting of extracellular vesicles flow cytometry experiments (MIFlowCyt-EV) [50].

The acquisition was performed at 100 μL of the total draw volume and 25 μL/min. Set options were set on 20,000 events. Control experiments for flow cytometric characterization were performed with a buffer control, an isotype control, and the single staining of EVs characterization markers (CD9 and CD63). Data were analyzed with the Attune NxT 3.2 Software.

4.5. RNA Extraction from Plasma EVs

miRNAs were isolated from 150 µL of EV pellet using the miRNeasy mini kit (Qiagen, Crawley, UK) according to the manufacturer's instructions. Spike-in control miRNA-39 (Applied Biosystem, ThermoFisher Scientific) from Caenorhabditis elegans solution (1.6×10^8 copies/µL) was added as an exogenous control for RNA extraction efficiency.

High-quality RNA, primarily miRNAs and other small RNA, was collected in the final elution volume of 20 µL of RNase-free water and stored at −80 °C.

4.6. Reverse Transcription

An amount of 2 µL of individual miRNA extracts was reverse-transcribed into complementary DNA (cDNA) using the TaqMan Advanced miRNA cDNA Synthesis Kit (Applied Biosystem, ThermoFisher Scientific) according to the manufacturer's instructions. Briefly, 5 µL of reverse transcription product were used for pre-amplification using a custom miR-Amp Primer Mix and the miR-Amp Master Mix (Applied Biosystem, ThermoFisher Scientific). Finally, 50 µL of pre-amplified cDNA were stored at −20 °C until further analysis for up to 2 months.

4.7. TaqMan Array

In the screening phase, pre-amplification cDNA samples were mixed into pools derived from five individual patient samples from BSPs and HSs in a final volume of 20 µL. qRT-PCR was set up using the TaqMan Fast Advanced Master Mix (Applied Biosystem, ThermoFisher Scientific) and pre-amplified cDNA pools from BSPs and HSs were diluted 1:10 in 0.1× TE buffer.

The expression profile of a panel of 754 human miRNAs was evaluated by TaqMan array human microRNA A + B cards (ThermoFisher Scientific) by loading each fill reservoir with 100 µL of the sample-specific PCR reaction mix and using the QuantStudio 12K Flex Real-Time PCR System (Applied Biosystem, ThermoFisher Scientific). Only the miRNAs found to be expressed in both replicates were considered.

Connect Data Analysis Apps (ThermoFisher Scientific) was used to calculate Raw C_t values, with an automatic baseline and threshold and to calculate RQ (2^{-ddC_t}) values. C_t values > 40 or with Amp score < 0.7 were excluded from the analysis.

4.8. qRT-PCR

In the validation phase, we performed single-tube assays on individual samples from each patient enrolled in the study using a QuantStudio 1 Real-Time PCR System (Applied Biosystem, ThermoFisher Scientific). Pre-amplified cDNA samples were diluted 1:10 in 0.1X TE buffer. Briefly, mastermix, assays, water, and diluted pre-amplified cDNA samples were placed in individual wells of an optical 96-well reaction plate. Each reaction was performed in triplicate. The utilized primers are listed in Table S3. Samples were run using the following parameters: 50 °C 2 min, 95 °C 10 min, 40 cycles of 95 °C 15 s and 60 °C 1 min, and a 4 °C hold.

The relative miRNA expression was calculated using the comparative cycle threshold (2^{-ddCt}) method normalized to cel-miR-39 levels (exogenous controls).

All calculations were performed using the QuantStudio Real-Time PCR Software v1.3 (Applied Biosystem, ThermoFisher Scientific).

4.9. Statistical Analysis

Descriptive statistics were reported as median (interquartile range, IQR) or mean (±standard error of mean, SEM), according to data distribution as assessed via the Shapiro–Wilk test. Comparison between groups was carried out via a Kruskal–Wallis one-way analysis of variance on ranks followed by Dunn's multiple comparison tests, or unpaired or paired Student's *t*-test, as appropriate. The diagnostic accuracy of each miRNA was calculated as the area under the receiver operating characteristic curve (AUC–ROC).

A *p*-value < 0.05 was considered significant.

Data were collected using an Excel spreadsheet (Microsoft Office 365 ProPlus) and analyses were conducted using the GraphPad Prism 9.0 software for Windows and Macintosh (GraphPad Software, La Jolla, CA, USA).

5. Conclusions

Our results suggest the potential utility of several circulating EV-miRNAs, namely miR-483-5p, -miR-193a-5p, and -miR-188-3p, as biomarkers for the diagnosis of sepsis in a heterogeneous population of burn patients at high risk of developing sepsis. Furthermore, we identified other EV-miRNAs, such as miR-34a-3p and miR-193a-5p, which are associated with the clinical severity of sepsis, whereas others (miR-1-3p, miR-34a-3p, and miR-193a-5p) vary according to the course of sepsis. In the future, these novel circulating biomarkers might serve as promising tools for the diagnosis of sepsis in burn patients and could aid in the prognostic stratification of these patients. In addition, our proof-of-concept findings establish an important step forward in developing our understanding of EV-miRNA's pathophysiology and of their potential contribution in ameliorating sepsis diagnosis.

Supplementary Materials: The following supporting information can be downloaded at: https://www.mdpi.com/article/10.3390/ijms26051844/s1.

Author Contributions: Conceptualization, M.S., G.M., F.M. (Filippo Mariano) and E.L.; methodology, M.S., O.B., B.V., A.S., A.P. and F.M. (Filippo Mariano); formal analysis, M.S.; investigation, M.S., F.M. (Filippo Mariano) and E.L.; resources, A.S., A.P., E.P., F.M. (Fulvio Morello), D.R. and F.M. (Filippo Mariano); data curation, M.S., O.B., B.V. and E.L.; writing—original draft preparation, M.S.; writing—review and editing, M.S. and E.L.; visualization, M.S. and O.B.; supervision, G.M, F.M. (Filippo Mariano) and E.L.; funding acquisition, G.M. and E.L. All authors have read and agreed to the published version of the manuscript.

Funding: This work was supported by the Ministero dell'Università e della Ricerca scientifica e Tecnologica (MURST) ex 60% to E.L. and G.M. and Research Projects of National Relevance (PRIN) prot. 2022BPNY3E to E.L.

Institutional Review Board Statement: The study was conducted in accordance with the Declaration of Helsinki, and approved by the Ethics Committee of A.O.U. "Città della Salute e della Scienza di Torino", University Hospital, Turin, Italy (n. CS2/815; 15 January 2020).

Informed Consent Statement: Informed consent was obtained from all subjects involved in the study.

Data Availability Statement: Deidentified participant data will be made available on a collaborative basis upon reasonable request. Data and research materials used in this study are available upon request to qualified researchers for purposes of replication, further analysis, and academic collaboration.

Acknowledgments: We would like to thank all the clinicians and staff members in Burn Center of CTO Hospital—A.O.U. Città della Salute e della Scienza di Torino, for their efforts in the enrollment of patients. We would also like to thank the Department of Medical Science—University of Turin—for the BioRender License provided to E.L.

Conflicts of Interest: The authors declare no conflicts of interest.

References

1. Hill, D.M.; Percy, M.D.; Velamuri, S.R.; Lanfranco, J.; Romero Legro, I.; Sinclair, S.E.; Hickerson, W.L. Predictors for Identifying Burn Sepsis and Performance vs. Existing Criteria. *J. Burn. Care Res.* **2018**, *39*, 982–988. [CrossRef] [PubMed]
2. Gomez, R.; Murray, C.K.; Hospenthal, D.R.; Cancio, L.C.; Renz, E.M.; Holcomb, J.B.; Wade, C.E.; Wolf, S.E. Causes of Mortality by Autopsy Findings of Combat Casualties and Civilian Patients Admitted to a Burn Unit. *J. Am. Coll. Surg.* **2009**, *208*, 348–354. [CrossRef]
3. Singer, M.; Deutschman, C.S.; Seymour, C.W.; Shankar-Hari, M.; Annane, D.; Bauer, M.; Bellomo, R.; Bernard, G.R.; Chiche, J.-D.; Coopersmith, C.M.; et al. The Third International Consensus Definitions for Sepsis and Septic Shock (Sepsis-3). *JAMA* **2016**, *315*, 801–810. [CrossRef] [PubMed]
4. Wayland, J.; Teixeira, J.P.; Nielsen, N.D. Sepsis in 2024: A Review. *Anaesth. Intensive Care Med.* **2024**, *25*, 642–651. [CrossRef]
5. Yan, J.; Hill, W.F.; Rehou, S.; Pinto, R.; Shahrokhi, S.; Jeschke, M.G. Sepsis Criteria versus Clinical Diagnosis of Sepsis in Burn Patients: A Validation of Current Sepsis Scores. *Surgery* **2018**, *164*, 1241–1245. [CrossRef]
6. Greenhalgh, D.G.; Hill, D.M.; Burmeister, D.M.; Gus, E.I.; Cleland, H.; Padiglione, A.; Holden, D.; Huss, F.; Chew, M.S.; Kubasiak, J.C.; et al. Surviving Sepsis After Burn Campaign. *Burns* **2023**, *49*, 1487–1524. [CrossRef]
7. Boehm, D.; Menke, H. Sepsis in Burns—Lessons Learnt from Developments in the Management of Septic Shock. *Medicina* **2021**, *58*, 26. [CrossRef] [PubMed]
8. Li, A.T.; Moussa, A.; Gus, E.; Paul, E.; Yii, E.; Romero, L.; Lin, Z.C.; Padiglione, A.; Lo, C.H.; Cleland, H.; et al. Biomarkers for the Early Diagnosis of Sepsis in Burns: Systematic Review and Meta-Analysis. *Ann. Surg.* **2022**, *275*, 654. [CrossRef]
9. Cabral, L.; Afreixo, V.; Santos, F.; Almeida, L.; Paiva, J.A. Procalcitonin for the Early Diagnosis of Sepsis in Burn Patients: A Retrospective Study. *Burns* **2017**, *43*, 1427–1434. [CrossRef]
10. Yoon, J.; Kym, D.; Cho, Y.S.; Hur, J.; Yoon, D. Advanced Biomarker Clustering Analysis Reveals Mortality Predictors in Burn Patients with Sepsis. *Sci. Rep.* **2024**, *14*, 22784. [CrossRef]
11. Schiavello, M.; Vizio, B.; Bosco, O.; Pivetta, E.; Mariano, F.; Montrucchio, G.; Lupia, E. Extracellular Vesicles: New Players in the Mechanisms of Sepsis- and COVID-19-Related Thromboinflammation. *Int. J. Mol. Sci.* **2023**, *24*, 1920. [CrossRef] [PubMed]
12. van Niel, G.; D'Angelo, G.; Raposo, G. Shedding Light on the Cell Biology of Extracellular Vesicles. *Nat. Rev. Mol. Cell Biol.* **2018**, *19*, 213–228. [CrossRef] [PubMed]
13. Im, Y.; Yoo, H.; Ko, R.-E.; Lee, J.Y.; Park, J.; Jeon, K. Exosomal CD63 in Critically Ill Patients with Sepsis. *Sci. Rep.* **2021**, *11*, 20300. [CrossRef]
14. Dakhlallah, D.A.; Wisler, J.; Gencheva, M.; Brown, C.M.; Leatherman, E.R.; Singh, K.; Brundage, K.; Karsies, T.; Dakhlallah, A.; Witwer, K.W.; et al. Circulating Extracellular Vesicle Content Reveals de Novo DNA Methyltransferase Expression as a Molecular Method to Predict Septic Shock. *J. Extracell. Vesicles* **2019**, *8*, 1669881. [CrossRef]
15. Yang, X.; Chatterjee, V.; Zheng, E.; Reynolds, A.; Ma, Y.; Villalba, N.; Tran, T.; Jung, M.; Smith, D.J.; Wu, M.H.; et al. Burn Injury-Induced Extracellular Vesicle Production and Characteristics. *Shock* **2022**, *57*, 228–242. [CrossRef] [PubMed]
16. O'Toole, H.J.; Lowe, N.; Arun, V.; Kolesov, A.V.; Palmieri, T.L.; Tran, N.K.; Carney, R.P. Plasma-Derived Extracellular Vesicles (EVs) as Biomarkers of Sepsis in Burn Patients via Label-Free Raman Spectroscopy. *bioRxiv* **2024**. [CrossRef] [PubMed]
17. Bartel, D.P. MicroRNAs: Genomics, Biogenesis, Mechanism, and Function. *Cell* **2004**, *116*, 281–297. [CrossRef]
18. Antonakos, N.; Gilbert, C.; Théroude, C.; Schrijver, I.T.; Roger, T. Modes of Action and Diagnostic Value of miRNAs in Sepsis. *Front. Immunol.* **2022**, *13*, 951798. [CrossRef]
19. Giza, D.E.; Fuentes-Mattei, E.; Bullock, M.D.; Tudor, S.; Goblirsch, M.J.; Fabbri, M.; Lupu, F.; Yeung, S.-C.J.; Vasilescu, C.; Calin, G.A. Cellular and Viral microRNAs in Sepsis: Mechanisms of Action and Clinical Applications. *Cell Death Differ.* **2016**, *23*, 1906–1918. [CrossRef] [PubMed]
20. Roderburg, C.; Luedde, M.; Vargas Cardenas, D.; Vucur, M.; Scholten, D.; Frey, N.; Koch, A.; Trautwein, C.; Tacke, F.; Luedde, T. Circulating MicroRNA-150 Serum Levels Predict Survival in Patients with Critical Illness and Sepsis. *PLoS ONE* **2013**, *8*, e54612. [CrossRef] [PubMed]
21. Tacke, F.; Roderburg, C.; Benz, F.; Cardenas, D.V.; Luedde, M.; Hippe, H.-J.; Frey, N.; Vucur, M.; Gautheron, J.; Koch, A.; et al. Levels of Circulating miR-133a Are Elevated in Sepsis and Predict Mortality in Critically Ill Patients. *Crit. Care Med.* **2014**, *42*, 1096–1104. [CrossRef] [PubMed]
22. Goodwin, A.J.; Guo, C.; Cook, J.A.; Wolf, B.; Halushka, P.V.; Fan, H. Plasma Levels of microRNA Are Altered with the Development of Shock in Human Sepsis: An Observational Study. *Crit. Care* **2015**, *19*, 440. [CrossRef] [PubMed]
23. Jeschke, M.G.; van Baar, M.E.; Choudhry, M.A.; Chung, K.K.; Gibran, N.S.; Logsetty, S. Burn Injury. *Nat. Rev. Dis. Primers* **2020**, *6*, 11. [CrossRef] [PubMed]
24. Zhang, P.; Zou, B.; Liou, Y.-C.; Huang, C. The Pathogenesis and Diagnosis of Sepsis Post Burn Injury. *Burn. Trauma* **2021**, *9*, tkaa047. [CrossRef] [PubMed]

25. Mariano, F.; Greco', D.; Depetris, N.; Mella, A.; Sciarrillo, A.; Stella, M.; Berardino, M.; Risso, D.; Gambino, R.; Biancone, L. CytoSorb® in Burn Patients with Septic Shock and Acute Kidney Injury on Continuous Kidney Replacement Therapy Is Associated with Improved Clinical Outcome and Survival. *Burns* **2024**, *50*, 1213–1222. [CrossRef]
26. Kibe, S.; Adams, K.; Barlow, G. Diagnostic and Prognostic Biomarkers of Sepsis in Critical Care. *J. Antimicrob. Chemother.* **2011**, *66*, ii33–ii40. [CrossRef]
27. Long, B.; Koyfman, A. Ready for Prime Time? Biomarkers in Sepsis. *Emerg. Med. Clin. N. Am.* **2017**, *35*, 109–122. [CrossRef] [PubMed]
28. Sandquist, M.; Wong, H.R. Biomarkers of Sepsis and Their Potential Value in Diagnosis, Prognosis and Treatment. *Expert Rev. Clin. Immunol.* **2014**, *10*, 1349–1356. [CrossRef]
29. Lim, J.; Park, C.; Kim, M.; Kim, H.; Kim, J.; Lee, D.-S. Advances in Single-Cell Omics and Multiomics for High-Resolution Molecular Profiling. *Exp. Mol. Med.* **2024**, *56*, 515–526. [CrossRef] [PubMed]
30. Huang, J.; Chen, Y.; Guo, Z.; Yu, Y.; Zhang, Y.; Li, P.; Shi, L.; Lv, G.; Sun, B. Prospective Study and Validation of Early Warning Marker Discovery Based on Integrating Multi-Omics Analysis in Severe Burn Patients with Sepsis. *Burn. Trauma* **2023**, *11*, tkac050. [CrossRef] [PubMed]
31. Kim, T.; Croce, C.M. MicroRNA: Trends in Clinical Trials of Cancer Diagnosis and Therapy Strategies. *Exp. Mol. Med.* **2023**, *55*, 1314–1321. [CrossRef] [PubMed]
32. Zhai, W.; Zhao, M.; Wei, C.; Zhang, G.; Qi, Y.; Zhao, A.; Sun, L. Biomarker Profiling to Determine Clinical Impact of microRNAs in Cognitive Disorders. *Sci. Rep.* **2024**, *14*, 8270. [CrossRef] [PubMed]
33. Mraz, M.; Malinova, K.; Mayer, J.; Pospisilova, S. MicroRNA Isolation and Stability in Stored RNA Samples. *Biochem. Biophys. Res. Commun.* **2009**, *390*, 1–4. [CrossRef] [PubMed]
34. Sanz-Rubio, D.; Martin-Burriel, I.; Gil, A.; Cubero, P.; Forner, M.; Khalyfa, A.; Marin, J.M. Stability of Circulating Exosomal miRNAs in Healthy Subjects. *Sci. Rep.* **2018**, *8*, 10306. [CrossRef] [PubMed]
35. Jang, J.Y.; Kim, Y.S.; Kang, K.N.; Kim, K.H.; Park, Y.J.; Kim, C.W. Multiple microRNAs as Biomarkers for Early Breast Cancer Diagnosis. *Mol. Clin. Oncol.* **2021**, *14*, 31. [CrossRef]
36. Rocci, A.; Hofmeister, C.; Geyer, S.; Stiff, A.; Gambella, M.; Cascione, L.; Guan, J.; Benson, D.; Efebera, Y.; Talabere, T.; et al. Circulating miRNA Markers Show Promise as New Prognosticators for Multiple Myeloma. *Leukemia* **2014**, *28*, 1922–1926. [CrossRef]
37. Li, C.; Zhou, T.; Chen, J.; Li, R.; Chen, H.; Luo, S.; Chen, D.; Cai, C.; Li, W. The Role of Exosomal miRNAs in Cancer. *J. Transl. Med.* **2022**, *20*, 6. [CrossRef] [PubMed]
38. Zheng, D.; Huo, M.; Li, B.; Wang, W.; Piao, H.; Wang, Y.; Zhu, Z.; Li, D.; Wang, T.; Liu, K. The Role of Exosomes and Exosomal MicroRNA in Cardiovascular Disease. *Front. Cell Dev. Biol.* **2021**, *8*, 616161. [CrossRef] [PubMed]
39. Leng, C.; Sun, J.; Xin, K.; Ge, J.; Liu, P.; Feng, X. High Expression of miR-483-5p Aggravates Sepsis-Induced Acute Lung Injury. *J. Toxicol. Sci.* **2020**, *45*, 77–86. [CrossRef] [PubMed]
40. Wang, H.; Zhang, P.; Chen, W.; Feng, D.; Jia, Y.; Xie, L. Serum microRNA Signatures Identified by Solexa Sequencing Predict Sepsis Patients' Mortality: A Prospective Observational Study. *PLoS ONE* **2012**, *7*, e38885. [CrossRef]
41. Reithmair, M.; Buschmann, D.; Märte, M.; Kirchner, B.; Hagl, D.; Kaufmann, I.; Pfob, M.; Chouker, A.; Steinlein, O.K.; Pfaffl, M.W.; et al. Cellular and Extracellular miRNAs Are Blood-Compartment-Specific Diagnostic Targets in Sepsis. *J. Cell. Mol. Med.* **2017**, *21*, 2403–2411. [CrossRef] [PubMed]
42. Pichler, M.; Stiegelbauer, V.; Vychytilova-Faltejskova, P.; Ivan, C.; Ling, H.; Winter, E.; Zhang, X.; Goblirsch, M.; Wulf-Goldenberg, A.; Ohtsuka, M.; et al. Genome-Wide miRNA Analysis Identifies miR-188-3p as a Novel Prognostic Marker and Molecular Factor Involved in Colorectal Carcinogenesis. *Clin. Cancer Res.* **2017**, *23*, 1323–1333. [CrossRef]
43. Mi, S.; Wang, P.; Lin, L. miR-188-3p Inhibits Vascular Smooth Muscle Cell Proliferation and Migration by Targeting Fibroblast Growth Factor 1 (FGF1). *Med. Sci. Monit.* **2020**, *26*, e924394-1–e924394-12. [CrossRef]
44. Cheng, D.-L.; Fang, H.-X.; Liang, Y.; Zhao, Y.; Shi, C.-S. MicroRNA-34a Promotes iNOS Secretion from Pulmonary Macrophages in Septic Suckling Rats through Activating STAT3 Pathway. *Biomed. Pharmacother.* **2018**, *105*, 1276–1282. [CrossRef] [PubMed]
45. Abdelaleem, O.O.; Mohammed, S.R.; El Sayed, H.S.; Hussein, S.K.; Ali, D.Y.; Abdelwahed, M.Y.; Gaber, S.N.; Hemeda, N.F.; El-Hmid, R.G.A. Serum miR-34a-5p and miR-199a-3p as New Biomarkers of Neonatal Sepsis. *PLoS ONE* **2022**, *17*, e0262339. [CrossRef] [PubMed]
46. Córdova-Rivas, S.; Fraire-Soto, I.; Mercado-Casas Torres, A.; Servín-González, L.S.; Granados-López, A.J.; López-Hernández, Y.; Reyes-Estrada, C.A.; Gutiérrez-Hernández, R.; Castañeda-Delgado, J.E.; Ramírez-Hernández, L.; et al. 5p and 3p Strands of miR-34 Family Members Have Differential Effects in Cell Proliferation, Migration, and Invasion in Cervical Cancer Cells. *Int. J. Mol. Sci.* **2019**, *20*, 545. [CrossRef]
47. Vincent, J.L.; de Mendonça, A.; Cantraine, F.; Moreno, R.; Takala, J.; Suter, P.M.; Sprung, C.L.; Colardyn, F.; Blecher, S. Use of the SOFA Score to Assess the Incidence of Organ Dysfunction/Failure in Intensive Care Units: Results of a Multicenter, Prospective Study. Working Group on "Sepsis-Related Problems" of the European Society of Intensive Care Medicine. *Crit. Care Med.* **1998**, *26*, 1793–1800. [CrossRef] [PubMed]

48. Deregibus, M.C.; Figliolini, F.; D'antico, S.; Manzini, P.M.; Pasquino, C.; De Lena, M.; Tetta, C.; Brizzi, M.F.; Camussi, G. Charge-Based Precipitation of Extracellular Vesicles. *Int. J. Mol. Med.* **2016**, *38*, 1359–1366. [CrossRef] [PubMed]
49. Welsh, J.A.; Goberdhan, D.C.I.; O'Driscoll, L.; Buzas, E.I.; Blenkiron, C.; Bussolati, B.; Cai, H.; Di Vizio, D.; Driedonks, T.A.P.; Erdbrügger, U.; et al. Minimal Information for Studies of Extracellular Vesicles (MISEV2023): From Basic to Advanced Approaches. *J. Extracell. Vesicles* **2024**, *13*, e12404. [CrossRef]
50. Welsh, J.A.; Van Der Pol, E.; Arkesteijn, G.J.A.; Bremer, M.; Brisson, A.; Coumans, F.; Dignat-George, F.; Duggan, E.; Ghiran, I.; Giebel, B.; et al. MIFlowCyt-EV: A Framework for Standardized Reporting of Extracellular Vesicle Flow Cytometry Experiments. *J. Extracell. Vesicles* **2020**, *9*, 1713526. [CrossRef]

International Journal of *Molecular Sciences*

MDPI

Article

Comparative Analysis of Hepatic Gene Expression Profiles in Murine and Porcine Sepsis Models

Fëllanza Halimi [1,†], Tineke Vanderhaeghen [2,3,†], Steven Timmermans [2,3], Siska Croubels [1], Claude Libert [2,3,*] and Jolien Vandewalle [2,3,*]

1 Department of Pathobiology, Pharmacology and Zoological Medicine, Faculty of Veterinary Medicine, Ghent University, 9820 Merelbeke, Belgium; fellanza.halimi@ugent.be (F.H.); siska.croubels@ugent.be (S.C.)
2 VIB Center for Inflammation Research, 9000 Ghent, Belgium; tineke.vanderhaeghen@irc.vib-ugent.be (T.V.); steven.timmermans@irc.vib-ugent.be (S.T.)
3 Department of Biomedical Molecular Biology, Ghent University, 9000 Ghent, Belgium
* Correspondence: claude.libert@irc.vib-ugent.be (C.L.); jolien.vandewalle@irc.vib-ugent.be (J.V.)
† These authors contributed equally to this work.

Abstract: Sepsis remains a huge unmet medical need for which no approved drugs, besides antibiotics, are on the market. Despite the clinical impact of sepsis, its molecular mechanism remains inadequately understood. Recent insights have shown that profound hepatic transcriptional reprogramming, leading to fatal metabolic abnormalities, might open a new avenue to treat sepsis. Translation of experimental results from rodents to larger animal models of higher relevance for human physiology, such as pigs, is critical and needs exploration. We performed a comparative analysis of the transcriptome profiles in murine and porcine livers using the following sepsis models: cecal ligation and puncture (CLP) in mice and fecal instillation (FI) in pigs, both of which induce polymicrobial septic peritonitis, and lipopolysaccharide (LPS)-induced endotoxemia in pigs, inducing sterile inflammation. Using bulk RNA sequencing, Metascape pathway analysis, and HOMER transcription factor motif analysis, we were able to identify key genes and pathways affected in septic livers. Conserved upregulated pathways in murine CLP and porcine LPS and FI generally comprise typical inflammatory pathways, except for ER stress, which was only found in the murine CLP model. Conserved pathways downregulated in sepsis comprise almost exclusively metabolic pathways such as monocarboxylic acid, steroid, biological oxidation, and small-molecule catabolism. Even though the upregulated inflammatory pathways were equally induced in the two porcine models, the porcine FI model more closely resembles the metabolic dysfunction observed in the CLP liver compared to the porcine LPS model. This comprehensive comparison focusing on the hepatic responses in mouse CLP versus LPS or FI in pigs shows that the two porcine sepsis models generally resemble quite well the mouse CLP model, with a typical inflammatory signature amongst the upregulated genes and metabolic dysfunction amongst the downregulated genes. The hepatic ER stress observed in the murine model could not be replicated in the porcine models. When studying metabolic dysfunction in the liver upon sepsis, the porcine FI model more closely resembles the mouse CLP model compared to the porcine LPS model.

Keywords: sepsis animal models; liver; cecal ligation and puncture; LPS infusion; fecal instillation; RNA sequencing

1. Introduction

Sepsis is defined as a life-threatening organ dysfunction resulting from a dysregulated host response to infection [1]. Both sepsis and septic shock (i.e., sepsis involving severe blood pressure decline) represent a major global healthcare challenge, being the predominant cause of morbidity and mortality among patients requiring admission to intensive care units (ICUs) and imposing a substantial economic burden on the healthcare system. Recent estimates reveal a staggering annual burden of 48.9 million sepsis cases and 11 million deaths worldwide in the human population [2], but sepsis is also of significant relevance in animals, e.g., in livestock [3]. Based on the epidemiological data, the World Health Organization (WHO) has declared sepsis as a global health priority [4]. The current management of septic patients is rather supportive than curative and relies on controlling the infection using antibiotics, fluid resuscitation combined with vasopressor treatment, and mechanical support of failing organs [5]. Despite five decades of intensive research, no innovative drugs have hit the market to treat sepsis patients [6]. The lack of successful therapies might be attributed to the following issues: (1) For decades, sepsis research has been focused on the inflammatory response, while recent studies have also described the occurrence of metabolic changes in the liver during sepsis [7,8]. (2) Because of practical and ethical constraints, research in sepsis patients is usually limited to serum, plasma, and white blood cells (WBCs). Therefore, it might be of great interest to study organ-specific processes in human sepsis patients; however, it is ethically difficult to obtain biopsies of live patients. In addition, postmortem human biopsies should be interpreted with caution since RNA and protein expression might be altered postmortem [9]. (3) Although rodent models have often yielded valuable information related to certain human diseases, in sepsis, however, translation of preclinical findings to human patients turns out to be difficult, as many promising therapeutic targets in preclinical studies have been disappointing in human clinical studies [6].

Therefore, it is important to close the gap between mouse data and sepsis patients by performing studies with larger animals. In preclinical models, rodents are often used due to their availability, size, low cost, and easy genetic manipulation. Using small animal models, especially transgenic models, allows researchers to gain insight into the proof-of-concept of the molecular mechanisms of diseases such as sepsis in a fast and cost-effective way. In rodent models, sepsis is often induced using cecal ligation and puncture (CLP), which is considered as the gold standard for experimental polymicrobial (peritoneal) sepsis [10]. CLP involves a combination of three insults: (1) tissue trauma due to laparotomy, (2) necrosis caused by ligation of the cecum, and (3) infection due to the leakage of enteric and cecal bacteria into the peritoneum. The latter results in peritonitis followed by translocation of microbial flora into the bloodstream and colonization of organs. It is characteristic of CLP that the pathogens originate from within the host, which is relevant in human septic peritonitis since this usually results from physical intestinal rupture or damage. However, the use of rodents as animal models is also associated with some weaknesses. Due to their small size, it is more difficult to apply regular clinical tools such as probes, catheters, multiple blood samplings, and source control. Moreover, their small size causes a relatively high surface-to-volume ratio, leading to very significant heat loss compared to larger animals and humans. Also, when compared to the human sepsis phenotype, significant differences exist in terms of their metabolic, inflammatory, and hemodynamic responses [11,12]. Therefore, there is a need for more clinically relevant, larger animal models that allow easy and reliable clinical translation [13,14].

The pig genome is related more closely to the human genome compared to the mouse genome, and pigs resemble humans in numerous anatomical and physiological aspects [15]. Due to the similar size of pigs and humans, a preclinical porcine sepsis model can profit from more extensive tools [16,17].

Three categories of experimental sepsis models are used in porcine models, namely (1) the endotoxemia model characterized by lipopolysaccharide (LPS) infusion [18], (2) intravenous administration of live bacterial strains such as *Pseudomonas aeruginosa*, and (3) inoculation of autologous feces (fecal instillation, FI). The use of pigs is, however, associated with higher costs and laborious handling during the experiments. Also, the availability of transgenic pig models is limited [14]. It is crucial to understand that the use of small and large animal models should be seen not as competitive but as complementary. This approach is essential for facilitating the optimal translation of findings from small animal models to large animal models, thereby enhancing the robustness and reliability of preclinical research outcomes.

In the current study, we compared the hepatic transcriptomic changes of CLP mice with those of the two most used porcine sepsis models, namely the porcine LPS and FI model. The CLP (mouse) model is considered the gold standard for studying sepsis, and we aim to determine which porcine model is most suitable for transitioning from CLP mice to pigs, thereby improving translatability in sepsis research.

2. Results

2.1. Literature Summary of Currently Used Porcine Sepsis Models

Today, the CLP model is considered the gold standard for sepsis studies and is typically induced in mice or rats. Analysis of the porcine sepsis models used in the last five years conducted using ISI Web of Knowledge database (using the query: *"sepsis model pig, article, 2019–2024"*) revealed that the LPS model is the most widely used porcine sepsis model (35%), followed by autologous FI (19%) and monobacterial infections such as *Escherichia coli*, *Streptococcus suis*, and *Pseudomonas aeruginosa* (Figure S1A). These porcine models are preferred by researchers, as these are relatively easy to perform—by infusion or instillation—and thus do not require complex surgery on the large animals. The group "other" in the pie chart of Figure S1A includes sepsis models such as anastomotic leak, ischemia reperfusion, and abdominal infusion of liver slurry. In this study, the aim was to investigate how closely the hepatic transcriptomic changes in CLP mice align with those observed in the most commonly used porcine sepsis models, specifically the LPS and FI models. Analysis was performed on available datasets, with focus on hepatic gene regulation given our recent observations pointing towards the essential role of the liver and its transcriptomic changes (particularly in relation to nuclear receptor transcription factors) during sepsis [19,20].

To identify differentially expressed genes (DEGs), we used a $p \leq 0.05$ cutoff and an LFC ≥ 1 or ≤ -1 to determine respectively up- or downregulated genes. Numbers of DEGs detected are summarized in Figure S1B. A total of 2019 and 2665 genes are up- and downregulated, respectively, in the mouse CLP model compared to sham mice, whereas the amount of DEGs is lower in the porcine models (683/756 and 761/1235 up/down in, respectively, LPS and FI). This might be attributed to the fact that the annotation of mouse genes is better compared to porcine genes. Indeed, the number of transcripts identified in mice is 2.5× times higher compared to pigs (149.194 gene transcripts are described in *Mus musculus* versus 60.273 in *Sus scrofa*, source: Ensembl). Next, the sepsis severity is higher in mice compared to pigs, as illustrated below. An overview of all DEGs per model and their associated *p*-values and LFCs is provided in Table S1.

2.2. Gene Expression Profiles in Liver from Murine CLP

To comprehensively explore hepatic changes at a genome-wide scale within the livers of septic mice, bulk RNA-seq analysis was conducted on liver tissue obtained 24 h after surgery from mice subjected to either the CLP or sham procedure (Figure 1A,B). To understand the functional implications of the dysregulated genes, a pathway analysis was performed using Metascape [21]. This analysis revealed a typical inflammatory signature being upregulated upon CLP that is characterized by different pathways involved in cell activation, migration, and cell death. Obviously, cytokines are involved, with pathways such as positive regulation of response to external stimulus and positive regulation of cell migration (Figure 1C).

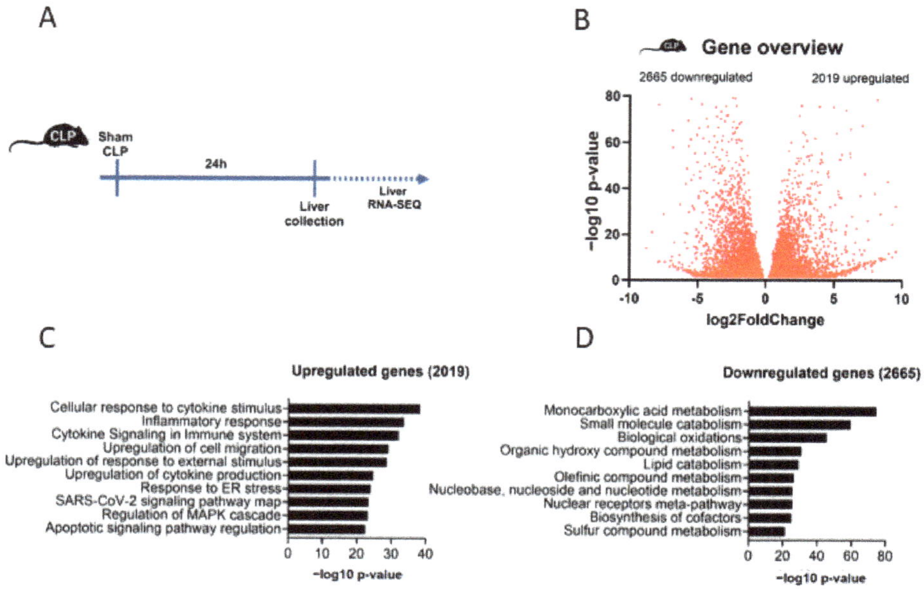

E

Name	p-val	#mots	#backgr	motif
Stat3+il21(Stat)	1×10^{-4}	421 (28.64%)	10,817.5 (24.02%)	
TATA-Box(TBP)	1×10^{-3}	619 (42.11%)	16,872.3 (37.47%)	
AP-1(bZIP)	1×10^{-3}	278 (18.91%)	7078.9 (15.72%)	
Hoxc9(Homeobox)	1×10^{-3}	230 (15.65%)	5744.0 (12.76%)	
Jun-AP1(bZIP)	1×10^{-3}	105 (7.14%)	2331.2 (5.18%)	

F

Name	p-val	#mots	#backgr	motif
HNF4a(NR),DR1	1×10^{-4}	358 (18.14%)	6592.2 (14.74%)	
Brachyury(T-box)	1×10^{-3}	166 (8.41%)	2817.5 (6.30%)	
PPARa(NR),DR1	1×10^{-3}	753 (38.17%)	15,438.8 (34.52%)	
Nkx2.2(Homeobox)	0.01	1108 (56.16%)	23,532.5 (52.62%)	
Bcl6(Zf)	0.01	859 (43.54%)	17,944.0 (40.12%)	

Figure 1. Genome-wide overview of the gene expression profile of the liver in CLP-induced polymicrobial sepsis in mice. (**A**) Male C57BL/6J mice were subjected to a sham or CLP procedure, and the livers were isolated 24 h after surgery for a genome-wide transcriptomics analysis via bulk RNA-seq. (**B**) Volcano plot depicting the differentially expressed genes ($p \leq 0.05$, LFC ≤ -1 or LFC ≥ 1) affected by CLP compared to sham. Genes with a $-$log10 p-value exceeding 80 were excluded for improved plot clarity. (**C**,**D**) Top ten enriched gene ontology (GO) terms for genes that are upregulated ($p \leq 0.05$, LFC ≥ 1) (**C**) or downregulated ($p \leq 0.05$, LFC ≤ -1) (**D**) in CLP mice compared to sham controls. Analyses were performed using the Metascape analysis interface. (**E**,**F**) HOMER motif analysis of CLP-induced genes (**E**) or genes downregulated by CLP (**F**) compared to sham controls (start offset: -1 kb, end offset: 50 bp downstream TSS) ($p \leq 0.05$). Enriched motifs with their name and p-value (p-val) are displayed. #mots = number of motifs found amongst the downregulated genes (absolute (relative %)); #background = number of motifs found amongst background genes (absolute (relative %)).

The downregulated genes reveal a profound influence of CLP on diverse metabolic pathways such as monocarboxylic acid metabolism, small-molecule catabolism, biological oxidations, and lipid catabolism (Figure 1D), all key processes within the organism.

To further determine the upstream regulators of the affected genes, HOMER motif analysis was applied. HOMER motif analysis on the upregulated DEGs unveiled factors such as Signal Transducer and Activator of Transcription 3 + Interleukin-21 (STAT3 + IL21), Activator Protein-1 (AP-1), and JUN-AP1 in the top five (Figure 1E), all factors known for their function in humoral immunity, regulation of cell proliferation, differentiation, and apoptosis [22–24]. HOMER motif analysis on the downregulated DEGs revealed Hepatic Nuclear Factor 4-alpha (HNF4α) as the top transcription factor being predicted to lose its transcriptional activity upon CLP surgery, followed by Brachyury (TBOX) and Peroxisome Proliferator-Activated Receptor Alpha (PPARα) (Figure 1E). Both HNF4α and PPARα are nuclear receptors known to be involved in processes such as the regulation of lipid metabolism, fatty acid oxidation, and control of energy homeostasis [20,25].

2.3. *Comparison Analysis: Predicted Common and Unique Affected Pathways in Liver from Murine CLP versus Porcine FI*

The porcine model studied here that clinically best resembles the mouse CLP model is the FI model, where, just as in the CLP model, peritonitis is induced through host-derived bacteria. We compared available RNA-seq datasets to explore the similarities and differences in altered pathways between these two septic peritonitis models (Figure 2A). Plotting the log2 fold change (LFC) of all DEGs in CLP mice ($p \leq 0.05$, LFC ≤ -1 or LFC ≥ 1) versus the LFC of the orthologues genes in the porcine FI model shows a reduced LFC in the porcine FI model. On average, gene expression changes by FI in pigs are limited to 15.17% of the level in CLP mice, as indicated by the slope of the red dotted line (Figure 2B). When overlapping the upregulated DEGs of both murine CLP and porcine FI, an overlap of 27% was found (206/761). Pathway analysis of the shared upregulated genes via Metascape revealed a typical inflammatory response with pathways involved in positive regulation of locomotion, burn wound healing, cytokine signaling in immune system, response to lipopolysaccharide, neutrophil degranulation, and NABA matrisome-associated pathway, the latter being linked to extra cellular matrix (ECM)-associated proteins (Figure 2C).

When overlapping the downregulated DEGs in murine CLP and porcine FI, an overlap of 33% was found (407/1235). Pathway analysis of the shared downregulated genes exclusively displayed an effect on metabolism with pathways involved in small-molecule catabolism, monocarboxylic acid metabolism, biological oxidations, steroid metabolism, and drug metabolism via cytochrome P450 (CYP450) (Figure 2D).

In concordance with the pathway analysis, motif analysis using HOMER of the overlapping upregulated DEGs displayed typical inflammatory-associated transcription factors such as AP-1, FBJ Osteosarcoma Oncogene (FOS), Activating Transcription Factor 3 (ATF3), and JUN, all being basic leucine zipper (bZIP) transcription factors (Figure 2E). HOMER motif analysis of the downregulated genes unveiled three nuclear receptors in the top five, namely HNF4α, PPARα, and Retinoid X Receptor (RXR), all being linked to metabolic pathways (Figure 2E). This comparison analysis shows strong concordance with the results obtained by the CLP only analysis in Figure 1, implicating potential towards a solidified translatability.

In the liver of CLP mice only, 1813 genes are upregulated (Figure 2C). These genes were found to be associated with response to endoplasmic reticulum (ER) stress, apoptotic signaling pathway regulation, regulation of MAPK cascade, and the unfolded protein response (UPR) and are thus more specifically affected in murine CLP. Furthermore, 2258 genes are specifically downregulated in the liver of CLP mice, and the unique pathways identified are, again, predominantly related to metabolism and to vascular processes in the circulatory system (Figure 2D).

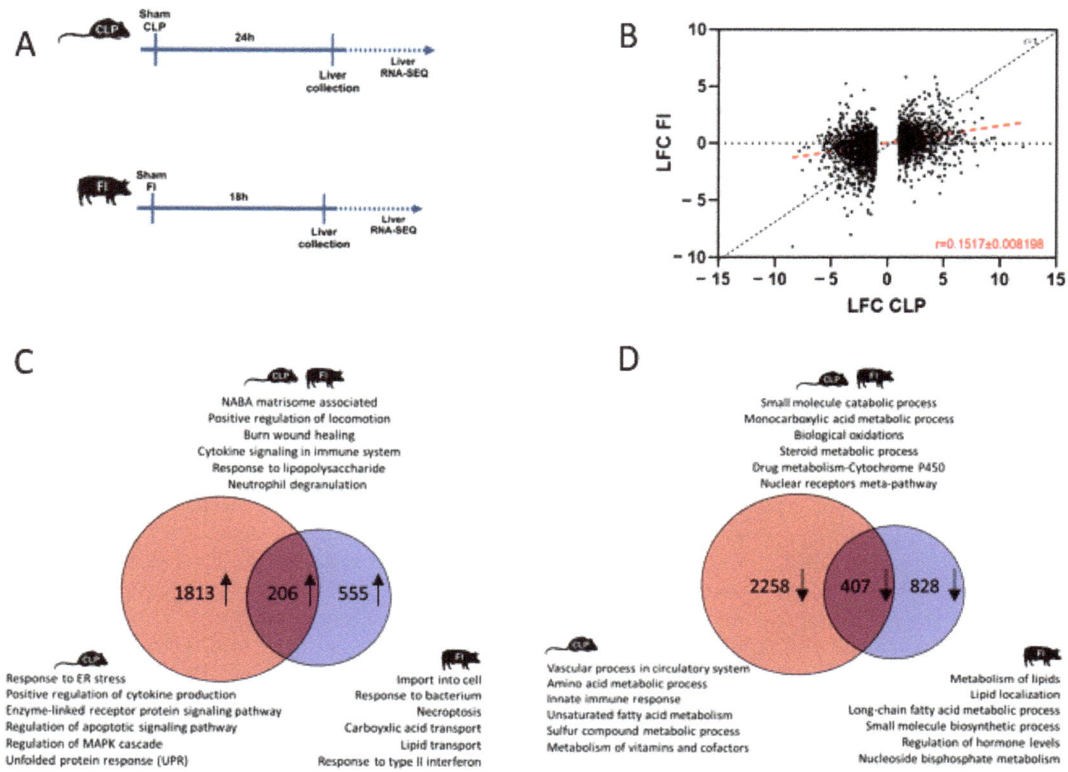

E

Upregulated genes (206)

Name	p-val	#mots	#backgr	motif
AP-1(bZIP)	1×10^{-3}	49 (25.65%)	7552.5 (16.42%)	
Fos(bZIP)	1×10^{-3}	42 (21.99%)	6182.7 (13.44%)	
Atf3(bZIP)	0.01	43 (22.51%)	6798.5 (14.78%)	
JunB(bZIP)	0.01	38 (19.90%)	5819.2 (12.65%)	
BATF(bZIP)	0.01	41 (21.47%)	6660.5 (14.48%)	

Downregulated genes (407)

Name	p-val	#mots	#backgr	motif
HNF4a(NR),DR1	1×10^{-6}	91 (25.07%)	6944.1 (15.02%)	
HNF1b(Homeobox)	1×10^{-4}	37 (10.19%)	2170.7 (4.70%)	
PPARa(NR),DR1	1×10^{-4}	164 (45.18%)	16,023.3 (34.66%)	
TCFL2(HMG)	1×10^{-3}	19 (5.23%)	954.9 (2.07%)	
RXR(NR),DR1	1×10^{-3}	171 (47.11%)	17,977 (38.89%)	

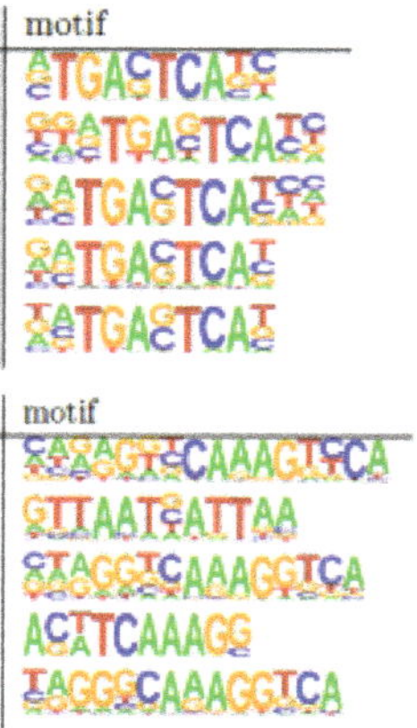

Figure 2. Comparative analysis of the gene expression profile in the liver of CLP-induced polymicrobial sepsis in mice and FI-induced polymicrobial sepsis in pigs. (**A**) Experimental set-up. Mice were subjected to a sham or CLP procedure, and pigs were subjected to a fecal peritonitis (FI) or control procedure. Livers were isolated, respectively, 24 h and 18 h after initiation for genome-wide transcriptomics analysis using bulk RNA-seq. (**B**) Scatter plot demonstrating LFC of all differentially expressed genes in CLP mice ($p \leq 0.05$, LFC ≤ -1 or LFC ≥ 1) versus the LFC of the orthologues genes in FI pigs. r = 1 depicts the slope if no difference in LFC can be observed between CLP or FI. The red dotted line indicates the real slope of the data. Data were analyzed with linear regression.

(**C**) Venn diagram depicting the overlap between the upregulated DEGs in murine CLP versus porcine FI. Selected condition-specific enriched Metascape pathways and biological functions are noted. For the separate DEGs in CLP or FI, only the unique pathways and biological functions are depicted. (**D**) Venn diagram depicting the overlap between the downregulated DEGs in murine CLP versus porcine FI. Selected condition-specific enriched Metascape pathways and biological functions are noted. For the separate DEGs in CLP or FI, only the unique pathways and biological functions are depicted. (**E**) HOMER motif analysis of the shared up- and downregulated DEGs in CLP mice and FI pigs compared to their appropriate controls (start offset: −1 kb, end offset: 50 bp downstream TSS) ($p \leq 0.05$ and genes with mouse orthologue). Enriched motifs with their name and p-value are depicted. #mots = number of motifs found amongst the downregulated genes (absolute (relative %)); #background = number of motifs found amongst background genes (absolute (relative %)).

Studying the pathways linked to the upregulated genes, specifically in the porcine FI model alone (Figure 2C), again show an inflammatory signature, with pathways involved in response to bacterium, necroptosis, and response to type II interferon. Unique pathways linked to the downregulated genes in the porcine FI model were related to regulation of metabolism of lipids and lipid localization, long-chain fatty acid metabolism, and small-molecule biosynthetic process (Figure 2D). An overview of the overlapping and unique genes shown in the Venn diagrams is provided in Table S2.

2.4. *Comparison Analysis: Predicted Common and Unique Affected Pathways in Liver from Murine CLP versus Porcine LPS*

In contrast to fecal peritonitis, which is a rather new sepsis induction method, the LPS-induced endotoxemia model is a more routinely used pig model to study sepsis. LPS is derived from the cell wall of Gram-negative bacteria and induces—in contrast to the CLP and FI models—sterile inflammation. While there are studies comparing the transcriptomic response in septic cardiomyopathy between CLP and LPS mice [26], the comparison of the effect of CLP in mice and LPS infusion in pigs on the hepatic gene expression levels has not been investigated so far (Figure 3A). Plotting the log2 fold change (LFC) of all DEGs in CLP mice ($p \leq 0.05$, LFC ≤ -1 or LFC ≥ 1) versus the LFC of these orthologues genes in the porcine LPS model showed a reduced LFC in the porcine LPS model. On average, gene expression changes by LPS in pigs are limited to 12.14% of the level in CLP mice, as indicated by the slope of the red dotted line (Figure 3B). When overlapping the upregulated DEGs found upon murine CLP and porcine LPS, an overlap of 30% was found (204/683). Pathway analysis of these shared upregulated genes with Metascape revealed a typical inflammatory response very similar to the previous overlap (i.e., CLP-FI) with pathways involved in inflammatory response, NABA matrisome-associated, external stimulus response upregulation, response to bacterium, burn wound healing, and neutrophil degranulation pathways (Figure 3C).

When overlapping the downregulated DEGs in murine CLP and porcine LPS, an overlap of 33% was found (247/756) (Figure 3D). Pathway analysis of the shared downregulated genes again displayed an effect on metabolism with pathways involved in monocarboxylic acid metabolism, steroid metabolism, biological oxidations, small-molecule catabolism, and the nuclear receptors meta-pathway. Motif analysis using HOMER of the overlapping upregulated DEGs displayed typical inflammatory-associated transcription factors such as RUNX, NF-κB-p65-Rel, and TEALD1. Motifs of the overlapping downregulated genes point towards Nuclear Factor (NF)1, HNF4α, and HNF1β (Figure 3E).

Analyzing the DEGs upregulated in the liver of CLP mice only, 1815 genes were identified (Figure 3C). These genes were found to be associated with response to ER stress, cytokine signaling in the immune system, positive regulation of cell migration, and UPR response, quite similar to the unique pathways identified in CLP mice when compared to the FI model. In contrast, 2418 genes are specifically downregulated in the liver of CLP mice, and the unique pathways identified are associated with lipid catabolism, vascular process in circulatory system, nucleobase-containing small-molecule metabolism, organic hydroxy compound metabolism, and the long-chain fatty acid metabolic process (Figure 3D).

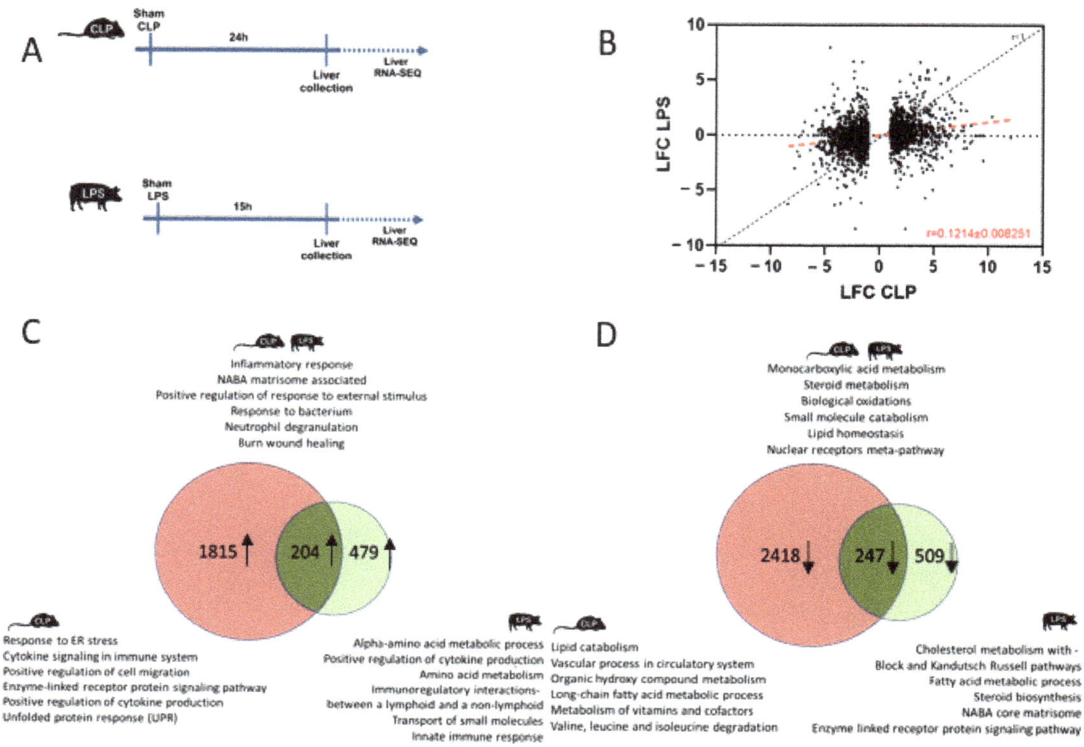

E

Upregulated genes (204)

Name	p-val	#mots	#backgr	motif
RUNX(Runt)	1×10^{-4}	60 (32.97%)	9196.4 (20.15%)	
RUNX-AML(Runt)	1×10^{-3}	55 (30.22%)	8829.6 (19.35%)	
NFkB-p65-Rel(RHD)	1×10^{-3}	14 (7.69%)	1187.2 (2.60%)	
TEAD1(TEAD)	1×10^{-3}	74 (40.66%)	13,479 (29.54%)	
RUNX2(Runt)	0.01	57 (31.32%)	9730 (21.32%)	

Downregulated genes (247)

Name	p-val	#mots	#backgr	motif
NF1(CTF)	1×10^{-4}	52 (23.96%)	6569.1 (14.13%)	
HNF4a(NR),DR1	1×10^{-3}	52 (23.96%)	6951.2 (14.95%)	
HNF1b(Homeobox)	1×10^{-3}	23 (10.60%)	2247.9 (4.84%)	
Tlx?(NR)	0.01	43 (19.82%)	6285.4 (13.52%)	
TEAD2(TEA)	0.01	48 (22.12%)	7258.7 (15.62%)	

Figure 3. Comparative analysis of the gene expression profile in the liver of CLP-induced polymicrobial sepsis in mice and LPS-induced endotoxemia in pigs. (**A**) Experimental set-up. Mice were subjected to a sham or CLP procedure, and pigs were subjected to a LPS infusion or control procedure. Livers were isolated, respectively, 24 h and 15 h after initiation for genome-wide transcriptomics analysis using bulk RNA-seq. (**B**) Scatter plot demonstrating LFC of all differentially expressed genes in CLP mice ($p \leq 0.05$, LFC ≤ -1 or LFC ≥ 1) versus the LFC of these orthologues genes in LPS pigs. r = 1 depicts the slope if no difference in LFC can be observed between CLP or LPS. The red dotted line indicates the real slope of the data. Data were analyzed with linear regression. (**C**) Venn diagram depicting the overlap between the upregulated DEGs in murine CLP versus porcine LPS. Selected condition-specific enriched Metascape pathways and biological functions are noted. For the separate DEGs in CLP or LPS, only the unique pathways and biological functions are depicted.

(**D**) Venn diagram depicting the overlap between the downregulated DEGs in murine CLP versus porcine LPS. Selected condition-specific enriched Metascape pathways and biological functions are noted. For the separate DEGs in CLP or LPS, only the unique pathways and biological functions are depicted. (**E**) HOMER motif analysis of the shared up- and downregulated DEGs in murine CLP versus porcine LPS compared to their appropriate controls (start offset: −1 kb, end offset: 50 bp downstream TSS) ($p \leq 0.05$ and genes with mouse orthologue). Enriched motifs with their name and *p*-value are depicted. #mots = number of motifs found amongst the downregulated genes (absolute (relative %)); #background = number of motifs found amongst background genes (absolute (relative %)).

Studying pathways linked to the upregulated DEGs specifically in the porcine LPS model, an inflammatory signature with positive regulation of cytokine production and innate immune response as well as metabolic pathways involved in amino acid metabolism were detected (Figure 3C). Unique pathways linked to the downregulated genes, specifically in the porcine LPS model, are related to metabolic pathways such as cholesterol metabolism with Block and Kandutsch Russell pathways, fatty acid metabolism, steroid biosynthesis, and NABA core matrisome (Figure 3D). An overview of the overlapping and unique genes shown in the Venn diagrams is provided in Table S2.

2.5. Comparison Analysis: Predicted Common and Unique Affected Pathways in Liver from Porcine FI versus Porcine LPS

To determine the common and unique pathways being affected in the two porcine animal sepsis models, we compared the DEGs upon porcine FI and porcine LPS (Figure S2A). To date, the hepatic gene response upon FI versus LPS in pigs has not yet been compared. An overlap of 35% was found (239/683) in the upregulated genes and 48% (360/756) in the downregulated genes (Figure S2B,C). These percentages are higher compared to the previous two comparison analysis with the murine CLP model and might be attributed to the higher amount of gene transcripts defined in mice compared to pigs. In the shared upregulated genes, the most important pathways identified are related to inflammation, characterized by cellular response to cytokine stimulus, inflammatory response, the NABA matrisome-associated pathway, neutrophil degranulation, and cytokine signaling in the immune system (Figure S2B). Pathway analysis of the shared downregulated genes again revealed a major impact on steroid, monocarboxylic acid metabolism, and biological oxidations, just as was observed in the pairwise analysis with the murine CLP model (Figure S2C). HOMER motif revealed, e.g., FOS and JUNB in the analysis of the common upregulated genes between porcine FI and LPS (Figure S2D). More significant differences were detected in the transcription factor hits of the shared downregulated genes. With the exception of HNF1β, V-maf Musculoaponeurotic Fibrosarcoma oncogene homolog B (MafB) and Broad complex-tramtrack-bric a brac And Cap'n'collar Homology 2 (BACH2) are newly identified transcription factors (Figure S2D), known to play a role in immune-related cells such as macrophages, monocytes, T cells, and B cells [27,28]. It is very striking that practically all motifs found in the porcine comparison analysis are bZIP transcription factors, which are one of the largest families of transcription factors. They are widely distributed and highly conserved in animals, plants, and microorganisms. All bZIP transcription factors contain leucine zippers that enable homo- or heterodimerization.

The FI model has the most unique DEGs among the two porcine models, especially when studying the downregulated genes. In total, 522 genes were found to be upregulated in the FI model only, and these genes belong to positive regulation of cell motility, actin filament-based process, nuclear receptors meta-pathway, and import into cell and tissue morphogenesis (Figure S2B). In contrast, 875 genes are specifically downregulated in the liver of FI pigs, and the unique pathways identified are associated with organic acid biosynthetic process, glycine, serine and threonine metabolism, amino acid metabolism, and the PPAR signaling pathway (Figure S2C). The unique pathways found to be upregulated in the porcine LPS model have a strong inflammation signature, whereas the 396 unique genes downregulated in the LPS porcine model are found to be involved in small-molecule biosynthetic process, SREBP signaling, fatty acid metabolic process, and lipid homeostasis (Figure S2B,C). An overview of the overlapping and unique genes shown in the Venn diagrams is provided in Table S2.

2.6. Side-by-Side Comparison of Affected Pathways Based on Target Gene Expression in the Three Different Sepsis Models

In previous comparison analysis, the three sepsis models were evaluated at the pathway level, focusing solely on significantly altered genes. This approach offers a general understanding of the types of pathways affected but does not indicate the extent of their alteration. In order to know to what extent the pathways in murine CLP are changed (shown in Figure 1C; comparable to the Z-score in Ingenuity Pathway Analysis (IPA)), the genes behind these pathways according to Metascape were retrieved.

By plotting the LFC of the affected genes within each pathway, we can better understand the extent to which each pathway is impacted across the models. For this analysis, only genes with a gene annotation present in all three models were included. Figure 4A reveals that for the top five upregulated pathways retrieved from the murine CLP model (see also Figure 1C), the CLP model induces the different gene sets the strongest, with an average LFC of ± 3 per pathway. Both the LPS and FI porcine models also induce these pathways but with an average LFC of ± 0.6 per pathway. Since these upregulated pathways are typically associated with inflammation, the data suggest that the CLP model induces the strongest inflammatory response, while the two porcine models exhibit a similar level of inflammation to each other, though it is less intense than that observed in the murine model.

When comparing the LFC of gene sets retrieved from the downregulated pathways detected in the CLP model (see also Figure 1D), the murine CLP model again has the strongest effect with an average LFC of ± -2.5 (Figure 4B). Interestingly, for each pathway that was found to be downregulated in the murine model, the FI model (average LFC ± -1) has a stronger effect compared to the LPS model (average LFC ± -0.5). As these downregulated pathways are typically related to metabolic functions, we can conclude from these data that the FI model is a better model to mimic the CLP-induced metabolic dysfunction in the liver compared to the porcine LPS model.

An illustration of these findings is the LFC of typical genes involved in metabolism, which are dependent on HNF4α or PPARα—two transcription factors predicted (Figure 1F) and shown to lose function in the murine liver following CLP surgery [20,29]. HNF4α is a transcriptional regulator of hepatocyte identity and controls genes that are essential for liver functions, such as *Cyp7a*, *Hes6*, *Nr1h4*, *Ppara*, and *Apoa2* (Figure 4C). All these genes were found to be downregulated in murine liver upon CLP compared to sham, and a similar trend was observed in the porcine FI model. The downregulation of these target genes is, however, less apparent in the porcine LPS model. Next, we focused on the target genes of PPARα (Figure 4D). PPARα is known to be involved in β-oxidation of free fatty acids (FFA) and ketogenesis by inducing, e.g., *Ehhadh*, *Hmgcs2*, *Hadha*, *Slc25a20*, *Cpt2*, and *Cpt1a*. Again, all these genes were found to be downregulated in murine liver upon CLP compared to sham, and a similar trend was observed in the porcine FI model, but no clear downregulation was observed in the porcine LPS model. *Hmgcs2*, known to be involved in ketogenesis, is even significantly upregulated upon LPS in the porcine model, a finding also observed in the murine LPS model. These data are in concordance with the HOMER analysis on the downregulated genes shown in Figures 2E and 3E, showing a stronger enrichment of these nuclear receptors in the FI model compared to the LPS model.

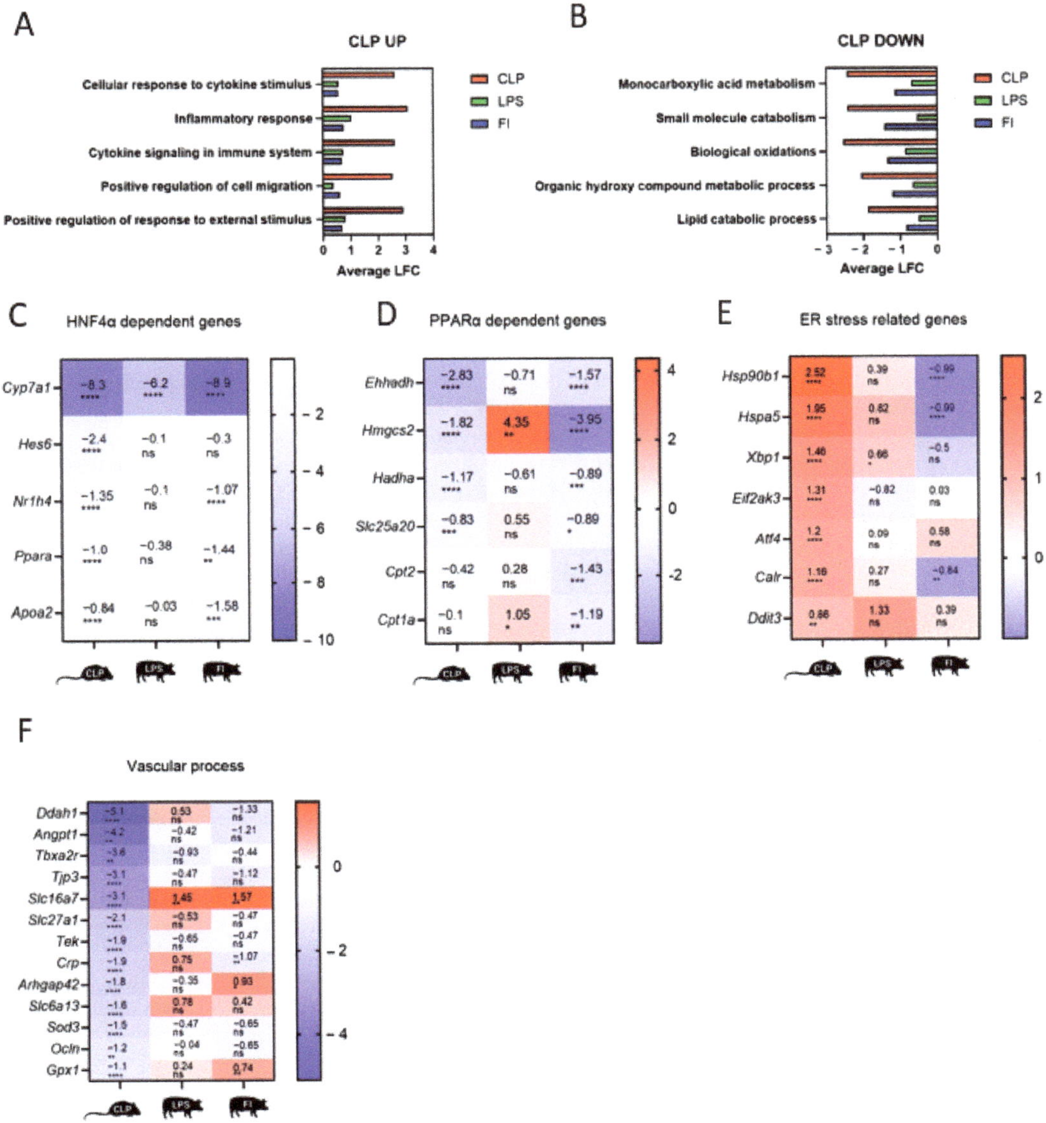

Figure 4. Side-by-side comparison of affected pathways based on target gene expression in the murine CLP and porcine LPS and FI model. (**A**) The top five affected pathways retrieved from the upregulated DEGs of the murine CLP model are depicted. The average LFC of genes belonging to the specified pathway is plotted for each sepsis model. (**B**) The top five affected pathways retrieved from the downregulated DEGs of the murine CLP model are depicted. The average LFC of genes belonging to the specified pathway is plotted for each sepsis model. (**C**) Heat map of selected HNF4α-dependent genes showing the LFC and significance of the specified gene compared to the respective control group for each animal model. (**D**) Heat map of selected PPARα-dependent genes showing the LFC and significance of the specified gene compared to the respective control group for each animal model.

(**E**) Heat map of selected ER stress-related genes showing the LFC and significance of the specified gene compared to the respective control group for each animal model. (**F**) Heat map of selected genes related to "vascular process in circulatory system" showing the LFC and significance of the specified gene compared to the respective control group for each animal model. **** $p \leq 0.0001$; *** $p \leq 0.001$; ** $p \leq 0.01$; * $p \leq 0.05$. ns, not significant.

Remarkably, the pathways "response to ER stress" and "UPR response" are uniquely affected among the upregulated genes in the mouse CLP model. These pathways were not identified by Metascape when analyzing the DEGs in either of the porcine models. When plotting the LFC of typical ER stress- and UPR-related genes (Figure 4E), we observe a strong upregulation of these genes in the murine sepsis model, a less pronounced induction in the porcine LPS model, and a decrease in gene expression in the FI porcine model. In contrast, one of the pathways uniquely affected amongst the downregulated genes in the mouse CLP model is "vascular process in circulatory system". This pathway was not retrieved by Metascape when entering the DEGs of either porcine model. When plotting the LFC of some typical genes involved in vascular function, as provided by Metascape, e.g., genes involved in regulation of endothelial permeability (*Angpt1*, *Tjp3*, *Tek*, and *Ocln*), platelet aggregation (*Tbxa2r*), transport of metabolites (*Slc* genes), complement activation (*Crp*), vascular tone (*Arhgap42*), antioxidant activity (*Sod3* and *Gpx1*), and nitric oxide generation (*Ddah1*), a strong downregulation of the genes in murine sepsis was observed. The two porcine models show similar behavior to each other in terms of LFC; however, unlike the CLP model, there is no clear downregulation of the described genes (Figure 4F). As vascular function is heavily affected by inflammation, the more pronounced effect of the murine CLP model on these vascular-related genes could be attributed to the higher inflammation that is detected in the mice. Of note, due to ethical considerations, there is a slight variation in timepoints amongst the different groups. To verify the robustness of the data, we also compared the LFC of the described genes in Figure 4C–F with another publicly available CLP dataset. This dataset was first described in Vandewalle et al. [19] and compared the hepatic transcriptome in sham or CLP mice 8 h after surgery. Interestingly, we confirmed that the genes depicted in the 24 h CLP dataset that were, respectively, up- (ER stress, Figure 4E) or downregulated (HNF4α, PPARα, and vascular process-related genes, Figure 4C,D,F) show a similar trend in the 8 h CLP dataset (Figure S3A–D). These data point towards the robustness of the data, irrespective of the timepoint chosen.

Overall, side-by-side comparisons between the three different animal models give a comparable overlap of genes shared between the murine CLP versus the two porcine sepsis models. The upregulated genes are typically associated with inflammatory processes, whereas the downregulated genes strongly indicate metabolic dysfunction in the liver. Upregulated genes that are not shared in the comparative analysis are similarly associated with inflammation and vice versa; downregulated genes that are not shared in the comparative analysis are still indicative for metabolic dysfunction. The murine CLP model has the strongest effect on both the up- and downregulated pathways. The two porcine models have a milder effect on the described pathways, with the porcine FI model most closely resembling the downregulated metabolic pathways found in the CLP model.

3. Discussion

Despite extensive research on sepsis, there is no real advancement in sepsis treatment, and many drugs have failed to show a clinical effect in human trials despite being successful in preclinical animal models [6]. Even worse, some therapies, such as TNFα neutralizing antibodies, were promising in preclinical studies but appeared to be harmful in sepsis patients. The animal model used to study drug efficacy has proven to be of utmost importance. Indeed, anti-TNF therapy reduced mortality in the LPS model, whereas TNF turned out to be essential for controlling the infection in the CLP model [30]. A similar disparity was observed when using TNFR1KO mice in murine LPS and CLP models [31]. Due to high similarities between the CLP model and human sepsis, the CLP model is regarded as the gold standard for studying sepsis [10]. Another major concern regarding the current sepsis research is that most studies examine the inflammatory aspect, with focus on serum, plasma, and WBCs. Of course, obtaining blood samples or determining blood parameters is the easiest way to study sepsis in human patients, but rather than investigating what happens in the blood, we need to focus on what happens in the organs, with the liver as the most promising organ based on our most recent insights [8,19,20]. The liver hosts, next to hepatocytes, a range of other cells, including endothelial, hepatic stellate, and Kupffer cells, which all play an essential role in a wide range of cellular processes, such as homeostasis, metabolism, and immunity. Some research has been conducted on postmortem liver samples of sepsis patients, but analysis of postmortem material is difficult owing to changes that occur within the body shortly after death [9]. Therefore, studies on animals such as mice and rats are indispensable, but to enhance translatability, research is warranted in larger animals that are more closely related to humans. Compared to the mouse genome, the pig genome is three times closer to that of a human, and its anatomy and physiology are also more comparable to humans [15]. Indeed, the macroscopic structure (subdivision in lobes and segments) and vascularization are comparable between pig and human livers. Unlike rodents, pigs have well-defined acinar structures with clear portal triads, similarly to humans [32]. In the current study, we examined whether the liver-specific gene expression profile in a murine CLP model reflects the profile seen in the two most routinely used porcine sepsis models. We sought to determine which porcine model is most suitable for follow-up studies based on findings from mouse research. Therefore, the hepatic transcriptomic changes of CLP mice were compared to the LPS and the FI porcine sepsis models. Analysis was carried out using Metascape, as this tool is very user friendly to analyze OMICs data.

A first view on the amount of DEGs (set as $p \leq 0.05$ and a LFC ≥ 1 or ≤ -1) showed 4684 DEGs in CLP mice compared to sham mice, whereas for the porcine LPS and FI model, this was, respectively, 1439 and 1996 genes. This reflects the higher number of transcripts identified in mice compared to pigs but could also be explained by the reduced variation and stronger effect size in mice. Throughout our comparative analysis, the major upregulated pathways point towards inflammation. However, the type of pathways activated in the different models used might differ. Unique to the CLP model is a strong response to ER stress and UPR, whereas this could not be detected in the liver of the two porcine models. The ER is involved in protein folding and post-translational modifications and is also a critical organelle of the secretory pathway. The burst of protein synthesis during the early phase of sepsis can lead to the accumulation of unfolded or misfolded proteins, a phenomenon also known as ER stress. ER stress can eventually activate the UPR response, an adaptive reaction that reduces unfolded protein load to maintain cell viability and function [33]. A closer look at typical ER stress-related genes indeed show a strong upregulation of these genes in the murine CLP model, whereas in the porcine LPS model and especially the porcine FI model, this was less apparent. This may indicate that the porcine model is not a good model to study hepatic ER stress during sepsis when making the transition from mice to larger sepsis models. In general, there are not many studies investigating the role of ER stress in liver during sepsis, and if so, these studies were performed in rodents. ER stress is activated upon sepsis in rodents, and inhibition of ER stress using 4-phenylbutyric acid could improve vital organ function in the liver, kidney, and intestinal barrier, resulting in improved survival following CLP in rats [34]. ER stress in septic pigs has not yet been reported in the literature. A potential reason for the lack of depiction of a strong ER stress response in porcine sepsis could be the comparatively lower inflammatory response observed in pigs compared to the CLP mouse model, as the inflammatory response and ER stress are strongly linked to each other. Indeed, it is known that inflammatory cytokines such as the pro-inflammatory cytokines IL1β, IL6, and TNFα induce ER stress, which further disrupts metabolic functions, thereby causing more inflammation. This vicious cycle exacerbates inflammatory signaling as well as metabolic deterioration [35]. Of note, compared to mice, the immune system of pigs generally more strongly resembles that of humans. Indeed, the lymphocyte % in blood is 75–90% in mice,

40–60% in pigs, and 20–50% in humans, whereas the neutrophil % in blood is 10–25% in mice, 30–50% in pigs, and 40–75% in humans [17,36]. These differences in immune composition might account for the stronger immune response to sepsis compared to pigs. In human sepsis patients, ER stress in skeletal muscle and immune cells has already been depicted [37]; yet, whether ER stress plays a role in the liver of human sepsis patients needs to be established. Based on the current data, it remains uncertain whether inhibiting ER stress would yield significant therapeutic benefits for human sepsis patients. While preclinical studies in mice suggest a role for ER stress in the pathophysiology of sepsis, translating these findings to humans is complex due to interspecies differences in immune response and disease progression. Further studies, including clinical trials, are needed to evaluate the potential efficacy and safety of ER stress inhibition in sepsis treatment.

Interestingly, the major downregulated pathways throughout our comparison analysis almost exclusively involve metabolic pathways. This observation supports recent findings showing that upon CLP surgery in mice, the liver loses activity of key transcription factors involved in metabolism [8], such as glucocorticoid receptor (GR) [19], PPARα [20], and HNF4α [29], eventually leading to metabolic failure. Indeed, upon CLP surgery, the liver acquires GR resistance. Since GR is involved in gluconeogenesis, GR functioning is essential for sepsis survival due to its role in lactate removal and glucose production [19]. The "monocarboxylic acid metabolism" pathway was found amongst the downregulated genes in all three models tested. Typical monocarboxylic acids includes lactate, pyruvate, and ketone bodies, and these metabolites are indeed all found to be increased upon sepsis. The GR motif was, however, not found by HOMER amidst the tested downregulated genes, which might be attributed to the initial corticosterone boost shortly after sepsis that first induces many GR-responsive genes [19]. PPARα is another major transcription factor involved in metabolism by coordinating the β-oxidation of FFAs in liver. Similar to that observed with GR, PPARα loses its transcriptional activity upon CLP surgery in mice, causing FFAs to accumulate in blood and organs eventually leading to lipotoxicity [20]. This finding was already confirmed in the porcine FI model [38], and in the current study, the porcine LPS model also presented with "fatty acid metabolic process" amongst the pathways retrieved from the downregulated genes. The PPARα motif was found amidst the downregulated DEGs of the murine CLP and porcine FI model according to HOMER but not in the porcine LPS model. In accordance with HOMER, *Ppara* gene expression and its target genes were less clearly downregulated upon LPS injection in pigs compared to the murine CLP and porcine FI model. This might explain why the "lipid catabolic process" is the least affected in the porcine LPS model compared to the two other models tested. Recently, it was demonstrated that PPARα mRNA and protein levels are downregulated upon sepsis due to HNF4α loss of function [29]. HNF4α is key regulator of hepatocyte identity by controlling genes involved in metabolism of lipids, glucose, bile acids, and xenobiotics. Transgenic mice with HNF4α-specific deletion in hepatocytes have severely reduced hepatic PPARα levels in steady state. Upon sepsis in wild-type mice, HNF4α is shown to lose its function, leading to PPARα reduction [29]. Next to its role in controlling PPARα expression and lipid metabolism, HNF4α also induces many CYP450-coding genes. CYP450 enzymes, encoded by the *Cyp* genes, are involved in the synthesis and metabolism of various compounds within cells. CYP450 enzymes are key phase I enzymes that metabolize many xenobiotics, such as drugs and environmental pollutants, and endogenous substances, such as toxins that are formed within cells. Interestingly, "drug or xenobiotic metabolism by cytochrome P450" was found by Metascape amongst the downregulated genes in all three sepsis models tested, and the HNF4α motif was also found amidst the downregulated genes in all three models. That metabolism reduced by CYP450 is a consequence of HNF4α loss of function seems logical but needs to be confirmed. Given the high similarities between pigs and humans in substrate selectivity and quantity-normalized activities for major drug-metabolizing CYP450 subfamilies in the liver [39], the porcine FI model thus seems a very good model when making the transition from mice to humans in studying CYP450 activity in septic liver. Just as observed with PPARα-dependent genes, other HNF4α target genes were also generally downregulated in both the murine CLP and porcine FI models, whereas the downregulation of these genes was less apparent in the porcine LPS model. This observation could be expanded to the top five downregulated pathways found in CLP mice, implicating that the FI model is a better model to mimic metabolic dysfunction in CLP mice compared to the porcine LPS model. Next to the global metabolic signature observed amongst the downregulated genes, "vascular process in circulatory system" was a typical pathway observed in the murine CLP model and not in the two porcine models when the downregulated DEGs were entered in Metascape. This might be related to the higher inflammation signature observed in the CLP mice compared to the two other models, as inflammation is a well-known inducer of vascular dysfunction.

The current study has some limitations. First, we made use of two published datasets to perform the comparative analysis in order to avoid unnecessary repetition of experiments, with only minor differences in isolation timing, in accordance with ethical considerations. This implies that the timepoints of liver collection are not exactly the same. For the murine CLP model, this was 24 h, whereas for the porcine LPS and FI model, this was, respectively, 15 h and 18 h after sepsis induction. Despite the later timepoint in the murine model, we had a greater inflammatory response in the murine model compared to the porcine models. This was inherent to the mouse model and not to the timepoint, as we observed the same finding when comparing the porcine datasets with our available 8 h CLP dataset. Interestingly, despite the slightly different timepoints between the two porcine models, the (inflammatory) upregulated pathways were equally induced in both models, suggesting a same degree of inflammation and sepsis severity. Second, it would have been interesting to compare sepsis severity not only based on transcriptional induction of inflammatory pathways but also based on the Sequential Organ Failure Assessment (SOFA) score. Clinical markers to score sepsis severity were, however, not measured in the porcine LPS model and murine CLP model, making it impossible to correlate the degree of affected pathways with sepsis severity. Third, the critical care provided to the animals was different amongst the three models. For the murine CLP model, this entailed antibiotics and fluid administration; for the porcine LPS model, no critical care was provided; and for the porcine FI model, this entailed an advanced intensive care that follows the MQTiPSS (Minimum Quality Threshold in Pre-Clinical Sepsis Studies) recommendations (including abdominal lavage, antimicrobial therapy, and early vasopressor introduction) in order to mimic human clinical care [40]. Lastly, we used the murine CLP model as the gold standard to study sepsis, but of course, ideally, we would have compared transcriptomic changes in the liver of animal models with those observed in human sepsis livers. We are currently conducting a clinical study to collect liver biopsies from (live) human peritoneal sepsis patients as well as controls to explore whether the observed results also apply to human patients (approved by ethical committee UZ Ghent (ONZ-2022-0520)).

Collectively, the pairwise analysis between the murine CLP–porcine LPS, murine CLP–porcine FI and porcine LPS–porcine FI generally showed an inflammatory pathway amongst the upregulated genes and metabolic failure amongst the downregulated genes. Focusing on the inflammatory pathways, ER stress and the UPR response were found to be induced in the liver of CLP mice, but this could not be confirmed in either of the porcine models. This might imply that ER stress does not occur in the porcine liver and—by extension—perhaps human sepsis livers. Focusing on the downregulated metabolic pathways, it was notable that the porcine FI model more closely resembles the murine CLP model than the porcine LPS model. Even though the LPS model is the most widely used sepsis model in pigs, it is thus advisable to use the porcine FI model, especially when studying the metabolic dysfunctions occurring in the liver following sepsis.

4. Materials and Methods

4.1. Animals

4.1.1. Mice

Male C57BL/6J mice at 8–12 weeks of age were purchased from Janvier (Le Genest-St. Isle, France). Mice were housed in a temperature-controlled, specific-pathogen-free (SPF), air-conditioned animal house with 14 h and 10 h light/dark cycles and received food and water ad libitum. All experiments were approved by the institutional ethics committee for animal welfare of the Faculty of Sciences, Ghent University, Belgium.

4.1.2. Pigs—LPS Infusion

Eight-week-old male pigs (Landrace × Large White, Seghers Hybrid®, RA-SE Genetics, Lokeren, Belgium) were group-housed in standard stables (2.30 m × 2.40 m) and provided with water and feed ad libitum. Throughout the entire experiment, the stable temperature was maintained at an average of 23.2 ± 0.45 °C, and the stables were enriched with rubber toys and cotton towels. The LPS infusion study was approved by the Ethical Committee of the Faculty of Veterinary Medicine and the Faculty of Bioscience Engineering of Ghent University (EC 2017/24).

4.1.3. Pigs—Fecal Instillation

Twelve pigs (seven male and five female, weighing 49 ± 5 kg) (RA-SE Genetics, Belgium), were kept in standard stables and provided with water and feed ad libitum. The study protocol followed the EU Directive (2010/63/EU) for animal experiments and was approved by the local animal ethics committee (Comité Ethique du Bien-Être Animal; protocol number 724N) from the Université Libre de Bruxelles (ULB) in Brussels, Belgium. These pig experiments were conducted in the Experimental Laboratory of Intensive Care of ULB (LA1230406), and the Minimum Quality Threshold in Preclinical Sepsis Studies (MQTiPSS) guidelines recommendations and ARRIVE guidelines for translational sepsis research were followed [40,41].

4.2. Experimental Procedures

4.2.1. Cecal Ligation and Puncture (CLP)

A detailed description of the experimental procedure to induce polymicrobial sepsis in mice was provided by Vandewalle et al. (2021) [19]. In short, polymicrobial sepsis was induced in mice using the CLP technique. For this, mice were anesthetized with isoflurane, and a midline abdominal incision was made to expose the cecum. Then, the cecum was ligated for 75%, and a double puncture using a 21-gauge needle was made. The abdominal muscles were sutured with running stitches, and the skin was closed using metallic clips. As a control group, the cecum was exposed in sham mice but neither ligated nor punctured. Mice were euthanized via cervical dislocation 24 h or 8 h (as detailed in text) after the onset of sepsis, and liver samples were collected for subsequent analysis.

4.2.2. LPS Infusion

A detailed description of the experimental procedure to induce endotoxemia in the pigs was provided by Dhondt et al. (2021) [42]. In short, following a 3-day acclimatization period, a double-lumen catheter was surgically implanted in the external jugular vein of piglets. After surgery, piglets were housed individually to prevent catheter displacement. To maintain catheter patency, regular flushing with a heparinized solution was performed, and bandages were replaced daily. Endotoxemia was induced after a recovery day, during which piglets received a continuous infusion of ultrapure LPS derived from *Escherichia coli* (O111) (Invitrogen, Toulouse, France) over a 15 h period at a rate of 5.0 μg/kg/h, alongside fluid therapy consisting of 0.9% NaCl at 6 mL/kg/h. Sham piglets were administered only the vehicle solution. After 15 h of LPS infusion, euthanasia was induced by an overdose of sodium pentobarbital (Sodium pentobarbital 20%®, Kela, Hoogstraten, Belgium), after which liver samples were collected for subsequent analysis.

4.2.3. Fecal Instillation

A detailed description of the experimental procedure to induce septic shock in the pigs was provided by Garcia et al. (2022) [43]. In short, prior to the start of the experiment, pigs were fasted for 18 h with free access to water. Fecal peritonitis resulting in septic shock was induced in 9 pigs (5 males and 4 females) by intraperitoneal instillation of 3 g/kg of autologous feces collected from the pig's enclosure and diluted in 300 mL of 5% glucose solution. Three sham pigs (two males and one female), consisting of anesthesia and surgical preparation without sepsis induction, were used as a control. The onset of septic shock was set at a mean arterial pressure (MAP) below 50 mmHg. A MAP between 45 and 50 mmHg was then maintained for 60 min to consolidate the multiple organ failure induction. Resuscitation fluids, norepinephrine (NE), antibiotics treatment, and abdominal lavage were applied to mimic human clinical care during the following 8 h. After 18 h of FI infusion, pigs were euthanized with 7.5% potassium chloride under deep anesthesia for organ isolation. Liver samples were isolated from the NE group at the end of the experiment (vasopressor 2 timepoint) for subsequent analysis.

4.2.4. RNA Sequencing

Mouse Liver—CLP Dataset

We used the liver murine CLP datasets GSE160795 (8 h timepoint) and GSE160830 (24 h timepoint) that was processed as described in Vandewalle et al. (2021) [19].

Pig Liver—LPS Dataset

Liver biopsies from the fourth segment were preserved in RNALater (AM7021, Invitrogen, Waltham, MA, USA) and subsequently processed for RNA extraction using the Aurum total RNA mini kit (732-6820, Bio-Rad, Temse, Belgium), following the manufacturer's protocol. The concentration and quality of the extracted RNA were analyzed using Agilent RNA 6000 Pico Kit (Agilent Technologies, Santa Clara, CA, USA). The RNA samples were sequenced by VIB Nucleomics Core (Leuven, Belgium). Libraries were prepared using the Illumina TruSeq3 stranded library prep protocol, and sequencing was performed with single-end reads (75 bp) on an Illumina NextSeq 550 platform. Pig reads were aligned to the Sscrofa11 reference genome using STAR 2.7.10a with the genequant option for direct read-count assignment to features. Differential gene expression analysis was conducted with DESeq2, and results were exported in Excel 2019 format. The RNA-seq data were deposited in the Gene Expression Omnibus (GEO) under accession number GSE250039 and are publicly accessible via the NCBI database.

Pig Liver—Fecal Instillation Dataset

We used the liver porcine FI dataset GSE218636 that was processed as described in Vandewalle et al. (2022) [38].

4.2.5. Processing of the RNA-Seq Results

The dataset under investigation was acquired in the form of Excel spreadsheets containing the genes associated with each sepsis model. To ensure the acquirement of statistically significant outcomes, we applied filters: adjusted p-value ≤ 0.05, log fold change (LFC) ≥ 1 for upregulated genes, and LFC ≤ -1 for downregulated genes. A comparative analysis between distinct sepsis models (CLP mouse versus porcine LPS, CLP mouse versus porcine FI, and porcine FI versus porcine LPS) was conducted. A considerable proportion of the genes associated with porcine sepsis lacked a designated name corresponding to their ENSG ID. To address this, genes lacking a specific name were filtered out. The refined gene lists were subsequently subjected to Ensembl Biomart analysis. We specifically focused on the Ensembl 110 genes database schema, selecting the dataset related to pig genes (Sscrofa11.1). Our criteria for this analysis included filtering by gene-stable ID (e.g., ENSSSCG00000000002) and extracting selected attributes such as homologues (up to six orthologues). The focus was on mouse orthologues, where we set our filters to receive the mouse gene names respective to the ENSG ID. The final gene lists were compared using Venn diagrams, juxtaposing the gene lists for distinct sepsis models (CLP mouse versus porcine LPS, CLP mouse versus porcine FI, and porcine FI versus porcine LPS). Each list was labeled with its corresponding designation and processed for intersection and independent region outcomes. These results were further subjected to pathway analysis using the Metascape analysis interface [21] (v3.5.20240101) with input as species "any species" and analysis as species "*H. sapiens*" and otherwise default settings. Motif finding for multiple motifs was carried out using the HOMER software version v4.11 [44]. We used the promoter region (start offset: −1 kb, end offset: 50 bp downstream of the transcription start site (TSS)) to explore known motif enrichment. HOMER motif enrichment *p*-values were determined using the whole genome promoter set as background. The reported *p*-values are those of the motif overrepresentation of the gene set of interest over background for each motif.

Supplementary Materials: The following supporting information can be downloaded at: https://www.mdpi.com/article/10.3390/ijms252011079/s1.

Author Contributions: Conceptualization, F.H., T.V., S.T., S.C., C.L. and J.V.; methodology, F.H., T.V., S.T., S.C., C.L. and J.V.; software, S.T.; formal analysis, F.H., T.V., S.T. and J.V.; investigation, F.H., T.V., S.T., S.C., C.L. and J.V.; resources, S.C. and C.L.; data curation, F.H., T.V., S.T. and J.V.; writing—original draft preparation, F.H., T.V., S.T. and J.V.; writing—review and editing, F.H., T.V., S.T., S.C., C.L. and J.V.; visualization, F.H., T.V., S.T. and J.V.; supervision, S.C., C.L. and J.V.; project administration, S.C. and C.L.; funding acquisition, S.C., C.L. and J.V. All authors have read and agreed to the published version of the manuscript.

Funding: This research was funded by a personal FWO grant to J.V. (1220924N) and by the Special Research Fund of Ghent University (GOA and Methusalem Program (BOF.MET.2021.0001.0) and BOF16/DOC/285) and FWO (S003122N). The APC was funded by FWO (S003122N).

Institutional Review Board Statement: The animal study involving LPS pigs was approved by the Ethical Committee of the Faculty of Veterinary Medicine and the Faculty of Bioscience Engineering of Ghent University (EC 2017/24). The mouse CLP and pig FI datasets were retrieved from publicly available datasets (see Section 4).

Data Availability Statement: RNA-seq data of the LPS pigs (these are newly deposited data) are deposited at the National Center for Biotechnology Information (NCBI) Gene Expression Omnibus public database (http://www.ncbi.nlm.nih.gov/geo/ accessed on 2 September 2024) under accession number GSE250039. The mouse CLP and pig FI datasets were retrieved from publicly available datasets (see Section 4).

Acknowledgments: We would like to thank Laura Dhondt for providing the porcine LPS liver samples.

Conflicts of Interest: The authors declare no conflict of interest.

References

1. Singer, M.; Deutschman, C.S.; Seymour, C.; Shankar-Hari, M.; Annane, D.; Bauer, M.; Bellomo, R.; Bernard, G.R.; Chiche, J.D.; Coopersmith, C.M.; et al. The Third International Consensus Definitions for Sepsis and Septic Shock (Sepsis-3). *JAMA—J. Am. Med. Assoc.* **2016**, *315*, 801–810. [CrossRef] [PubMed]
2. Rudd, K.E.; Johnson, S.C.; Agesa, K.M.; Shackelford, K.A.; Tsoi, D.; Kievlan, D.R.; Colombara, D.V.; Ikuta, K.S.; Kissoon, N.; Finfer, S.; et al. Global, Regional, and National Sepsis Incidence and Mortality, 1990–2017: Analysis for the Global Burden of Disease Study. *Lancet* **2020**, *395*, 200. [CrossRef] [PubMed]
3. Pas, M.L.; Bokma, J.; Lowie, T.; Boyen, F.; Pardon, B. Sepsis and Survival in Critically Ill Calves: Risk Factors and Antimicrobial Use. *J. Vet. Intern. Med.* **2023**, *37*, 374–389. [CrossRef] [PubMed]
4. Global Report on the Epidemiology and Burden of Sepsis: Current Evidence, Identifying Gaps and Future Directions—World | ReliefWeb. Available online: https://reliefweb.int/report/world/global-report-epidemiology-and-burden-sepsis-current-evidence-identifying-gaps-and?gad_source=1&gclid=Cj0KCQiAgqGrBhDtARIsAM5s0_lIRiWZJSWGwqYk2ER4WAKHctkvT-KTQn2z9WL1EsmwDHRgGDZtgmYaAgoVEALw_wcB (accessed on 30 November 2023).
5. Evans, L.; Rhodes, A.; Alhazzani, W.; Antonelli, M.; Coopersmith, C.M.; French, C.; Machado, F.R.; Mcintyre, L.; Ostermann, M.; Prescott, H.C.; et al. Surviving Sepsis Campaign: International Guidelines for Management of Sepsis and Septic Shock 2021. *William Schweickert* **2021**, *47*, 62. [CrossRef]

6. Cavaillon, J.; Singer, M.; Skirecki, T. Sepsis Therapies: Learning from 30 Years of Failure of Translational Research to Propose New Leads. *EMBO Mol. Med.* **2020**, *12*, e10128. [CrossRef] [PubMed]
7. Van Wyngene, L.; Vandewalle, J.; Libert, C. Reprogramming of Basic Metabolic Pathways in Microbial Sepsis: Therapeutic Targets at Last? Introduction: Sepsis Pathophysiology. *EMBO Mol. Med.* **2018**, *10*, 8712. [CrossRef]
8. Vandewalle, J.; Libert, C. Sepsis: A Failing Starvation Response. *Trends Endocrinol. Metab.* **2022**, *33*, 292–304. [CrossRef]
9. Van Der Linden, A.; Blokker, B.M.; Kap, M.; Weustink, A.C.; Riegman, P.H.J.; Oosterhuis, J.W.; Cappello, F. Post-Mortem Tissue Biopsies Obtained at Minimally Invasive Autopsy: An RNA-Quality Analysis. *PLoS ONE* **2014**, *9*, e0115675. [CrossRef]
10. Dejager, L.; Pinheiro, I.; Dejonckheere, E.; Libert, C. Cecal Ligation and Puncture: The Gold Standard Model for Polymicrobial Sepsis? *Trends Microbiol.* **2011**, *19*, 198–208. [CrossRef]
11. Alverdy, J.C.; Keskey, R.; Thewissena, R. Can the Cecal Ligation and Puncture Model Be Repurposed to Better Inform Therapy in Human Sepsis. *Infect. Immun.* **2020**, *88*, 10-1128. [CrossRef]
12. Wang, N.; Lu, Y.; Zheng, J.; Liu, X. Of Mice and Men: Laboratory Murine Models for Recapitulating the Immunosuppression of Human Sepsis. *Front. Immunol.* **2022**, *13*, 956448. [CrossRef] [PubMed]
13. Zurek-Leffers, F.M.; Lehmann, F.; Brabenec, L.; Kintrup, S.; Hellenthal, K.E.M.; Mersjann, K.; Kneifel, F.; Hessler, M.; Arnemann, P.H.; Kampmeier, T.G.; et al. A Model of Porcine Polymicrobial Septic Shock. *Intensive Care Med. Exp.* **2023**, *11*, 31. [CrossRef]
14. Vintrych, P.; Al-Obeidallah, M.; Horák, J.; Chvojka, J.; Valešová, L.; Nalos, L.; Jarkovská, D.; Matějovič, M.; Štengl, M. Modeling Sepsis, with a Special Focus on Large Animal Models of Porcine Peritonitis and Bacteremia. *Front. Physiol.* **2023**, *13*, 1094199. [CrossRef] [PubMed]
15. Walters, E.M.; Prather, R.S. Advancing Swine Models for Human Health and Diseases. *Mo. Med.* **2013**, *110*, 212.
16. Parker, S.J.; Watkins, P.E. Experimental Models of Gram-Negative Sepsis. *Br. J. Surg.* **2000**, *88*, 22–30. [CrossRef]
17. Lunney, J.K.; Van Goor, A.; Walker, K.E.; Hailstock, T.; Franklin, J.; Dai, C. Importance of the Pig as a Human Biomedical Model. *Sci. Transl. Med.* **2021**, *13*, eabd5758. [CrossRef]
18. Gasthuys, E.; Vandecasteele, T.; De Bruyne, P.; Vande Walle, J.; De Backer, P.; Cornillie, P.; Devreese, M.; Croubels, S. The Potential Use of Piglets as Human Pediatric Surrogate for Preclinical Pharmacokinetic and Pharmacodynamic Drug Testing. *Curr. Pharm. Des.* **2016**, *22*, 4069–4085. [CrossRef]
19. Vandewalle, J.; Timmermans, S.; Paakinaho, V.; Vancraeynest, L.; Dewyse, L.; Vanderhaeghen, T.; Wallaeys, C.; Van Wyngene, L.; Van Looveren, K.; Nuyttens, L.; et al. Combined Glucocorticoid Resistance and Hyperlactatemia Contributes to Lethal Shock in Sepsis. *Cell Metab.* **2021**, *33*, 1763–1776.e5. [CrossRef]
20. Van Wyngene, L.; Vanderhaeghen, T.; Timmermans, S.; Vandewalle, J.; Van Looveren, K.; Souffriau, J.; Wallaeys, C.; Eggermont, M.; Ernst, S.; Van Hamme, E.; et al. Hepatic PPARα Function and Lipid Metabolic Pathways Are Dysregulated in Polymicrobial Sepsis. *EMBO Mol. Med.* **2020**, *12*, e11319. [CrossRef]
21. Zhou, Y.; Zhou, B.; Pache, L.; Chang, M.; Khodabakhshi, A.H.; Tanaseichuk, O.; Benner, C.; Chanda, S.K. Metascape Provides a Biologist-Oriented Resource for the Analysis of Systems-Level Datasets. *Nat. Commun.* **2019**, *10*, 1523. [CrossRef]
22. Berglund, L.J.; Avery, D.T.; Ma, C.S.; Moens, L.; Deenick, E.K.; Bustamante, J.; Boisson-Dupuis, S.; Wong, M.; Adelstein, S.; Arkwright, P.D.; et al. IL-21 Signalling via STAT3 Primes Human Näive B Cells to Respond to IL-2 to Enhance Their Differentiation into Plasmablasts. *Blood* **2013**, *122*, 3940–3950. [CrossRef] [PubMed]
23. Karin, M.; Liu, Z.G.; Zandi, E. AP-1 Function and Regulation. *Curr. Opin. Cell Biol.* **1997**, *9*, 240–246. [CrossRef] [PubMed]
24. Manna, P.R.; Dyson, M.T.; Stocco, D.M. Role of Basic Leucine Zipper Proteins in Transcriptional Regulation of the Steroidogenic Acute Regulatory Protein Gene HHS Public Access. *Mol. Cell Endocrinol.* **2009**, *302*, 1–11. [CrossRef]
25. Paumelle, R.; Haas, J.T.; Hennuyer, N.; Baugé, E.; Deleye, Y.; Mesotten, D.; Langouche, L.; Vanhoutte, J.; Cudejko, C.; Wouters, K.; et al. Hepatic PPARa Is Critical in the Metabolic Adaptation to Sepsis. *J. Hepatol.* **2019**, *70*, 963–973. [CrossRef]
26. Ullah, K.; Li, Y.; Lin, Q.; Pan, K.; Nguyen, T.; Aniruddhsingh, S.; Su, Q.; Sharp, W.; Wu, R. Comparative Analysis of Whole Transcriptome Profiles in Septic Cardiomyopathy: Insights from CLP- and LPS-Induced Mouse Models. *Genes* **2023**, *14*, 1366. [CrossRef]
27. Sun, Y.; Liu, T.; Bai, W. MAF BZIP Transcription Factor B (MAFB) Protected Against Ovalbumin-Induced Allergic Rhinitis via the Alleviation of Inflammation by Restoring the T Helper (Th) 1/Th2/Th17 Imbalance and Epithelial Barrier Dysfunction. *J. Asthma Allergy* **2022**, *15*, 267–280. [CrossRef]
28. Oyake, T.; Itoh, K.; Motohashi, H.; Hayashi, N.; Hoshino, H.; Nishizawa, M.; Yamamoto, M.; Igarashi, K. Bach Proteins Belong to a Novel Family of BTB-Basic. Leucine Zipper Transcription Factors That Interact with MafK and Regulate Transcription through the NF-E2 Site. *Mol. Cell. Biol.* **1996**, *16*, 6083–6095. [CrossRef]
29. Van Dender, C.; Timmermans, S.; Paakinaho, V.; Vanderhaeghen, T.; Vandewalle, J.; Claes, M.; Garcia, B.; Roman, B.; De Waele, J.; Croubels, S.; et al. A Critical Role for HNF4α in Polymicrobial Sepsis-Associated Metabolic Reprogramming and Death. *EMBO Mol. Med.* **2024**, *in press*. [CrossRef]
30. Moldawer, L.; Manohar, P.; Bolgos, G.; Rodriguez, J.; Wollenberg, G. Blockade of Tumor Necrosis Factor Reduces Lipopolysaccharide Lethality, but Not the Lethality of Cecal Ligation and Puncture. *Shock* **1995**, *4*, 89–95. [CrossRef]
31. Vandewalle, J.; Steeland, S.; Van Ryckeghem, S.; Eggermont, M.; Van Wonterghem, E.; Vandenbroucke, R.E.; Libert, C. A Study of Cecal Ligation and Puncture-Induced Sepsis in Tissue-Specific Tumor Necrosis Factor Receptor 1-Deficient Mice. *Front. Immunol.* **2019**, *10*, 2574. [CrossRef]

32. Swindle, M.M.; Makin, A.; Herron, A.J.; Clubb, F.J.; Frazier, K.S. Swine as Models in Biomedical Research and Toxicology Testing. *Vet. Pathol.* **2012**, *49*, 344–356. [CrossRef]
33. Almanza, A.; Carlesso, A.; Chintha, C.; Creedican, S.; Doultsinos, D.; Leuzzi, B.; Luís, A.; McCarthy, N.; Montibeller, L.; More, S.; et al. Endoplasmic Reticulum Stress Signalling—From Basic Mechanisms to Clinical Applications. *FEBS J.* **2019**, *286*, 241–278. [CrossRef] [PubMed]
34. Liu, L.; Wu, H.; Zang, J.T.; Yang, G.; Zhu, Y.; Wu, Y.; Chen, X.; Lan, D.; Li, T. 4-Phenylbutyric Acid Reveals Good Beneficial Effects on Vital Organ Function via Anti-Endoplasmic Reticulum Stress in Septic Rats. *Crit. Care Med.* **2016**, *44*, e689–e701. [CrossRef] [PubMed]
35. Zhang, K.; Kaufman, R.J. From Endoplasmic-Reticulum Stress to the Inflammatory Response. *Nature* **2008**, *454*, 455–462. [CrossRef]
36. Mestas, J.; Hughes, C.C.W. Of Mice and Not Men: Differences between Mouse and Human Immunology. *J. Immunol.* **2004**, *172*, 2731–2738. [CrossRef] [PubMed]
37. Metzing, U.B.; von Loeffelholz, C.; Steidl, R.; Romeike, B.; Winkler, R.; Rauchfuß, F.; Settmacher, U.; Stoppe, C.; Coldewey, S.M.; Weinmann, C.; et al. Endoplasmic Reticulum Stress and the Unfolded Protein Response in Skeletal Muscle of Subjects Suffering from Peritoneal Sepsis. *Sci. Rep.* **2022**, *12*, 504. [CrossRef]
38. Vandewalle, J.; Garcia, B.; Timmermans, S.; Vanderhaeghen, T.; Van Wyngene, L.; Eggermont, M.; Dufoor, H.; Van Dender, C.; Halimi, F.; Croubels, S.; et al. Hepatic Peroxisome Proliferator-Activated Receptor Alpha Dysfunction in Porcine Septic Shock. *Cells* **2022**, *11*, 4080. [CrossRef]
39. Schelstraete, W.; De Clerck, L.; Govaert, E.; Millecam, J.; Devreese, M.; Deforce, D.; Van Bocxlaer, J.; Croubels, S. Characterization of Porcine Hepatic and Intestinal Drug Metabolizing CYP450: Comparison with Human Orthologues from A Quantitative, Activity and Selectivity Perspective. *Sci. Rep.* **2019**, *9*, 9233. [CrossRef]
40. Osuchowski, M.F.; Ayala, A.; Bahrami, S.; Bauer, M.; Boros, M.; Cavaillon, J.M.; Chaudry, I.H.; Coopersmith, C.M.; Deutschman, C.; Drechsler, S.; et al. International Expert Consensus for Pre-Clinical Sepsis Studies. Minimum Quality Threshold in Pre-Clinical Sepsis Studies (Mqtipss): An International Expert Consensus Initiative for Improvement of Animal Modeling in Sepsis. *Shock* **2018**, *50*, 377–380. [CrossRef]
41. du Sert, N.P.; Hurst, V.; Ahluwalia, A.; Alam, S.; Avey, M.T.; Baker, M.; Browne, W.J.; Clark, A.; Cuthill, I.C.; Dirnagl, U.; et al. The Arrive Guidelines 2.0: Updated Guidelines for Reporting Animal Research. *PLoS Biol.* **2020**, *18*, 703181. [CrossRef]
42. Dhondt, L.; Croubels, S.; Temmerman, R.; De Cock, P.; Meyer, E.; Van Den Broeck, W.; De Paepe, P.; Devreese, M. The Development of a Juvenile Porcine Augmented Renal Clearance Model Through Continuous Infusion of Lipopolysaccharides: An Exploratory Study. *Front. Vet. Sci.* **2021**, *8*, 639771. [CrossRef] [PubMed]
43. Garcia, B.; Su, F.; Dewachter, L.; Favory, R.; Khaldi, A.; Moiroux-Sahraoui, A.; Annoni, F.; Vasques-Nóvoa, F.; Rocha-Oliveira, E.; Roncon-Albuquerque, R.; et al. Myocardial Effects of Angiotensin II Compared to Norepinephrine in an Animal Model of Septic Shock. *Crit. Care* **2022**, *26*, 281. [CrossRef] [PubMed]
44. Heinz, S.; Benner, C.; Spann, N.; Bertolino, E.; Lin, Y.C.; Laslo, P.; Cheng, J.X.; Murre, C.; Singh, H.; Glass, C.K. Article Simple Combinations of Lineage-Determining Transcription Factors Prime Cis-Regulatory Elements Required for Macrophage and B Cell Identities. *Mol. Cell* **2010**, *38*, 576–589. [CrossRef] [PubMed]

International Journal of
Molecular Sciences

MDPI

Article

C5a Induces Inflammatory Signaling and Apoptosis in PC12 Cells through C5aR-Dependent Signaling: A Potential Mechanism for Adrenal Damage in Sepsis

Lucas Mrozewski [1], Sujeenthar Tharmalingam [1,2], Paul Michael [1], Aseem Kumar [1,2] and T. C. Tai [1,2,*]

1 School of Natural Sciences, Laurentian University, Sudbury, ON P3E 2C6, Canada; lmrozewski@laurentian.ca (L.M.); sutharmalingam@nosm.ca (S.T.); pmichael@laurentian.ca (P.M.); akumar@laurentian.ca (A.K.)
2 Medical Science Division, NOSM University, Sudbury, ON P3E 2C6, Canada
* Correspondence: tc.tai@nosm.ca

Abstract: The complement system is critically involved in the pathogenesis of sepsis. In particular, complement anaphylatoxin C5a is generated in excess during sepsis, leading to cellular dysfunction. Recent studies have shown that excessive C5a impairs adrenomedullary catecholamine production release and induces apoptosis in adrenomedullary cells. Currently, the mechanisms by which C5a impacts adrenal cell function are poorly understood. The PC12 cell model was used to examine the cellular effects following treatment with recombinant rat C5a. The levels of caspase activation and cell death, protein kinase signaling pathway activation, and changes in inflammatory protein expression were examined following treatment with C5a. There was an increase in apoptosis of PC12 cells following treatment with high-dose C5a. Ten inflammatory proteins, primarily involved in apoptosis, cell survival, and cell proliferation, were upregulated following treatment with high-dose C5a. Five inflammatory proteins, involved primarily in chemotaxis and anti-inflammatory functions, were downregulated. The ERK/MAPK, p38/MAPK, JNK/MAPK, and AKT protein kinase signaling pathways were upregulated in a C5aR-dependent manner. These results demonstrate an apoptotic effect and cellular signaling effect of high-dose C5a. Taken together, the overall data suggest that high levels of C5a may play a role in C5aR-dependent apoptosis of adrenal medullary cells in sepsis.

Keywords: complement C5a; catecholamines; sepsis; adrenal gland; adrenal insufficiency

1. Introduction

1.1. Sepsis

Sepsis, as defined by the Third International Consensus Definitions for Sepsis and Septic Shock, is a life-threatening condition caused by a dysregulated host response to infection [1]. Sepsis is characterized by high levels of inflammation and, upon disease progression, organ failure and potentially death if treatment is unsuccessful [2].

Sepsis is typically incurred through bacterial infection, with Gram-positive bacteria such as Staphylococcus aureus being the most common cause; however, fungal infections are an increasingly common cause [3]. The response to infection includes the activation, transcription, and expression of a large set of cytokines and other signaling molecules involved in promoting inflammation, activating immune tissue, and inducing immune cell chemotaxis [4–6]. Anti-inflammatory cytokines are also released to help modulate the effect caused by an influx of pro-inflammatory cytokines. While this response is typical of many infections, in septic environments this response extends and propagates outside the local microenvironment, inducing an uncontrolled systemic response [7]. One system associated with the promotion of the inflammatory response that is upregulated in sepsis is known as the complement system.

1.2. The Complement System

The complement system is composed of over 30 plasma proteins, found predominantly in an inactive, zymogen form, which are present throughout the circulatory system. The complement system is highly interconnected with three separate initiation pathways: classical, lectin, and alternative [8,9]. Each pathway is activated by its own respective stimulus, and they play an integral role in the immune system's response to infection [8,9]. The complement system also plays a role in the mediation of inflammation, and its activation induces the release of various inflammatory cytokines, which results in both localized and systemic inflammation, depending upon the degree of complement activation [10,11]. The complement system also has important auto-immune functions such as apoptotic cell clearance, and dysfunction of this system has been proposed as a mechanism of systemic lupus erythematosus [12]. The functions of the complement system are driven primarily by its effector molecules, namely the anaphylatoxins, C3a and C5a, with C5a being the more potent of the two [13].

1.3. Complement C5a

C5a is a glycosylated protein that is part of the terminal complement pathway. C5a was first reported to only be a leukocyte attractant; however, it has since been shown to be involved in a broad range of immune and inflammatory functions. The two known receptors that bind C5a are complement component 5a receptor 1 (C5aR), also known as CD88, and complement component 5a receptor 2 (C5L2), also known as GPR77 [14]. C5aR is a G protein-coupled receptor (GPCR), and the interaction of C5a and C5aR results in the activation of the mitogen-activated protein kinase (MAPK)/extracellular signal-regulated kinase (ERK) pathway and induces the oxidative burst in immune cells [15,16]. In contract, C5L2 is not a GPCR, and understanding of its function remains unclear [17–19].

C5a levels are routinely elevated in septic individuals. In healthy human subjects, plasma levels of C5a are observed at approximately 5 ng/mL ($\approx$0.5 nM), while in septic shock, C5a concentrations can increase to over 100 nM and remain elevated for many days following the event [17,20–22]. The release of C5a, while helping to generate an immune response, can also result in undesirable, damaging effects for various cell types, including both immune and non-immune cells [23–26].

C5a may also play a role in adrenal dysfunction and has been shown to impair the production of norepinephrine (NE) and dopamine (DA) in a time- and dose-dependent manner [23]. Following incubation with relatively high concentrations of C5a, there was an increase in PI and Annexin V staining, which was inhibited by the pan-caspase inhibitor Z-VAD-FMK [23]. The effects of C5a on cellular function and viability may be related to the decrease in mitochondrial function. Incubation of PC12 cells with C5a decreased mitochondrial respiration, dehydrogenase, and cytochrome c oxidase activities [27]. In addition, the mitochondrial repair protein chaperonin 60 was upregulated, demonstrating the occurrence of mitochondrial damage. In the context of secondary adrenal dysfunction, both forms of C5a receptors are expressed by the pituitary gland and the adrenal gland, and activation of these receptors is known to stimulate protein kinase signaling pathways, suggesting a possible role for C5a in the regulation of HPA [28–30]. Currently, the literature examining the impact of C5a on adrenal cells suggests cellular dysfunction; however, the molecular mechanisms underlying this phenotype have not yet been elucidated.

1.4. Primary Adrenal Dysfunction

The adrenal medulla is responsible for the synthesis of catecholamines, namely dopamine (DA), norepinephrine (NE), and epinephrine (EPI) [31]. Catecholamines are integral to the body's response to external threats, known as the "fight-or-flight" response, which results in an increase in blood pressure and cardiac output, smooth muscle relaxation, and increased blood glucose concentrations [32,33].

Sepsis has also been shown to be associated with abnormal circulating levels of catecholamines [34–36]. Adrenal insufficiency is commonly observed in sepsis and may be associated with a higher mortality rate in patients [37]. Proper adrenal function has also been shown to be an important factor in the survival of mice in an endotoxin-induced sepsis model [38]. In particular, primary adrenal dysfunction, which occurs when the adrenal glands are damaged and produce inadequate levels of catecholamines, is one of the main causes of adrenal dysfunction in sepsis [39].

In vivo studies of sepsis have shown evidence of damage and dysfunction of the adrenal glands during experimentally induced sepsis. Adrenal necrosis, hemorrhage, and thrombi were identified in 37 of 46 calves suffering from bacterially caused endotoxic shock [40]. A recent study reported significant damage and apoptosis in various regions of the adrenal medulla and high levels of mRNA of inflammatory cytokines (IL-1β, IL-6, and TNF-α) in sepsis models using intraperitoneal injection of *Pseudomonas aeruginosa*, a Gram-negative bacterium [41]. Clinical evidence also shows a strong relationship between sepsis and adrenal damage. Septic patients generally have enlarged adrenal glands, approximately double the volume of the control group [42]. In addition, in a cohort of intensive care patients with septic shock, lack of adrenal gland enlargement was associated with an increase in day 28 mortality [43].

PC12 cells, derived from a rat pheochromocytoma (tumor of adrenal medullary chromaffin cells), provide an effective in vitro model of adrenal functionality and can also provide a model for analysis of neuronal function and differentiation, which is induced by exposing cells to neuronal growth factor (NGF) [44]. Numerous studies have shown that the incubation of PC12 cells with LPS induces significant cell death in both differentiated and undifferentiated PC12 cells [45,46]. This apoptotic effect was seen to be inhibited by inactivation of the caspase 3/nuclear factor kappa beta (NF-$\kappa\beta$) pathway via TLR-4 following pre-incubation in low concentrations of LPS [45].

1.5. Research Objectives and Hypothesis

As discussed, the relationship between sepsis and C5a has been well established, as has the relationship between sepsis and adrenal dysregulation. However, the molecular mechanisms by which C5a regulates adrenal cell function are poorly understood. Moreover, the cellular signaling pathways seen in C5a-treated adrenal cells have not been elucidated. In the current study, an in vitro model with PC12 cells, derived from a rat pheochromocytoma, was utilized to examine the effect of complement C5a on cellular signaling, inflammatory response, and apoptosis in rat adrenal medullary cells. It is hypothesized that exposure to septic levels of C5a will induce cell death in PC12 cells. The overall scientific objective of this study is to identify C5a cytotoxicity on PC12 cells. The secondary objective is to identify cellular signaling pathways related to the effect of C5a on PC12 cells.

2. Results

2.1. Complement C5a Induces Caspase Activation and Apoptosis in PC12 Cells

The level of caspase activation, PI staining, and overall cell staining was determined following treatment of cells with 0 (control), 0.001, 0.01, 0.1, 1, and 10 nM C5a for 30 min. The level of caspase activation was increased following 30 min treatment of cells with 10 nM C5a and H_2O_2 (Figure 1a). The level of cell death as indicated by PI staining was significantly elevated only in the H_2O_2 positive control (Figure 1b). The cell count did not differ between any of the treatment conditions (Figure A1). This demonstrated an increase in caspase 3/7 activity, but not apoptosis, following a 30 min treatment of PC12 cells with 10 nM C5a.

The level of caspase activation, PI staining, and overall cell staining was also determined following treatment of PC12 cells with C5a for 24 h. There was no significant change in caspase activation for any of the treatment conditions relative to the no-treatment control (Figure 2a). The level of cell death was significantly elevated in the 10 nM treatment (Figure 2b). The cell count did not differ between any of the treatments (Figure A2). The H_2O_2 positive control was not used at the 24 h timepoint because following the H_2O_2 treatment the cells were completely degraded and there was no signal detectable above background. This demonstrated an increase in cell death, but not caspase 3/7 activity, following a 24 h treatment of PC12 cells with 10 nM C5a.

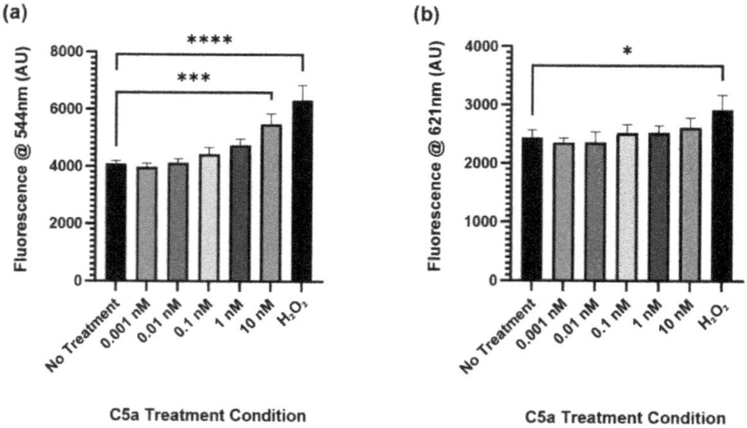

Figure 1. Caspase Activity and PI Staining following 30 min Treatment with C5a. (**a**) The level of caspase activation was measured by detecting the fluorescence at an excitation wavelength of 495 ± 20 nm and an emission wavelength of 544 ± 25 nm. The level of caspase activation was increased in the 10 nM C5a treatment and H_2O_2 positive control. (**b**) The level of PI staining was determined by measuring the fluorescence using an excitation wavelength of 586 ± 15 nm and a read wavelength of 621 ± 25 nm. The level of cell death was only elevated in the H_2O_2 positive control. One-way ANOVA with Dunnett's post hoc test were used for statistical analysis. * $p < 0.05$, *** $p < 0.001$, **** $p < 0.0001$. $n = 3$.

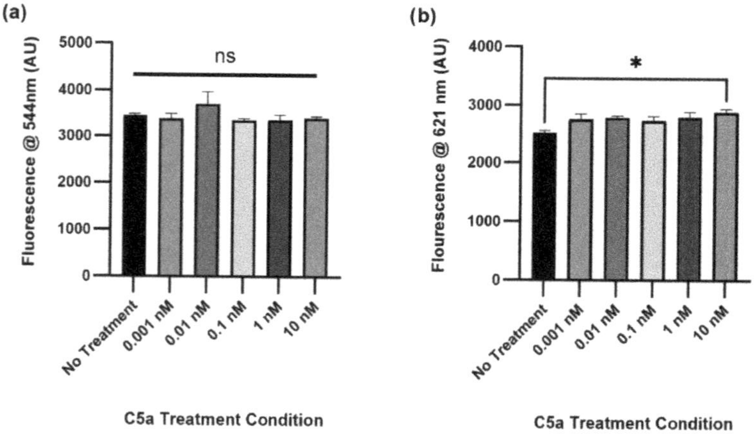

Figure 2. Caspase Activity and PI Staining following 24 h Treatment with C5a. (**a**) The level of caspase activation was measured by detecting the fluorescence at an excitation wavelength of 495 ± 20 nm and an emission wavelength of 544 ± 25 nm. There was no significant change in caspase activation at this timepoint. (**b**) The level of PI staining was determined by measuring the fluorescence using an excitation wavelength of 586 ± 15 nm and a read wavelength of 621 ± 25 nm. There was increased cell death in the 10 nM C5a treatment relative to the no-treatment condition. One-way ANOVA with Dunnett's post hoc test were used for statistical analysis. * $p < 0.05$. ns = non significant. $n = 3$.

2.2. PMX-53 Inhibits C5a-Induced Caspase Upregulation

After identifying increased caspase activation and PI staining as a result of 10 nM C5a treatment, the C5aR inhibitor, PMX-53, was utilized to identify whether this receptor is involved in the cell death response mediated by C5a. PC12 cells were treated with 10 nM C5a or 50 nM PMX-53 alone or in combination (50 nM PMX-53 + 10 nM C5a). Following incubation in 10 nM C5a, caspase activation was increased compared to the no-treatment condition. This response was inhibited by pre-treatment with 50 nM PMX-53, a C5aR inhibitor (Figure 3). Treatment with 50 nM PMX-53 alone did not induce an increase in caspase activation. The cell count did not differ between the different treatment conditions (Figure A3). This demonstrated that the increase in caspase 3/7 activity following 30 min treatment of PC12 cells with 10 nM C5a was C5aR-dependent.

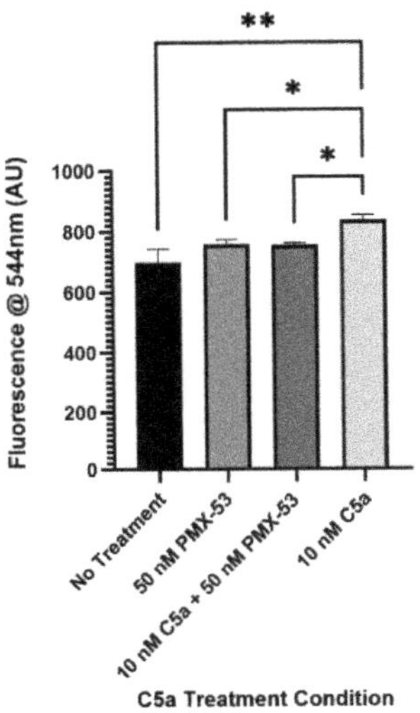

Figure 3. Effect of C5aR Inhibitor on Caspase Activation. The level of caspase activation following a 30 min incubation with various concentrations of C5a and 50 nM PMX-53 was examined. This was measured by detecting the fluorescence at an excitation wavelength of 495 ± 20 nm and an emission wavelength of 544 ± 25 nm. There was an increase in the level of caspase activation for the 10 nM C5a treatment compared to the no treatment, 50 nM PMX-53, and 10 nM C5a + 50 nM PMX-53 treatments. Treatment with 50 nM PMX-53 alone or 10 nM C5a/50nM PMX-53 did not induce an upregulation in caspase activation relative to the control. One-way ANOVA with Dunnett's post hoc test were used for statistical analysis. * $p < 0.05$, ** $p < 0.01$. $n = 3$.

2.3. C5a Induces Inflammatory Signaling in PC12 Cells

The level of inflammation induced by PC12 cell exposure to C5a was measured by detecting the levels of various inflammatory cytokines related to inflammatory signaling using an antibody array (Figure 4). The cells were examined following a 24 h incubation in 10 nM C5a and compared to a no-treatment control. There was a total of 10 proteins that were determined to be upregulated and 5 that were significantly downregulated following treatment with 10 nM C5a (Tables 1 and 2). The general function of the individual proteins is detailed in Tables 1 and 2. The general functions of the proteins that were upregulated are apoptosis, inflammatory processes, and cell health/proliferation. The proteins that were downregulated were generally involved in chemotaxis, immune cell differentiation, and anti-inflammation.

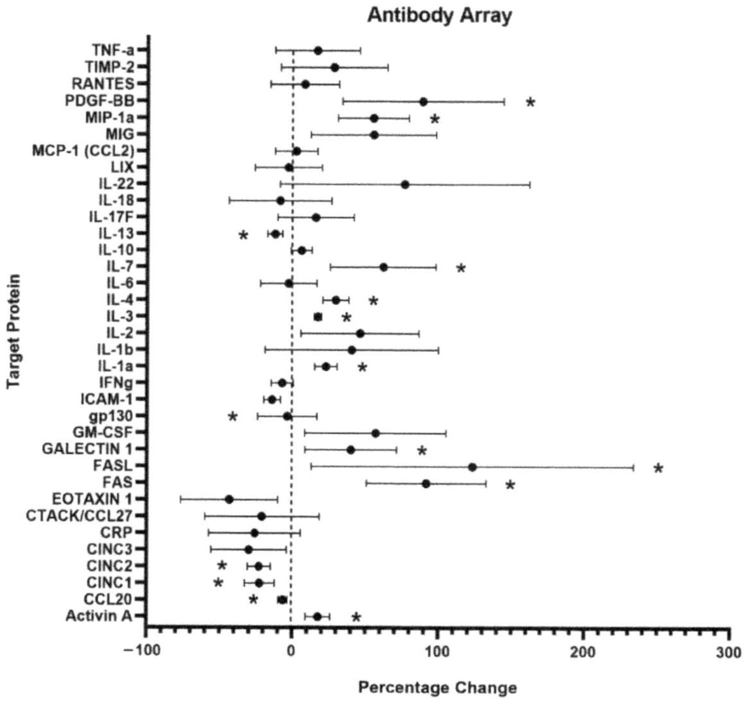

Figure 4. Inflammatory Antibody Array Analysis. An antibody array labelled with 36 unique protein targets was used to examine the levels of inflammatory protein produced by PC12 following a 24 h incubation in 10 nM C5a. $n = 3$. An unpaired t-test used for statistical analysis. For significance information, see Tables 1 and 2. * $p < 0.05$. $n = 3$.

Table 1. Upregulated Inflammatory Proteins After C5a Treatment.

Protein	Percentage Change	SEM (%)	Significant ($p < 0.05$)	Function
Activin A	17.59	4.868	Yes	Cell Cycle Progression, Cell Proliferation, and Apoptosis [47]
FAS	91.74	23.7	Yes	Induction of Apoptosis [48]
FASL	99.56	50.96	Yes	
GALECTIN 1	39.95	11.54	Yes	Regulation of Cell Cycle [49]
IL-1α	22.68	4.439	Yes	Alarmin and Inflammatory Process [50]
IL-3	17.01	1.369	Yes	Inflammatory processes, Cell Growth, and Differentiation [51]
IL-4	29.42	5.13	Yes	Proliferation and Cell Survival [52]
IL-7	61.77	19.08	Yes	Proliferation and Cell Survival [53]
MIP-1a	54.91	12.89	Yes	Immune Cell Activation and Chemotaxis [54]
PDGF-BB	88.81	20.92	Yes	Proliferation, Immune Cell Activation, and Differentiation [55]

Table 2. Downregulated Inflammatory Protein After C5a Treatment.

Protein	Percentage Change	SEM (%)	Significant ($p < 0.05$)	Function
CCL20	−6.356	1.787	Yes	Immune Migration and Chemotaxis [56]
CINC1	−22.5	6.018	Yes	Neutrophil Chemoattractant [57]
CINC2	−22.68	4.599	Yes	Immune Cell Recruitment and Chemotaxis [58]
ICAM-1	−14.18	3.261	Yes	Cell Adhesion and Immune Cell Recruitment [59]
IL-13	−12.33	2.959	Yes	Anti-inflammatory Effects [60]

2.4. Complement C5a Induces Protein Kinase Signaling in PC12 Cells

The level of phosphorylation of target proteins in specific intracellular signaling pathways was determined using ELISA kits. This was performed to better understand the signaling pathways inducing caspase activation and the apoptotic response. The cells were examined following 30 min of incubation with C5a (0.1 nM, 10 nM), PMX-53 inhibitor (50 nM) alone, or in combination (10 nM C5a + 50 nM PMX53). Increased phosphorylation of JNK1/2 (Figure 5a), ERK1/2 (Figure 5b), p38 (Figure 5c), and AKT (Figure 5d) was observed following treatment with 10 nM C5a for 30 min. Pre-treatment of PC12 cells with 50 nM PMX-53 inhibited this response for all analytes. Neither the 0.1 nM C5a nor the 50 nM PMX-53 treatment alone showed an increased level of phosphorylation. These results demonstrate a C5aR-dependent increase in JNK1/2, ERK1/2, p38, and AKT phosphorylation following 30 min treatment of PC12 cells with 10 nM C5a.

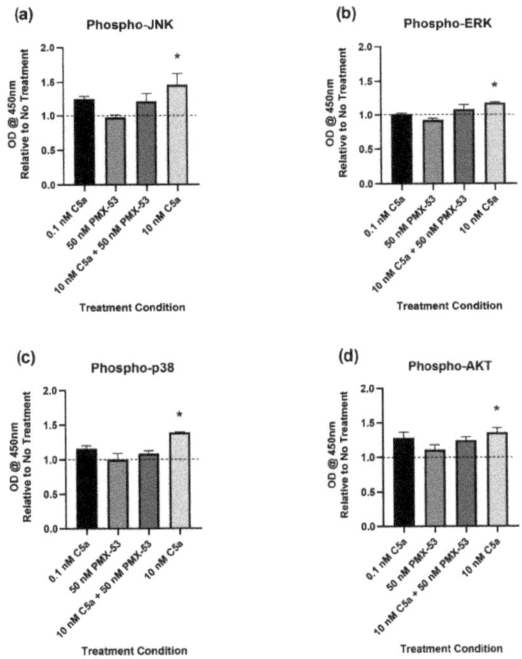

Figure 5. Phosphorylated Protein Kinase Pathway Analysis. Phosphorylation of (**a**) JNK1/2, (**b**) ERK1/2, (**c**) p38 (pT180/pY182), and (**d**) AKT (PI3K) was analyzed by ELISA. The cells were incubated in 0.1 nM C5a, 10 nM C5a, 10 nM C5a + 50 nM PMX-53, and 50 nM PMX-53. The OD at 450 nm was determined, and the data were graphed relative to the no-treatment control (dashed line). Following treatment with 10 nM C5a, the activations of JNK1/2, ERK1/2, p38, and AKT were all upregulated relative to the control. * $p < 0.05$. $n = 3$.

3. Discussion

3.1. C5a and Apoptosis

Inflammation in sepsis is known to induce adrenal gland damage; furthermore, complement C5a has been suggested to induce apoptosis in PC12 cells [23,61,62]. The current study further investigated and characterized the mechanisms involved in C5a-induced apoptosis.

The viability of PC12 cells was decreased following incubation with elevated concentrations of C5a (10 nM). Incubations with lower ($\leq$1 nM) C5a concentrations did not induce a decrease in cell viability. These results are interesting since concentrations of C5a are measured at >10 nM in septic conditions [63]. The decrease in cell viability at 10 nM of C5a provides an argument for the cytotoxic effect of C5a on adrenal tissue in sepsis [22]. The caspase activation assay showed a significant increase in the activation of caspases following 10 nM C5a incubation at the 30 min timepoint. This increase in caspase activation is in accordance with what has been previously reported in the literature. Previous studies show that C5a induces caspase 3/7 activation in PC12 cells and that this apoptotic response was inhibited with a caspase inhibitor [23]. The current study demonstrates a novel result where this caspase activation was also inhibited by pre-treatment with the C5aR inhibitor PMX-53. This finding indicates that the apoptotic response is dependent on C5aR signaling. PI staining has previously been used to examine cell viability in PC12 cells; however, only treatment with 10 nM C5a has been examined [23]. In addition, the previous studies that implemented PI to study C5a-induced apoptosis in PC12 cells only presented images of the staining without any quantified data analysis. Despite this lack of quantitation, the increase in propidium iodide staining seen in the paper following exposure to 10 nM for 30 min is drastic, further suggesting an apoptotic response of PC12 cells by 10 nM C5a [23]. Also of note, only the 30 min timepoint was previously examined, and the long-term effects of this incubation were not examined. Overall, the results of this study are in accordance with, and expand upon, the current literature on C5a cytotoxicity in adrenal cells.

Incubation with 10 nM C5a for 24 h induced an increase in FAS, FASL, and activin A expression in PC12. The increased expressions of FAS and FASL were the largest significant changes in the assessed proteins. The FAS receptor and its ligand (FASL) have been repeatedly shown to be involved in apoptosis in PC12 cells [64–66]. The increase in FAS/FASL in PC12 cells is supported by observations reported in other cell lines. C5a plays a role in activating the FAS/FASL axis, with C5a-induced FAS playing a role in brain vascular cell apoptosis and caspase activation in an experimental lupus model [25]. Additionally, C5a exposure was shown to increase the expression of the FAS ligand in B-lymphoblasts [67].

Activin A has also been repeatedly shown to induce an apoptotic response in numerous cell lines [68–70]. In NGF-differentiated PC12 cells, however, it had a neuroprotective and anti-apoptotic effect [71,72]. Activin A has been shown to activate p38 signaling in undifferentiated PC12 cells, which, as discussed later, has potential implications for apoptotic signaling [73]. To date, activin A and apoptosis have not been extensively examined in undifferentiated PC12 cells and are a potential area for further investigation.

While there are some other studies examining C5a cytotoxicity, they primarily examine the effect on immune cells; however, there is an increasing body of research demonstrating the cytotoxic effects of septic levels of C5a in non-immune tissues. To date, these effects at elevated C5a concentrations have been examined mainly in endothelial tissue models [25,74]. Overall, the results of this study help to corroborate the growing body of evidence suggesting an apoptotic effect of elevated concentrations of C5a, with the induction of apoptotic signaling mediated by C5aR.

3.2. C5a and Cellular Signaling

The activation of JNK1/2, ERK1/2, p38, and AKT1/2/3 pathways was increased following treatment with 10 nM C5a for 30 min. The phosphorylation ELISA method was used because the activity of these pathways is mediated by post-transcriptional modifications, namely phosphorylation, on established sites of the proteins [75,76]. Characterizing the level of phosphorylated proteins allowed for the determination of the levels of activation of each of the respective pathways.

The activation of all four pathways was inhibited by pre-treatment with 50 nM PMX-53, a C5aR inhibitor, demonstrating that C5a signaling occurred in a C5aR-dependent manner. Our data are consistent with previous reports that the activation of all four of the studied protein kinase pathways by C5a is dependent on the C5a/C5aR pathway, while C5a/C5L2 does not appear to result in activation of these pathways [77–81]. As previously discussed, the function of C5L2, which is not a GPCR, is not clearly elucidated, and more research is needed to understand its role in C5a signaling.

3.2.1. JNK

A member of the MAPK family, the JNK pathway is an important regulator of cell function, primarily apoptosis, gene transcription, and cellular survival [82]. It is also notable for its role in modulating neuronal function [83]. In PC12 cells, JNK is associated with the induction of apoptosis following exposure to various stressors [84–86]. In some models of apoptosis in PC12 cells, the JNK and p38 pathways are both necessary for the induction of apoptosis [87]. In septic conditions, JNK has been identified as a target for drug treatments due to the hyperactivation of JNK and its role in stimulating inflammation and apoptosis [88,89]. The apparent pro-apoptotic effects of JNK activation may be a potential explanation for the apoptosis observed in PC12 cells in this study.

3.2.2. ERK

The ERK kinases are a member of the MAPK family and are generally involved in cell growth, proliferation, and differentiation [90]. Additionally, ERK signaling is known to induce signaling in response to inflammatory stimuli and has been implicated in the Fas-induced cell death pathway in certain cell types [91–94]. In contrast, ERK signaling may be activated to counteract cell death pathways and promote cell proliferation and survival [95]. In accordance with this previous literature on immune cells, ERK activation was increased in response to C5a [96].

3.2.3. p38

The third member of the MAPK family, p38, plays an important role in various cellular processes, including inflammation, proliferation, and apoptosis [97]. In PC12 cells, p38 has been shown to be involved in the apoptotic response to various stressors [98–100]. In addition, p38 has been shown to be involved in the recruitment and cleavage of caspases in cell death [101,102]. Furthermore, p38 is involved in the previously discussed mitochondrial-dependent pathway of apoptosis [103]. The inflammatory response in sepsis is largely dependent on p38 activation, which in turn has been shown to be activated by C5a [104–106]. p38, along with the other MAPK pathways, plays an important role in inflammation regulation through the production of various cytokines and other inflammatory molecules [107]. This role in inflammatory molecule production may help to explain the results seen in the antibody array (Table 1).

3.2.4. AKT

AKT (also known as PKB) is a serine/threonine kinase involved in cell cycle regulation, metabolism, apoptosis, and the regulation of various gene targets [108]. In PC12 cells, AKT is often upregulated in response to stressors [109–111]. In other tissues, C5a-induced MAPK and AKT activation is linked to damage to cardiac and liver tissues in various stress states and has been argued to provide a protective effect [112,113]. Moreover, in septic conditions, C5a-induced activation of MAPK and AKT signaling has been linked to cardiac dysfunction [114]. When this activation was inhibited by a p38 inhibitor, inflammatory cytokine release was decreased, suggesting a role for MAPK and AKT in inflammatory signaling in non-immune tissues. AKT has also been shown to induce Cyclin E2, and this may be a mechanism by which Cyclin E2 was upregulated following C5a treatment in this study [115].

3.2.5. Intercellular and Inflammatory Signaling

Treatment of PC12 cells with 10 nM C5a induced an increase in the production of 10 inflammatory proteins (Table 1) and a decrease in the production of 5 inflammatory proteins (Table 2). FAS and FASL have previously been shown to be upregulated by C5a in other cell types and are involved in the FAS-apoptotic pathway. Various immune cell types have been shown to upregulate the levels of the identified inflammatory cytokines in response to C5a, including IL-1α, IL-4, and MIP-1α. Other cytokines showed differential responses in PC12 cells than in immune cells, such as IL-13, which was downregulated but has been shown to be upregulated in response to C5a/Il-3 treatment in basophils [116].

3.2.6. Chemotaxis

The decrease in expression of chemotaxis-associated proteins is systematically observed in this experimental model. It is worth noting that C5a is a potent chemotactic agent for immune cells and is commonly cited as one of the primary effector functions of C5a in neutrophils and macrophages [117–119]. C5a has also been shown to aid in CCL20-dependent T-cell recruitment [120].

Interestingly, some of the proteins that are downregulated, such as IL-13 and CCL20, are upregulated in other cell types following exposure to C5a [117,121]. This contradiction helps to support the argument for differential C5a signaling effects across cell types. This has been described in the effect of C5a on mast cells, where the induced signaling effects were shown to vary between different variants of mast cells [122]. Recently, this line of research was expanded to suggest that C5a responsiveness is cell-type-dependent [123]. This differential response may help to explain differences in the expression levels of various proteins in cell lines following exposure to C5a.

3.3. *Clinical Relevance and Future Directions*

Currently, there are a small number of drugs targeting complement C5a and C5aR. Avacopan is a C5aR antagonist that was approved in 2021 in the United States for the treatment of antineutrophil cytoplasmic antibody (ANCA)-associated vasculitis [124]. Eculizumab is an antibody that binds to complement C5, inhibiting the cleavage of C5 to C5a and C5b, and is approved for the treatment of paroxysmal nocturnal hemoglobinuria [125]. Therapeutics targeting C5a in sepsis have been explored in animal models but have not been examined extensively in human studies. However, Eculizumab was used in a study investigating ICU patients with severe COVID-19 and increased the survival rate from 62.2% (48.1–76.4%) to 82.9% (95% CI: 70.4–95.3%). The results of the current study, coupled with the increased usage of therapeutics targeting C5a and C5aR, suggest a promising potential area for investigation in the treatment of sepsis. Future studies should examine a potentially protective effect of inhibiting C5a/C5aR signaling in septic conditions.

4. Materials and Methods

4.1. *Materials*

Dulbecco's modified Eagle's medium (DMEM), bovine calf serum, and equine serum were purchased from Medi-Res Corporation (Sudbury, ON, Canada). Rat recombinant C5a (Asp1-Arg77) was purchased from Abbexa (Cambridge, UK). The C5a inhibitor PMX-53 was purchased from Cayman Chemical Company (Ann Arbor, MI, USA). Propidium Iodide (PI), the CellEvent™ Caspase-3/7 Detection Reagent, NucBlue™ nuclear probe, FluoroBrite™ DMEM, and the white-walled 96-well tissue-culture treated plate were purchased from Thermo Fisher Scientific (Nepean, ON, Canada). The rat inflammation array (C3) was purchased from Raybiotech (Peachtree Corners, GA, USA). The phosphorylation arrays were purchased from Thermo Fisher Scientific. All other reagents were purchased from Medi-Res Corporation.

4.2. Cell Culture

PC12 cells (Dr. Sushil Mahata, Department of Medicine, University of California, San Diego, CA, USA) were cultured in DMEM supplemented with 5% equine serum, 5% bovine calf serum, and gentamycin sulfate (50 µg/mL). The cells were maintained in a humidified incubator at 37 °C in an atmosphere of 5% CO_2. Prior to experimentation, cells were transferred to FluoroBrite™ DMEM containing charcoal-treated serum.

4.3. C5a Treatment

The C5a was reconstituted to a concentration of 2.5 µM in accordance with the manufacturer's specifications. In the experiments requiring treatments, PC12 cells were treated with varied concentrations of C5a (0.001, 0.01, 0.1, 1, and 10 nM) and a no-treatment control. The cells were treated for either 30 min or 24 h, depending on the experimental protocol.

4.4. Caspase Activation and Cell Death Assay

Cells were seeded at a density of 2×10^4 cells/well in white-walled 96-well plates. The cells were treated with C5a for specific treatment times: (1) 30 min, to examine the level of caspase activation following treatment; and (2) 24 h, which examined potential continued caspase activation and late-stage apoptosis in PC12 cells. A subset of samples was also pre-treated with 10 nM PMX-53 for 30 min. The cells were incubated with the Caspase 3/7 detection reagent, PI, and nuclear probe in accordance with the manufacturer's protocol. A positive H_2O_2 control was used to induce cell death, and the data were compared to the no-treatment negative control. The well fluorescence was measured using a Biotek Cytation 5 Multimode Reader (Agilent Technologies, Santa Clara, CA, USA).

4.5. Antibody Array

Cells were seeded at a density of 5×10^5 cells/well in 6-well plates. The cells were treated with 10 nM C5a for 24 h. The media were aspirated from the plate, and the cells were trypsinized, resuspended in media, and then transferred to a 1.5 mL tube. The protein cell lysate was prepared by centrifuging the sample at 1000× g for 5 min at 4 °C and aspirating the supernatant. The pellet was resuspended in 100 uL of RIPA lysis buffer (150 mM NaCl, 1% Nonidet P-40, 0.5% DOC, 0.25% SDS, 50 mM Tris [pH = 7.4]) containing a protease inhibitor (87785, Thermo Fisher Scientific) and stored at −80 °C overnight. The cell lysate was thawed and then sonicated (Branson 150, Thermo Fisher Scientific) for 4 s (5×), with a 1 min rest between each pulse. The samples were then incubated for 15 min on ice, with vortexing every 3 min. The samples were centrifuged for 10 min at 20,000× g at 4 °C. The protein lysate was then analyzed using the antibody array in accordance with the manufacturer's specifications. The array was imaged using the ChemiDoc Imaging System (Biorad, Hercules, CA, USA) and analyzed using ImageJ software (Version 1.54g) with the DotBlot Plugin (http://image.bio.methods.free.fr/dotblot.html [accessed on 12 April 2024]).

4.6. Phosphorylation ELISA

PC12 cells were treated with 0.1 and 10 nM C5a, and a subset of cells was also pre-treated with 50 nM PMX-53 for 30 min. The levels of phosphorylated AKT, JNK1/2, ERK1/2, and p38 were determined following the manufacturer's protocol. The optical density at 450 nm with a reference wavelength of 650 nm was determined using the Biotek Cytation 5 Multimode Reader.

4.7. Statistical Analysis

Statistics were performed using GraphPad Prism software (Version 10.0.3) (La Jolla, CA, USA) and were analyzed using one-way analysis of variance analysis (ANOVA) with Dunnett's post hoc test or unpaired t-test. All data are presented as the mean ± standard error of mean (SEM) of at least three independent experiments.

5. Conclusions

The current study investigated the impact of C5a on PC12 signaling and apoptosis. Incubation with 10 nM C5a triggered caspase activation in PC12 cells through a C5aR-dependent mechanism. Exposure to septic levels of C5a (10 nM) induced C5aR-dependent JNK/MAPK, ERK/MAPK, p38/MAPK, and AKT (PI3K) signaling. Furthermore, exposure to 10 nM C5a for 24 h induced an increase in the expression of proteins associated with cell survival, inflammatory processes, and apoptosis and a decrease in the expression of proteins associated with chemotaxis, adhesion, and anti-inflammatory effects. These results provide insight into the mechanism of C5a-induced apoptosis and cellular signaling in PC12 cells. These findings suggest that elevated levels of complement C5a may play an important role in the mechanism of adrenal dysfunction in sepsis.

Author Contributions: Conceptualization, T.C.T., L.M. and A.K.; methodology, L.M.; validation, S.T. and P.M.; formal analysis, L.M.; investigation, L.M.; resources, T.C.T., S.T. and L.M.; data curation, T.C.T. and A.K.; writing—original draft preparation, L.M.; writing—review and editing, A.K., S.T., P.M. and T.C.T.; visualization, L.M.; supervision, T.C.T., A.K. and S.T.; project administration, T.C.T.; funding acquisition, T.C.T. All authors have read and agreed to the published version of the manuscript.

Funding: This research was funded by a NOSMUFA Research Development Grant. Lucas Mrozewski was supported by the Natural Sciences and Engineering Research Council of Canada (NSERC), [CGS-M].

Institutional Review Board Statement: Not applicable.

Informed Consent Statement: Not applicable.

Data Availability Statement: The raw data supporting the conclusions of this article will be made available by the authors on request.

Conflicts of Interest: The authors declare no conflicts of interest. The funders had no role in the design of the study; in the collection, analyses, or interpretation of data; in the writing of the manuscript; or in the decision to publish the results.

Appendix A

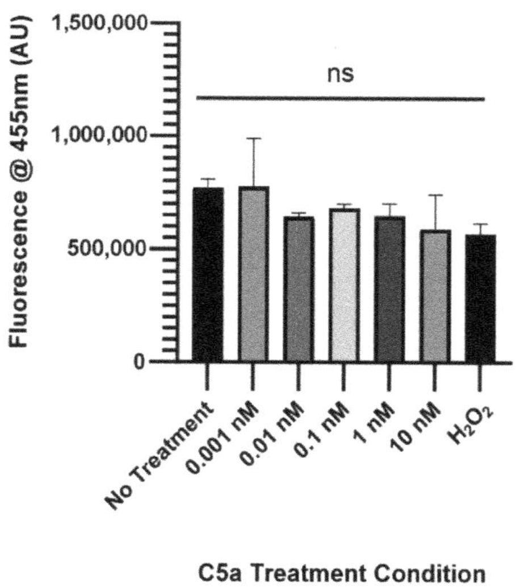

Figure A1. Nuclear Staining following 24 h Treatment with C5a. Cell count did not change following 30 min 0.001, 0.01, 0.1, 1, or 10 nM treatment in C5a. One-way ANOVA with Dunnett's post hoc test were used for statistical analysis. ns = non significant.

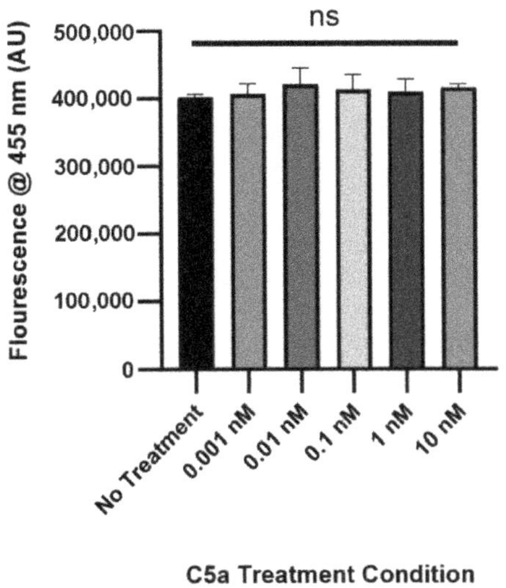

Figure A2. Nuclear Staining following 24 h Treatment with C5a. Cell count did not change following 24 h 0.001, 0.01, 0.1, 1, or 10 nM treatment in C5a. One-way ANOVA with Dunnett's post hoc test were used for statistical analysis. ns = non significant.

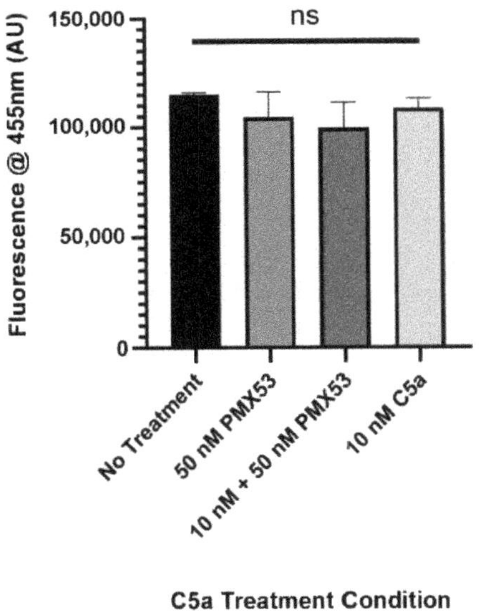

Figure A3. Effect of C5aR Inhibitor on Caspase Activation. Pre-treatment of PC12 cells with 50 nM PMX-53 and treatment with C5a for 30 min did not impact cell count. One-way ANOVA with Dunnett's post hoc test were used for statistical analysis. ns = non significant.

References

1. Singer, M.; Deutschman, C.S.; Seymour, C.W.; Shankar-Hari, M.; Annane, D.; Bauer, M.; Bellomo, R.; Bernard, G.R.; Chiche, J.-D.; Coopersmith, C.M.; et al. The Third International Consensus Definitions for Sepsis and Septic Shock (Sepsis-3). *JAMA* **2016**, *315*, 801–810. [CrossRef] [PubMed]
2. Abraham, E.; Singer, M. Mechanisms of Sepsis-Induced Organ Dysfunction. *Crit. Care Med.* **2007**, *35*, 2408–2416. [CrossRef] [PubMed]
3. Martin, G.S.; Mannino, D.M.; Eaton, S.; Moss, M. The Epidemiology of Sepsis in the United States from 1979 through 2000. *N. Engl. J. Med.* **2003**, *348*, 1546–1554. [CrossRef] [PubMed]

4. Janeway, C.A.; Medzhitov, R. Innate Immune Recognition. *Annu. Rev. Immunol.* **2002**, *20*, 197–216. [CrossRef] [PubMed]
5. Ming, W.J.; Bersani, L.; Mantovani, A. Tumor Necrosis Factor Is Chemotactic for Monocytes and Polymorphonuclear Leukocytes. *J. Immunol.* **1987**, *138*, 1469–1474. [CrossRef]
6. Vidya, M.K.; Kumar, V.G.; Sejian, V.; Bagath, M.; Krishnan, G.; Bhatta, R. Toll-like Receptors: Significance, Ligands, Signaling Pathways, and Functions in Mammals. *Int. Rev. Immunol.* **2018**, *37*, 20–36. [CrossRef]
7. Munoz, C.; Carlet, J.; Fitting, C.; Misset, B.; Blériot, J.P.; Cavaillon, J.M. Dysregulation of In Vitro Cytokine Production by Monocytes During Sepsis. *J. Clin. Investig.* **1991**, *88*, 1747. [CrossRef]
8. Walport, M.J. Complement. *N. Engl. J. Med.* **2001**, *344*, 1058–1066. [CrossRef]
9. Sarma, J.V.; Ward, P.A. The Complement System. *Cell Tissue Res.* **2011**, *343*, 227–235. [CrossRef]
10. Halstensen, T.S.; Brandtzaeg, P. Local Complement Activation in Inflammatory Bowel Disease. *Immunol. Res.* **1991**, *10*, 485–492. [CrossRef]
11. Mannes, M.; Schmidt, C.Q.; Nilsson, B.; Ekdahl, K.N.; Huber-Lang, M. Complement as Driver of Systemic Inflammation and Organ Failure in Trauma, Burn, and Sepsis. *Semin. Immunopathol.* **2021**, *43*, 773–788. [CrossRef] [PubMed]
12. Korb, L.C.; Ahearn, J.M. C1q Binds Directly and Specifically to Surface Blebs of Apoptotic Human Keratinocytes: Complement Deficiency and Systemic Lupus Erythematosus Revisited. *J. Immunol.* **1997**, *158*, 4525–4528. [CrossRef]
13. El-Lati, S.G.; Dahinden, C.A.; Church, M.K. Complement Peptides C3a- and C5a-Induced Mediator Release from Dissociated Human Skin Mast Cells. *J. Investig. Dermatol.* **1994**, *102*, 803–806. [CrossRef] [PubMed]
14. Ohno, M.; Hirata, T.; Enomoto, M.; Araki, T.; Ishimaru, H.; Takahashi, T.A. A Putative Chemoattractant Receptor, C5L2, Is Expressed in Granulocyte and Immature Dendritic Cells, but Not in Mature Dendritic Cells. *Mol. Immunol.* **2000**, *37*, 407–412. [CrossRef]
15. Mollnes, T.E.; Brekke, O.-L.; Fung, M.; Fure, H.; Christiansen, D.; Bergseth, G.; Videm, V.; Lappegård, K.T.; Köhl, J.; Lambris, J.D. Essential Role of the C5a Receptor in E Coli–Induced Oxidative Burst and Phagocytosis Revealed by a Novel Lepirudin-Based Human Whole Blood Model of Inflammation. *Blood* **2002**, *100*, 1869–1877. [CrossRef] [PubMed]
16. Zhang, J.X.; Zha, W.s.; Ye, L.p.; Wang, F.; Wang, H.; Shen, T.; Wu, C.h.; Zhu, Q.x. Complement C5a-C5aR Interaction Enhances MAPK Signaling Pathway Activities to Mediate Renal Injury in Trichloroethylene Sensitized BALB/c Mice. *J. Appl. Toxicol.* **2016**, *36*, 271–284. [CrossRef]
17. Klos, A.; Wende, E.; Wareham, K.J.; Monk, P.N. International Union of Basic and Clinical Pharmacology. LXXXVII. Complement Peptide C5a, C4a, and C3a Receptors. *Pharmacol. Rev.* **2013**, *65*, 500–543. [CrossRef]
18. Li, X.X.; Lee, J.D.; Kemper, C.; Woodruff, T.M. The Complement Receptor C5aR2: A Powerful Modulator of Innate and Adaptive Immunity. *J. Immunol.* **2019**, *202*, 3339–3348. [CrossRef]
19. Scola, A.M.; Johswich, K.O.; Morgan, B.P.; Klos, A.; Monk, P.N. The Human Complement Fragment Receptor, C5L2, Is a Recycling Decoy Receptor. *Mol. Immunol.* **2009**, *46*, 1149–1162. [CrossRef]
20. Bengtson, A.; Holmberg, P.; Heideman, M. The Ischaemic Leg as a Source of Complement Activation. *Br. J. Surg.* **2005**, *74*, 697–700. [CrossRef]
21. Solomkin, J.S.; Jenkins, M.K.; Nelson, R.D.; Chenoweth, D.; Simmons, R.L. Neutrophil Dysfunction in Sepsis. II. Evidence for the Role of Complement Activation Products in Cellular Deactivation. *Surgery* **1981**, *90*, 319–327. [PubMed]
22. Nakae, H.; Endo, S.; Inada, K.; Yoshida, M. Chronological Changes in the Complement System in Sepsis. *Surg. Today* **1996**, *26*, 225–229. [CrossRef]
23. Flierl, M.A.; Rittirsch, D.; Chen, A.J.; Nadeau, B.A.; Day, D.E.; Sarma, J.V.; Huber-Lang, M.S.; Ward, P.A. The Complement Anaphylatoxin C5a Induces Apoptosis in Adrenomedullary Cells during Experimental Sepsis. *PLoS ONE* **2008**, *3*, e2560. [CrossRef] [PubMed]
24. Hu, R.; Chen, Z.F.; Yan, J.; Li, Q.F.; Huang, Y.; Xu, H.; Zhang, X.; Jiang, H. Complement C5a Exacerbates Acute Lung Injury Induced through Autophagy-Mediated Alveolar Macrophage Apoptosis. *Cell Death Dis.* **2014**, *5*, e1330. [CrossRef] [PubMed]
25. Mahajan, S.D.; Tutino, V.M.; Redae, Y.; Meng, H.; Siddiqui, A.; Woodruff, T.M.; Jarvis, J.N.; Hennon, T.; Schwartz, S.; Quigg, R.J.; et al. C5a Induces Caspase-dependent Apoptosis in Brain Vascular Endothelial Cells in Experimental Lupus. *Immunology* **2016**, *148*, 407. [CrossRef] [PubMed]
26. Nishiura, H.; Nonaka, H.; Revollo, I.S.; Semba, U.; Li, Y.; Ota, Y.; Irie, A.; Harada, K.; Kehrl, J.H.; Yamamoto, T. Pro- and Anti-Apoptotic Dual Functions of the C5a Receptor: Involvement of Regulator of G Protein Signaling 3 and Extracellular Signal-Regulated Kinase. *Lab. Investig.* **2009**, *89*, 676–694. [CrossRef]
27. Martinus, R.D.; Cook, C.J. The Effect of Complement C5a on Mitochondrial Functions of PC12 Cells. *Neuroreport* **2011**, *22*, 581–585. [CrossRef]
28. Francis, K.; Lewis, B.; Monk, P.; Scanlon, M.; Ham, J. Complement C5a Receptors Are Expressed Throughout the Anterior Pituitary Gland. *Endocr. Abstr.* **2005**, *9*, 126.
29. Chiou, W.F.; Tsai, H.R.; Yang, L.M.; Tsai, W.J. C5a Differentially Stimulates the ERK1/2 and P38 MAPK Phosphorylation Through Independent Signaling Pathways to Induced Chemotactic Migration in RAW264.7 Macrophages. *Int. Immunopharmacol.* **2004**, *4*, 1329–1341. [CrossRef]
30. Uhlén, M.; Fagerberg, L.; Hallström, B.M.; Lindskog, C.; Oksvold, P.; Mardinoglu, A.; Sivertsson, Å.; Kampf, C.; Sjöstedt, E.; Asplund, A.; et al. Tissue-Based Map of the Human Proteome. *Science* **2015**, *347*, 1260419. [CrossRef]

31. Kvetnansky, R.; Sabban, E.L.; Palkovits, M. Catecholaminergic Systems in Stress: Structural and Molecular Genetic Approaches. *Physiol. Rev.* **2009**, *89*, 535–606. [CrossRef] [PubMed]
32. Barth, E.; Albuszies, G.; Baumgart, K.; Matejovic, M.; Wachter, U.; Vogt, J.; Radermacher, P.; Calzia, E. Glucose Metabolism and Catecholamines. *Crit. Care Med.* **2007**, *35*, S518. [CrossRef] [PubMed]
33. Motiejunaite, J.; Amar, L.; Vidal-Petiot, E. Adrenergic Receptors and Cardiovascular Effects of Catecholamines. *Ann. Endocrinol.* **2021**, *82*, 193–197. [CrossRef] [PubMed]
34. Prigent, H.; Maxime, V.; Annane, D. Clinical Review: Corticotherapy in Sepsis. *Crit. Care* **2004**, *8*, 122–129. [CrossRef]
35. Hahn, P.Y.; Wang, P.; Tait, S.M.; Ba, Z.F.; Reich, S.S.; Chaudry, I.H. Sustained Elevation in Circulating Catecholamine Levels During Polymicrobial Sepsis. *Shock* **1995**, *4*, 269–273. [CrossRef]
36. Epstein, F.H.; Parrillo, J.E. Pathogenetic Mechanisms of Septic Shock. *New Engl. J. Med.* **2010**, *328*, 1471–1477. [CrossRef]
37. Dalegrave, D.; Silva, R.L.; Becker, M.; Gehrke, L.V.; Friedman, G. Relative Adrenal Insufficiency as a Predictor of Disease Severity and Mortality in Severe Septic Shock. *Rev. Bras. Ter. Intensiv.* **2012**, *24*, 362. [CrossRef]
38. McKechnie, K.; Dean, H.G.; Furman, B.L.; Parratt, J.R. Plasma Catecholamines during Endotoxin Infusion in Conscious Unrestrained Rats: Effects of Adrenal Demedullation and/or Guanethidine Treatment. *Circ. Shock* **1985**, *17*, 85–94.
39. Prigent, H.; Maxime, V.; Annane, D. Science Review: Mechanisms of Impaired Adrenal Function in Sepsis and Molecular Actions of Glucocorticoids. *Crit. Care* **2004**, *8*, 243–252. [CrossRef]
40. Hoffmann, R. Adrenal Lesions in Calves Dying from Endotoxin Shock, with Special Reference to the Waterhouse-Friderichsen Syndrome. *J. Comp. Pathol.* **1977**, *87*, 231–239. [CrossRef]
41. Cherkasova, M.N.; Borovaya, T.G.; Zhukhovitskii, V.G.; Pukhalskaia, V.G. Results of Structural and Bacteriological Analysis of the Mouse Adrenal Glands in a Sepsis Model. *Bull. Exp. Biol. Med.* **2022**, *173*, 67–71. [CrossRef] [PubMed]
42. Nougaret, S.; Jung, B.; Aufort, S.; Chanques, G.; Jaber, S.; Gallix, B. Emergency Radiology—Adrenal Gland Volume Measurement in Septic Shock and Control Patients: A Pilot Study. *Eur. Radiol.* **2010**, *20*, 2348–2357. [CrossRef] [PubMed]
43. Jung, B.; Nougaret, S.; Chanques, G.; Mercier, G.; Cisse, M.; Aufort, S.; Gallix, B.; Annane, D.; Jaber, S. The Absence of Adrenal Gland Enlargement during Septic Shock Predicts MortalityA Computed Tomography Study of 239 Patients. *Anesthesiology* **2011**, *115*, 334–343. [CrossRef] [PubMed]
44. Greene, L.A.; Tischler, A.S. Establishment of a Noradrenergic Clonal Line of Rat Adrenal Pheochromocytoma Cells Which Respond to Nerve Growth Factor. *Proc. Natl. Acad. Sci. USA* **1976**, *73*, 2424–2428. [CrossRef] [PubMed]
45. Sangaran, P.G.; Ibrahim, Z.A.; Chik, Z.; Mohamed, Z.; Ahmadiani, A. Lipopolysaccharide Pre-Conditioning Attenuates Pro-Inflammatory Responses and Promotes Cytoprotective Effect in Differentiated PC12 Cell Lines via Pre-Activation of Toll-Like Receptor-4 Signaling Pathway Leading to the Inhibition of Caspase-3/Nuclear Factor-Kappa B Pathway. *Front. Cell. Neurosci.* **2021**, *14*, 469. [CrossRef]
46. Hui, W.; Xu, Y.S.; Miao Lin, W.; Chao, C.; Bian, R.; Yuan, H.; Yi, W.; Guo, T.; Zhu, L.L.; Zhou, H. Protective Effect of Naringin Against the LPS-Induced Apoptosis of PC12 Cells: Implications for the Treatment of Neurodegenerative Disorders. *Int. J. Mol. Med.* **2017**, *39*, 819–830. [CrossRef]
47. Bloise, E.; Ciarmela, P.; Dela Cruz, C.; Luisi, S.; Petraglia, F.; Reis, F.M. Activin A in Mammalian Physiology. *Physiol. Rev.* **2019**, *99*, 739–780. [CrossRef]
48. Guicciardi, M.E.; Gores, G.J. The Fas/FasL Signaling Pathway. In *Signaling Pathways in Liver Diseases*; Dufour, J.-F., Clavien, P.-A., Eds.; Springer: Berlin, Germany, 2005; pp. 129–138. ISBN 978-3-540-27194-9.
49. Camby, I.; Le Mercier, M.; Lefranc, F.; Kiss, R. Galectin-1: A Small Protein with Major Functions. *Glycobiology* **2006**, *16*, 137R–157R. [CrossRef]
50. Malik, A.; Kanneganti, T.D. Function and Regulation of IL-1α in Inflammatory Diseases and Cancer. *Immunol. Rev.* **2018**, *281*, 124. [CrossRef]
51. Dougan, M.; Dranoff, G.; Dougan, S.K. GM-CSF, IL-3, and IL-5 Family of Cytokines: Regulators of Inflammation. *Immunity* **2019**, *50*, 796–811. [CrossRef]
52. Lindemann, A.; Mertelsmann, R. Interleukin-3: Structure and Function. *Cancer Investig.* **1993**, *11*, 609–623. [CrossRef] [PubMed]
53. Brown, M.A.; Hural, J. Functions of IL-4 and Control of Its Expression. *Crit. Rev. Immunol.* **1997**, *17*, 1–32. [CrossRef] [PubMed]
54. Bhavsar, I.; Miller, C.S.; Al-Sabbagh, M. Macrophage Inflammatory Protein-1 Alpha (MIP-1 Alpha)/CCL3: As a Biomarker. *General. Methods Biomark. Res. Their Appl.* **2015**, *1–2*, 223. [CrossRef]
55. Fredriksson, L.; Li, H.; Eriksson, U. The PDGF Family: Four Gene Products Form Five Dimeric Isoforms. *Cytokine Growth Factor. Rev.* **2004**, *15*, 197–204. [CrossRef] [PubMed]
56. Schutyser, E.; Struyf, S.; Van Damme, J. The CC Chemokine CCL20 and Its Receptor CCR6. *Cytokine Growth Factor. Rev.* **2003**, *14*, 409–426. [CrossRef]
57. Campbell, S.J.; Hughes, P.M.; Iredale, J.P.; Wilcockson, D.C.; Waters, S.; Docagne, F.; Perry, V.H.; Anthony, D.C. CINC-1 Is an Acute-Phase Protein Induced by Focal Brain Injury Causing Leukocyte Mobilization and Liver Injury. *FASEB J.* **2003**, *17*, 1168–1170. [CrossRef]
58. Takano, K.; Nakagawa, H. Contribution of Cytokine-Induced Neutrophil Chemoattractant CINC-2 and CINC-3 to Neutrophil Recruitment in Lipopolysaccharide-Induced Inflammation in Rats. *Inflamm. Res.* **2001**, *50*, 503–508. [CrossRef]
59. Van De Stolpe, A.; Van Der Saag, P.T. Intercellular Adhesion Molecule-1. *J. Mol. Med.* **1996**, *74*, 13–33. [CrossRef]
60. Wynn, T.A. IL-13 Effector Functions. *Annu. Rev. Immunol.* **2003**, *21*, 425–456. [CrossRef]

61. Kanczkowski, W.; Zacharowski, K.; Wirth, M.P.; Ehrhart-Bornstein, M.; Bornstein, S.R. Differential Expression and Action of Toll-like Receptors in Human Adrenocortical Cells. *Mol. Cell. Endocrinol.* **2009**, *300*, 57–65. [CrossRef]
62. Jennewein, C.; Tran, N.; Kanczkowski, W.; Heerdegen, L.; Kantharajah, A.; Dröse, S.; Bornstein, S.; Scheller, B.; Zacharowski, K. Mortality of Septic Mice Strongly Correlates with Adrenal Gland Inflammation. *Crit. Care Med.* **2016**, *44*, e190–e199. [CrossRef] [PubMed]
63. Ward, P.A. The Dark Side of C5a in Sepsis. *Nat. Rev. Immunol.* **2004**, *4*, 133–142. [CrossRef] [PubMed]
64. Dermitzaki, E.; Tsatsanis, C.; Gravanis, A.; Margioris, A.N. Corticotropin-Releasing Hormone Induces Fas Ligand Production and Apoptosis in PC12 Cells via Activation of P38 Mitogen-Activated Protein Kinase. *J. Biol. Chem.* **2002**, *277*, 12280–12287. [CrossRef]
65. Zheng, Y.; You, F.; Li, Q.; Chen, J.; Yang, H. The Effect of Geniste on Aβ25–35-Induced PC12 Cell Apoptosis through the JNK-Dependent Fas Pathway. *Food Funct.* **2016**, *7*, 4702–4708. [CrossRef]
66. Luo, Z.; Zhang, Z.; Zhang, F.; Liu, Y.; Zhang, Y.; Sun, X.; Sang, M.; Luo, H. Ropivacaine Mesylate Exerts Neurotoxicity via Up-Regulation of Fas/FasL Expression in Rat Pheochromocytoma PC12 Cells. *Am. J. Transl. Res.* **2019**, *11*, 1626.
67. Shivshankar, P.; Li, Y.D.; Mueller-Ortiz, S.L.; Wetsel, R.A. In Response to Complement Anaphylatoxin Peptides C3a and C5a, Human Vascular Endothelial Cells Migrate and Mediate the Activation of B-Cells and Polarization of T-Cells. *FASEB J.* **2020**, *34*, 7540–7560. [CrossRef] [PubMed]
68. Chen, W.; Woodruff, T.K.; Mayo, K.E. Activin A-Induced HepG2 Liver Cell Apoptosis: Involvement of Activin Receptors and Smad Proteins. *Endocrinology* **2000**, *141*, 1263–1272. [CrossRef]
69. Zhang, F.; Qi, Y.; Li, J.; Liu, B.; Liu, Z.; Cui, X. Activin A Induces Apoptosis of Human Lung Adenocarcinoma A549 Cells Through Endoplasmic Reticulum Stress Pathway. *Oncol. Rep.* **2024**, *51*, 29. [CrossRef]
70. Zhang, Y.; Qi, Y.; Zhao, Y.; Sun, H.; Ge, J.; Liu, Z. Activin A Induces Apoptosis of Mouse Myeloma Cells Via the Mitochondrial Pathway. *Oncol. Lett.* **2018**, *15*, 2590. [CrossRef]
71. Xue, L.X.; Liu, H.Y.; Cui, Y.; Dong, Y.; Wang, J.Q.; Ji, Q.Y.; He, J.T.; Yao, M.; Wang, Y.Y.; Shao, Y.K.; et al. Neuroprotective Effects of Activin A on Endoplasmic Reticulum Stress-Mediated Apoptotic and Autophagic PC12 Cell Death. *Neural Regen. Res.* **2017**, *12*, 779. [CrossRef]
72. Xu, G.H.; He, J.T.; Guo, H.L.; Mei, C.L.; Wang, J.Q.; Li, Z.S.; Chen, H.; Mang, J.; Yang, H.; Xu, Z.X. Activin A Prevents Neuron-like PC12 Cell Apoptosis after Oxygen-Glucose Deprivation. *Neural Regen. Res.* **2013**, *8*, 1016. [CrossRef] [PubMed]
73. Iwasaki, S.; Iguchi, M.; Watanabe, K.; Hoshino, R.; Tsujimoto, M.; Kohno, M. Specific Activation of the P38 Mitogen-Activated Protein Kinase Signaling Pathway and Induction of Neurite Outgrowth in PC12 Cells by Bone Morphogenetic Protein-2. *J. Biol. Chem.* **1999**, *274*, 26503–26510. [CrossRef] [PubMed]
74. Tsai, I.J.; Lin, W.C.; Yang, Y.H.; Tseng, Y.L.; Lin, Y.H.; Chou, C.H.; Tsau, Y.K. High Concentration of C5a-Induced Mitochondria-Dependent Apoptosis in Murine Kidney Endothelial Cells. *Int. J. Mol. Sci.* **2019**, *20*, 4465. [CrossRef]
75. Chang, L.; Karin, M. Mammalian MAP Kinase Signalling Cascades. *Nature* **2001**, *410*, 37–40. [CrossRef]
76. Ardito, F.; Giuliani, M.; Perrone, D.; Troiano, G.; Lo Muzio, L. The Crucial Role of Protein Phosphorylation in Cell Signaling and Its Use as Targeted Therapy (Review). *Int. J. Mol. Med.* **2017**, *40*, 271–280. [CrossRef]
77. An, L.L.; Gorman, J.V.; Stephens, G.; Swerdlow, B.; Warrener, P.; Bonnell, J.; Mustelin, T.; Fung, M.; Kolbeck, R. Complement C5a Induces PD-L1 Expression and Acts in Synergy with LPS Through Erk1/2 and JNK Signaling Pathways. *Sci. Rep.* **2016**, *6*, 33346. [CrossRef] [PubMed]
78. Lei, Y.C.; Lu, C.L.; Chen, L.; Ge, K.; Yang, L.L.; Li, W.; Wu, Y.H. C5a/C5aR Pathway Is Essential for Up-Regulating SphK1 Expression Through P38-MAPK Activation in Acute Liver Failure. *World J. Gastroenterol.* **2016**, *22*, 10148–10157. [CrossRef]
79. Zhang, Z. Association of C5a/C5aR Pathway to Activate ERK1/2 and P38 MAPK in Acute Kidney Injury—A Mouse Model. *Rev. Rom. Med. Lab.* **2022**, *30*, 31–40. [CrossRef]
80. Xu, G.; Chen, J.; Yang, F.; Li, G.; Zheng, L.; Wu, Y. C5a/C5aR Pathway Is Essential for the Pathogenesis of Murine Viral Fulminant Hepatitis by Way of Potentiating Fgl2/Fibroleukin Expression. *Hepatology* **2014**, *60*, 114–124. [CrossRef]
81. Chen, J.; Li, G.q.; Zhang, L.; Tang, M.; Cao, X.; Xu, G.l.; Wu, Y.Z. Complement C5a/C5aR Pathway Potentiates the Pathogenesis of Gastric Cancer by Down-Regulating P21 Expression. *Cancer Lett.* **2018**, *412*, 30–36. [CrossRef]
82. Zeke, A.; Misheva, M.; Reményi, A.; Bogoyevitch, M.A. JNK Signaling: Regulation and Functions Based on Complex Protein-Protein Partnerships. *Microbiol. Mol. Biol. Rev.* **2016**, *80*, 793–835. [CrossRef] [PubMed]
83. Coffey, E.T. Nuclear and Cytosolic JNK Signalling in Neurons. *Nat. Rev. Neurosci.* **2014**, *15*, 285–299. [CrossRef]
84. Hirata, Y.; Adachi, K.; Kiuchi, K. Activation of JNK Pathway and Induction of Apoptosis by Manganese in PC12 Cells. *J. Neurochem.* **1998**, *71*, 1607–1615. [CrossRef]
85. Zheng, G.; Luo, W.; Zhang, X.; Zhao, F.; Wang, J.; Chen, Y.; Chen, J. Effect of JNK Pathway in Apoptosis of PC12 Cell by MPP+. *J. Hyg. Res.* **2011**, *40*, 109–111.
86. Zhang, H.; Wang, S.; Wang, Y.; Lu, A.; Hu, C.; Yan, C. DHA Ameliorates MeHg-induced PC12 Cell Apoptosis by Inhibiting the ROS/JNK Signaling Pathway. *Mol. Med. Rep.* **2021**, *24*, 558. [CrossRef] [PubMed]
87. Shacka, J.J.; Sahawneh, M.A.; Gonzalez, J.D.; Ye, Y.Z.; D'Alessandro, T.L.; Estévez, A.G. Two Distinct Signaling Pathways Regulate Peroxynitrite-Induced Apoptosis in PC12 Cells. *Cell Death Differ.* **2006**, *13*, 1506–1514. [CrossRef] [PubMed]
88. Pizzino, G.; Bitto, A.; Pallio, G.; Irrera, N.; Galfo, F.; Interdonato, M.; Mecchio, A.; De Luca, F.; Minutoli, L.; Squadrito, F.; et al. Blockade of the JNK Signalling as a Rational Therapeutic Approach to Modulate the Early and Late Steps of the Inflammatory Cascade in Polymicrobial Sepsis. *Mediat. Inflamm.* **2015**, *2015*, 591572. [CrossRef] [PubMed]

89. Lou, L.; Hu, D.; Chen, S.; Wang, S.; Xu, Y.; Huang, Y.; Shi, Y.; Zhang, H. Protective Role of JNK Inhibitor SP600125 in Sepsis-Induced Acute Lung Injury. *Int. J. Clin. Exp. Pathol.* **2019**, *12*, 528.
90. Schramek, H. MAP Kinases: From Intracellular Signals to Physiology and Disease. *News Physiol. Sci.* **2002**, *17*, 62–67. [CrossRef]
91. Zhang, L.; Jope, R.S. Oxidative Stress Differentially Modulates Phosphorylation of ERK, P38 and CREB Induced by NGF or EGF in PC12 Cells. *Neurobiol. Aging* **1999**, *20*, 271–278. [CrossRef]
92. Goillot, E.; Raingeaud, J.; Ranger, A.; Tepper, R.I.; Davis, R.J.; Harlow, E.D.; Sanchez, I. Mitogen-Activated Protein Kinase-Mediated Fas Apoptotic Signaling Pathway. *Proc. Natl. Acad. Sci. USA* **1997**, *94*, 3302–3307. [CrossRef] [PubMed]
93. Yang, L.Y.; Ko, W.C.; Lin, C.M.; Lin, J.W.; Wu, J.C.; Lin, C.J.; Cheng, H.H.; Shih, C.M. Antioxidant N-Acetylcysteine Blocks Nerve Growth Factor-Induced H_2O_2/ERK Signaling in PC12 Cells. *Ann. N. Y. Acad. Sci.* **2005**, *1042*, 325–337. [CrossRef] [PubMed]
94. Park, H.J.; Park, K.H.; Shin, K.S.; Lee, M.K. The Roles of Cyclic AMP–ERK–Bad Signaling Pathways on 6-Hydroxydopamine-Induced Cell Survival and Death in PC12 Cells. *Toxicol. Vitr.* **2013**, *27*, 2233–2241. [CrossRef] [PubMed]
95. Mebratu, Y.; Tesfaigzi, Y. How ERK1/2 Activation Controls Cell Proliferation and Cell Death Is Subcellular Localization the Answer? *Cell Cycle* **2009**, *8*, 1168. [CrossRef] [PubMed]
96. Hao, J.; Meng, L.Q.; Xu, P.C.; Chen, M.; Zhao, M.H. P38MAPK, ERK and PI3K Signaling Pathways Are Involved in C5a-Primed Neutrophils for ANCA-Mediated Activation. *PLoS ONE* **2012**, *7*, e38317. [CrossRef]
97. Ono, K.; Han, J. The P38 Signal Transduction Pathway Activation and Function. *Cell. Signal.* **2000**, *12*, 1–13. [CrossRef]
98. Yamamoto, T.; Yuyama, K.; Yamamoto, H. Low Concentrations of Nitric Oxide (NO) Induced Cell Death in PC12 Cells through Activation of P38 Mitogen-Activated Protein Kinase (P38 MAPK) but Not via Extracellular Signal-Regulated Kinases (ERK1/2) or c-Jun N-Terminal Protein Kinase (JNK). *Neurosci. Lett.* **2006**, *392*, 170–173. [CrossRef]
99. Liu, J.; Zhu, Y.; Chen, S.; Shen, B.; Yu, F.; Zhang, Y.; Shen, R. Apocynin Attenuates Cobalt Chloride-Induced Pheochromocytoma Cell Apoptosis by Inhibiting P38-MAPK/Caspase-3 Pathway. *Cell. Physiol. Biochem.* **2018**, *48*, 208–214. [CrossRef]
100. Chen, Y.; Wang, E.; Sun, Z.; Song, Z.; Ye, Z.; Zhang, Z. P38 MAPK Inhibitor SB203580 Attenuates the Toxicity of Ropivacaine on PC12 Cells. *J. Cent. S. Univ. Med. Sci.* **2019**, *44*, 985–989. [CrossRef]
101. Zhuang, S.; Demirs, J.T.; Kochevar, I.E. P38 Mitogen-Activated Protein Kinase Mediates Bid Cleavage, Mitochondrial Dysfunction, and Caspase-3 Activation during Apoptosis Induced by Singlet Oxygen but Not by Hydrogen Peroxide. *J. Biol. Chem.* **2000**, *275*, 25939–25948. [CrossRef]
102. Alvarado-Kristensson, M.; Melander, F.; Leandersson, K.; Rönnstrand, L.; Wernstedt, C.; Andersson, T. P38-MAPK Signals Survival by Phosphorylation of Caspase-8 and Caspase-3 in Human Neutrophils. *J. Exp. Med.* **2004**, *199*, 449. [CrossRef] [PubMed]
103. Speidel, D. Transcription-Independent P53 Apoptosis: An Alternative Route to Death. *Trends Cell Biol.* **2010**, *20*, 14–24. [CrossRef] [PubMed]
104. O'Sullivan, A.W.; Wang, J.H.; Redmond, H.P. NF-KB and P38 MAPK Inhibition Improve Survival in Endotoxin Shock and in a Cecal Ligation and Puncture Model of Sepsis in Combination With Antibiotic Therapy. *J. Surg. Res.* **2009**, *152*, 46–53. [CrossRef] [PubMed]
105. Yang, Y.; Kim, S.C.; Yu, T.; Yi, Y.S.; Rhee, M.H.; Sung, G.H.; Yoo, B.C.; Cho, J.Y. Functional Roles of P38 Mitogen-Activated Protein Kinase in Macrophage-Mediated Inflammatory Responses. *Mediat. Inflamm.* **2014**, *2014*, 352371. [CrossRef]
106. Fattahi, F.; Zetoune, F.S.; Ward, P.A. Complement as a Major Inducer of Harmful Events in Infectious Sepsis. *Shock* **2020**, *54*, 595–605. [CrossRef]
107. Moens, U.; Kostenko, S.; Sveinbjørnsson, B. The Role of Mitogen-Activated Protein Kinase-Activated Protein Kinases (MAPKAPKs) in Inflammation. *Genes* **2013**, *4*, 101. [CrossRef]
108. Manning, B.D.; Toker, A. AKT/PKB Signaling: Navigating the Network. *Cell* **2017**, *169*, 381–405. [CrossRef]
109. Weihl, C.C.; Ghadge, G.D.; Kennedy, S.G.; Hay, N.; Miller, R.J.; Roos, R.P. Mutant Presenilin-1 Induces Apoptosis and Downregulates Akt/PKB. *J. Neurosci.* **1999**, *19*, 5360–5369. [CrossRef]
110. Alvarez-Tejado, M.; Naranjo-Suárez, S.; Jiménez, C.; Carrera, A.C.; Landázuri, M.O.; Del Peso, L. Hypoxia Induces the Activation of the Phosphatidylinositol 3-Kinase/Akt Cell Survival Pathway in PC12 Cells: Protective Role in Apoptosis. *J. Biol. Chem.* **2001**, *276*, 22368–22374. [CrossRef]
111. Zhang, L.; Ding, W.; Sun, H.; Zhou, Q.; Huang, J.Q.; Li, X.; Xie, Y.; Chen, J. Salidroside Protects PC12 Cells from MPP+-Induced Apoptosis via Activation of the PI3K/Akt Pathway. *Food Chem. Toxicol.* **2012**, *50*, 2591–2597. [CrossRef]
112. Toledo-Pereyra, L.H.; Lopez-Neblina, F.; Reuben, J.S.; Toledo, A.H.; Ward, P.A. Selectin Inhibition Modulates Akt/MAPK Signaling and Chemokine Expression After Liver Ischemia–Reperfusion. *J. Investig. Surg.* **2004**, *17*, 303–313. [CrossRef] [PubMed]
113. Chen, Y.; Ba, L.; Huang, W.; Liu, Y.; Pan, H.; Mingyao, E.; Shi, P.; Wang, Y.; Li, S.; Qi, H.; et al. Role of Carvacrol in Cardioprotection against Myocardial Ischemia/Reperfusion Injury in Rats through Activation of MAPK/ERK and Akt/ENOS Signaling Pathways. *Eur. J. Pharmacol.* **2017**, *796*, 90–100. [CrossRef] [PubMed]
114. Fattahi, F.; Kalbitz, M.; Malan, E.A.; Abe, E.; Jajou, L.; Huber-Lang, M.S.; Bosmann, M.; Russell, M.W.; Zetoune, F.S.; Ward, P.A. Complement-Induced Activation of MAPKs and Akt during Sepsis: Role in Cardiac Dysfunction. *FASEB J.* **2017**, *31*, 4129–4139. [CrossRef] [PubMed]
115. Mullany, L.K.; Nelsen, C.J.; Hanse, E.A.; Goggin, M.M.; Anttila, C.K.; Peterson, M.; Bitterman, P.B.; Raghavan, A.; Crary, G.S.; Albrecht, J.H. Akt-Mediated Liver Growth Promotes Induction of Cyclin E through a Novel Translational Mechanism and a P21-Mediated Cell Cycle Arrest. *J. Biol. Chem.* **2007**, *282*, 21244–21252. [CrossRef] [PubMed]

116. Eglite, S.; Plüss, K.; Dahinden, C.A. Requirements for C5a Receptor-Mediated IL-4 and IL-13 Production and Leukotriene C4 Generation in Human Basophils. *J. Immunol.* **2000**, *165*, 2183–2189. [CrossRef]
117. Snyderman, R.; Phillips, J.; Mergenhagen, S.E. Polymorphonuclear Leukocyte Chemotactic Activity in Rabbit Serum and Guinea Pig Serum Treated with Immune Complexes: Evidence for C5a as the Major Chemotactic Factor. *Infect. Immun.* **1970**, *1*, 521. [CrossRef]
118. Becker, E.L. The Relationship of the Chemotactic Behavior of the Complement-Derived Factors, C3a, C5a, C567, and a Bacterial Chemotactic Factor to Their Ability to Activate the Proesterase 1 of Rabbit Polymorphonuclear Leukocytes. *J. Exp. Med.* **1972**, *135*, 376. [CrossRef]
119. Snyderman, R.; Pike, M.C.; McCarley, D.; Lang, L. Quantification of Mouse Macrophage Chemotaxis in Vitro: Role of C5 for the Production of Chemotactic Activity. *Infect. Immun.* **1975**, *11*, 488. [CrossRef]
120. Deng, S.; Zhou, F.; Wang, F.; Jiang, Y.; Tang, J.; Hu, X.; Luo, L.; Jin, Y.; Huang, L.; Sun, D.; et al. C5a Enhances Vδ1 T Cells Recruitment via the CCL2-CCR2 Axis in IgA Nephropathy. *Int. Immunopharmacol.* **2023**, *125*, 111065. [CrossRef]
121. Skei, J.M.; Fingert, J.H.; Russell, S.R.; Stone, E.M.; Mullins, R.F. Complement Component C5a Activates ICAM-1 Expression on Human Choroidal Endothelial Cells. *Investig. Ophthalmol. Vis. Sci.* **2010**, *51*, 5336–5342. [CrossRef]
122. Lawrence, I.D.; Warner, J.A.; Cohan, V.L.; Hubbard, W.C.; Kagey-Sobotka, A.; Lichtenstein, L.M. Purification and Characterization of Human Skin Mast Cells. Evidence for Human Mast Cell Heterogeneity. *J. Immunol.* **1987**, *139*, 3062–3069. [CrossRef] [PubMed]
123. Oskeritzian, C.A.; Zhao, W.; Min, H.K.; Xia, H.Z.; Pozez, A.; Kiev, J.; Schwartz, L.B. Surface CD88 Functionally Distinguishes the MCTC from the MCT Type of Human Lung Mast Cell. *J. Allergy Clin. Immunol.* **2005**, *115*, 1162. [CrossRef] [PubMed]
124. Thorley, J. FDA Approves Avacopan for ANCA-Associated Vasculitis. *Lancet Rheumatol.* **2022**, *4*, e21. [CrossRef]
125. Dubois, E.A.; Cohen, A.F. Eculizumab. *Br. J. Clin. Pharmacol.* **2009**, *68*, 318. [CrossRef]

International Journal of
Molecular Sciences

Review

Biomarkers as Beacons: Illuminating Sepsis-Associated Hepato-Renal Injury

Maria-Antoanela Pasare [1,2], Cristian Sorin Prepeliuc [1,3], Maria Gabriela Grigoriu [2], Ionela-Larisa Miftode [2,4,*] and Egidia Gabriela Miftode [2,4]

1 Doctoral School, "Grigore T. Popa" University of Medicine and Pharmacy, 700115 Iasi, Romania; antoanela.pasare@gmail.com (M.-A.P.); cristiprep94@gmail.com (C.S.P.)
2 "Sf Parascheva" Clinical Hospital of Infectious Diseases, 700116 Iasi, Romania; grigoriumaria.mg@gmail.com (M.G.G.); emiftode@yahoo.co.uk (E.G.M.)
3 Emergency Hospital "Mavromati", 710221 Botosani, Romania
4 Department of Infectious Diseases, Faculty of Medicine, "Grigore T. Popa" University of Medicine and Pharmacy, 700115 Iasi, Romania
* Correspondence: ionela-larisa.miftode@umfiasi.ro; Tel.: +40-747-337-968

Abstract: Sepsis, defined as a dysregulated host response to infection, is one of the leading causes of mortality worldwide. It unleashes in the organism a cascade of molecules, cytokines, and proteins which leads to an inflammatory storm. If this response to infection is uncontrolled, any organ is susceptible to damage. Acute kidney injury (AKI) is one of the most frequent organ dysfunctions in septic patients, and while it can be reversible, its presence leads to a higher burden of morbidity and mortality. While serum creatinine is essential in evaluating kidney function, the pathophysiology of AKI is not completely elucidated, and a plethora of novel biomarkers have been studied in the hope of an early diagnosis and fast treatment. While the liver is not as affected by sepsis, it plays an important role as a guardian by providing acute-phase proteins, activating neutrophils, and controlling iron balance. Acute liver failure (ALF) could impair the organism's capacity to contain and eliminate pathogens. Some molecules have been associated with either AKI or ALF, although biomarkers specific for organ dysfunction are difficult to validate. The aim of this review is to understand the role of several molecules in the pathophysiology of sepsis and their clinical ability for diagnosing or predicting sepsis-induced hepato-renal dysfunction.

Keywords: sepsis; acute kidney injury; acute liver failure; IL-18; hepcidin; ferritin; IL-27

1. Introduction

To our best understanding today, sepsis represents a life-threatening organ dysfunction that is caused by a dysregulated host response to infection [1]. The task force that was appointed to define sepsis recommends using the SOFA (sequential organ failure assessment) scoring system to evaluate organ dysfunction in a patient with a suspected or confirmed infection [2].

Sepsis is one of the major contributors to the global health burden, alongside stroke, heart disease, and kidney disease [3,4]. Recent data indicate that sepsis incidence rates vary between 500 and 1500 cases per 100,000 people. Mortality rates are lower in high-income countries, between 15 and 25%, and can reach up to 40% in low- and middle-income countries [5]. Further epidemiological studies will elucidate sepsis's incidence and health impact through the coronavirus disease (COVID-19) pandemic years, as some have categorized sepsis while referring to viral sepsis and some as a bacterial infection associated with COVID-19 [6].

On a cellular level, sepsis starts with the recognition of pathogen-derived molecular patterns (PAMPs) and damage-associated molecular patterns (DAMPs), which bind to receptors of antigen-presenting cells. Immune cells release a plethora of cytokines, both pro-inflammatory: such as interleukin (IL)-1, IL-6, IL-12, IL-18, and tumor necrosis factor alpha (TNF-α), and anti-inflammatory: IL-10, IL-27, and transforming growth factor beta 1 (TGFβ1). Inflammation leads to the release of acute-phase proteins by the liver, which in turn determines immune cell recruitment, activation of the complement system, the coagulation pathway, and iron regulation. Following the response from the innate immune system, the adaptive immune system comes into play as the organism tries to resolve the disease [7,8]. Part of the pathophysiology of sepsis and the interplay of various molecules is synthesized in Figure 1.

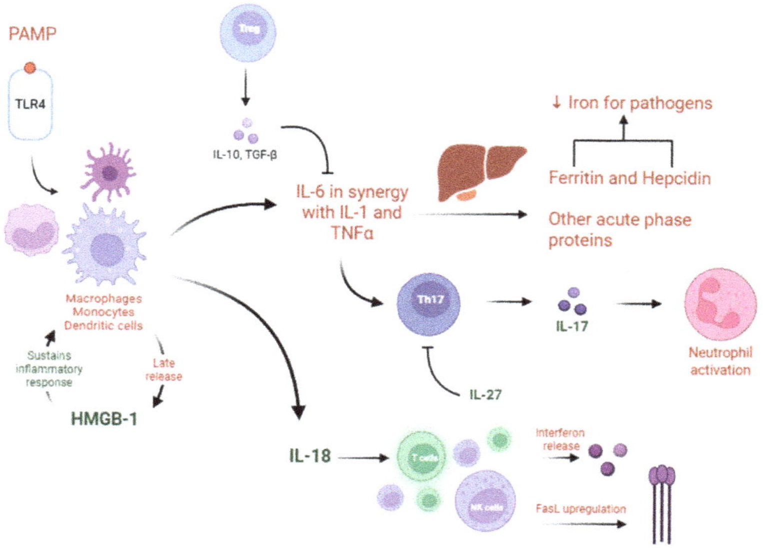

Figure 1. Overview of sepsis pathophysiology. FasL: Fas Ligand; HMGB1: high-mobility group box-1; NK: natural killer; Th: T helper cells; TLR: Toll-like Receptor; Treg: Regulatory T cell. Created in BioRender. Pasare, A. (2025) https://BioRender.com/0fgjo31. Accessed on 1 May 2025.

The delicate balance of inflammation and anti-inflammation is disrupted in sepsis, and while both pathways are upregulated, the resulting inflammation triggers progressive tissue damage and multi-organ dysfunction [7]. The kidneys and the liver are highly susceptible to microcirculatory dysfunction, and sepsis complicated with either hepatic or renal injury leads to high mortality rates, from 38% to almost 50% [8,9]. Hepato-renal dysfunction can exacerbate injury to other organs and can lead to an influx of toxins into the central nervous system. Additionally, coagulopathy can produce cerebral ischemia or hemorrhage [10]. Therefore, it is imperative to recognize sepsis-associated acute kidney injury (SA-AKI) and sepsis-associated liver injury (SALI) in a timely manner. Classical methods to detect kidney injury, such as creatinine and urine output, are not sufficiently sensitive, and their changes do not occur early enough to detect declines in renal function [11]. Liver biomarkers, such as bilirubin, aminotransferases, and alkaline phosphatase, are not satisfactory in their ability to reflect liver dysfunction, to differentiate acute from chronic injury, and to predict mortality [12].

As a result, in the last decades, research has been focused on finding biomarkers that aid in predicting diagnosis and prognosis. Although many molecules have been proposed, only a few are used in practice today. Biomarkers are objective indicators that characterize normal to pathogenic processes or pharmacological responses to therapeutic intervention. An ideal biomarker must be highly sensitive and specific to the provided data, reproducible, and cost-effective [13].

The scope of this review is to examine certain interleukins and molecules that show promising diagnostic or prognostic values related to sepsis-specific hepatic or renal injury, but whose clinical utility is still under investigation. We have excluded biomarkers that have been extensively reviewed in recent years, such as IL-6, interferons (IFNs), neutrophil gelatinase-associated lipocalin (NGAL), kidney injury molecule 1 (KIM-1), and presepsin.

2. Sepsis Phenotypes and Endotypes

Given that sepsis is a highly heterogeneous syndrome, the concepts of sepsis phenotypes and endotypes have emerged. Various phenotype categories divide sepsis based on temperature, hemodynamics, and organ dysfunction. Temperature profiling identified three different groups: hypothermic, normothermic, and hyperthermic, with the highest mortality among those with a greater deviation from normal temperature, either below or above. As a distinction, patients in the hypothermic group exhibit an inclination towards a tempered anti-inflammatory response compared to febrile patients, who exhibit higher plasma concentrations of both pro- and anti-inflammatory cytokines. (IL-6, TNF-α, granulocyte colony-stimulating factor, IL-10, IL-27). Hemodynamic profiling distinguishes the highest mortality among patients with a mean systolic blood pressure (SBP) around 80 mmHg. For organ dysfunction, multiple research groups have identified distinct phenotypes, with the highest mortality among patients with cardiogenic dysfunction/shock associated with either renal impairment or altered mental status [14–16]. One study on a substantially large cohort categorized patients into: "α phenotype" with less organ dysfunction and lower median values compared to the entire study group for IL-10, IL-6, IL-8, procalcitonin, and TNF-α; "β phenotype" with renal injury and greater comorbidities; "γ phenotype" with associated cardiovascular, hematologic, and inflammatory abnormalities, and "δ phenotype", linked to cardiovascular and hepatic injury and which associated the highest values for IL-10, IL-6, IL-8, procalcitonin, D-dimer, and plasminogen activator inhibitor 1 (PAI-1) [17].

Concerning endotypes, multiple research groups have defined various categories, without any scholarly consensus. One proposed classification denotes the following endotypes: neutrophilic-suppressive (upregulation of innate system pathways); inflammatory (increased inflammatory response); innate host defense (moderate regulation of interleukin signaling); interferon (high expression of interferons); and adaptive (upregulation of adaptive immune pathways) [18]. Another classification indicates two extremes: macrophage activation-like syndrome (MALS) and immuno-paralysis. In MALS, a high concentration of pro-inflammatory cytokines leads to liver dysfunction, disseminated intravascular coagulation (DIC), and pancytopenia. Ferritin levels exceed 4420 nanograms/milliliter (ng/mL) and are associated with increased concentrations of IL-6, IL-18, and soluble cluster of differentiation 163 (sCD163), and a decreased ratio of IL-10/TNF-α. Immuno-paralysis is defined by a low percentage of monocytes that express human leucocyte antigen (HLA)-DR and therefore present a weak ability to initiate adaptive immune responses. Patients who did not meet either criterion were considered to fall between the two groups [19,20].

3. The Liver and Kidney in Sepsis

3.1. Acute Kidney Injury

Acute kidney injury is increasingly frequent in patients with sepsis or septic shock, contributing to worse outcomes and longer hospitalization [21]. AKI is defined by KDIGO criteria, which rely on creatinine or urine output, and in the absence of baseline information, clinicians use eGFR [9]. Crucial roles of the kidneys are maintaining fluid and electrolyte balance and filtering waste, such as exogenous drugs. Administration of intravenous fluids and antibiotics can contribute to adverse renal outcomes due to fluid overload and toxicity [22]. Sepsis-associated AKI pathogenesis (Figure 2) is not completely elucidated, but the most relevant theories are related to circulatory dysfunction, immune response, and metabolic changes. Microcirculatory dysfunction determines the loss of nurturing capillaries, microthrombi formation, and endothelial injury due to shedding of the glycocalyx and hyperpermeability. The inflammatory response in the kidneys is managed by renal tubular epithelial cells (TECs) that bind to DAMPs and PAMPs, triggering the expression of pro-inflammatory cytokines and immune cell recruitment. The complement system is mainly composed of C1–C9 components and their subunits. The activation of the complement cascade induces the formation of the membrane attack complex (C5b-C9), causing cell lysis [23,24].

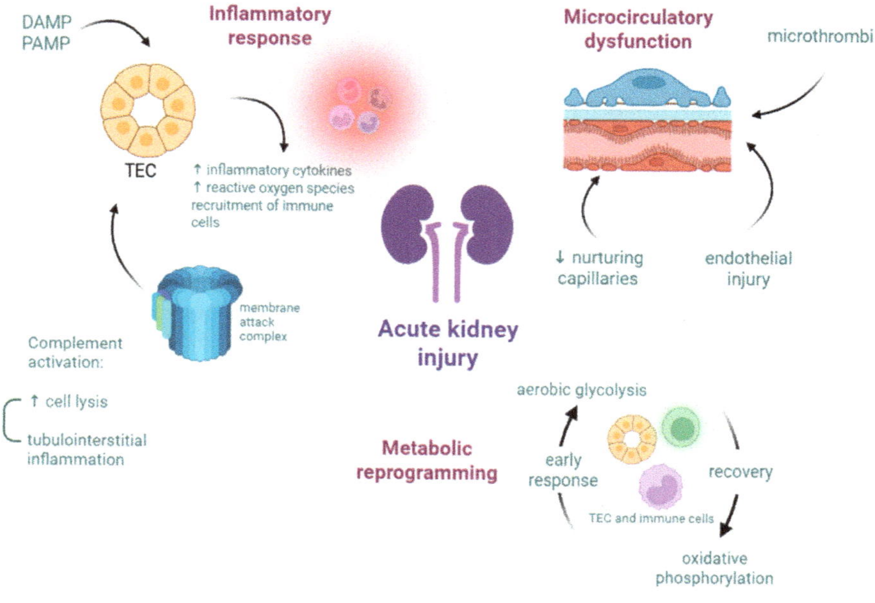

Figure 2. Overview of SA-AKI pathophysiology. Created in BioRender. Pasare, A. (2025) https://BioRender.com/1f9k56c. Accessed on 11 May 2025.

3.2. Acute Liver Failure and Liver Dysfunction

Although the liver is less affected by sepsis, with an incidence of 11–12% sepsis-associated liver failure [12,25], its importance in pathophysiology is greater. Some of the mechanisms by which the liver protects the organism are related but not limited to: Kupffer cells that release pro-inflammatory cytokines and prevent the entrance of bacteria in the circulatory system, the recruitment and activation of neutrophils, the synthesis of complement factors, and acute-phase proteins [26]. Controlling iron metabolism is also part of liver defenses, as many microbes require iron. Sepsis-associated liver dysfunction can arise from either hypoxic hepatitis (hypoxic cell death leads to a serum increase in aminotransferases) or cholestasis (inflammation of bile ducts leads to impaired bile flow). Liver dysfunction in sepsis can progress to acute liver failure [8,26].

Another way the liver acts as a guardian is by producing clotting factors to help limit pathogens in a fibrin network. Sepsis-induced coagulopathy (SIC) represents the disruption in the fine balance of the coagulation pathway, leading to hypercoagulability in the early stages, followed by the depletion of clotting factors. After immune cells are activated by pathogens, and cytokines are released, monocytes and endothelial cells respond by releasing tissue factor (TF). TF activates the extrinsic coagulation pathway, and as sepsis progresses, anticoagulants decrease, leading to their inability to control clot formation. Fibrinolytic activity is also impaired due to elevated levels of PAI-1, which accentuates the formation of microthrombi [26,27]. SIC is an important contributor to organ injury through microthrombi, and in later stages, through the risk of bleeding due to consumption of clotting factors. Around 29% of critically ill septic patients are diagnosed with SIC [7].

4. Biomarkers That Pertain to AKI or ALF

4.1. IL-18

Interleukin-18 is part of the interleukin-1 family, and its precursor is found in Kupffer cells and other hematopoietic and non-hematopoietic cells. As a cytokine, it plays different roles depending on the receptor or other interleukins. Combined with interleukin-12, it helps T cells and natural killer cells to produce IFN-gamma. Without IL-12 or IL-15, it can lead to the differentiation of naive T cells into T helper-2 cells. Similar to other cytokines, it increases nitric oxide (NO) synthesis and cell adhesion molecules, but one specific property is Fas ligand induction, which leads to cell apoptosis. In order to minimize the immune response, IL-18 binding protein (IL-18BP) serves as the main regulatory mechanism, reducing the plasmatic levels of IL-18 [28,29].

Animal studies concluded that IL-18 not only increases cytokine levels but also helps promote serum immunoglobulin M (IgM) levels. Research has demonstrated that mice injected with *Escherichia coli* have increased serum IgM levels after multiple IL-18 injections compared to control mice, but a single shot of IL-18 only increases IFN-gamma levels [30]. Similar results were found in a study with mice that sustained burn injuries and were injected with *Pseudomonas aeruginosa.* IL-18 injections increased the mice survival rate, and serum IgM levels were higher [31].

Regarding its clinical significance, IL-18 has been shown to play a role in various diseases that display an inflammatory component. High concentrations of IL-18 have been found in patients with Crohn's disease, asthma, chronic obstructive pulmonary disease, systemic juvenile idiopathic arthritis, and Still's disease [28]. Given that sepsis and inflammatory disorders could clinically overlap, evidence suggests significant differences in IL-18 plasma levels between a small cohort of patients diagnosed with Still's disease and septic patients, as the molecule displayed higher values in patients with active inflammatory disease [32].

The value of IL-18 as a mortality predictor in sepsis is disputed, as there are varying results from clinical and in vitro studies. In a study involving 40 sepsis and septic shock patients, the authors found that although IL-18 was higher at all study times in septic patients compared to healthy volunteers, there was no difference between survivors and non-survivors [33]. However, in another study involving 65 septic patients, the authors showed that patients with elevated IL-18 levels have about a 90% higher risk of death [34].

Concerning AKI, a study involving approximately 1400 patients from intensive care units found that IL-18 performed poorly to moderately regarding its ability to predict new AKI or progression of kidney injury. However, only 6.2% of those patients were diagnosed with sepsis [35]. Given that interleukin-18 is expressed in renal tubular cells, one meta-analysis shows that in patients with cirrhosis, it can differentiate between acute tubular necrosis and hepatorenal syndrome with high specificity and sensitivity [36]. SA-AKI has a complicated pathophysiology, and it is believed that it is characterized by reversible injury of the tubular cells and not by necrosis [37]. One study showed that IL-18, alongside KIM-1 and the renal resistive index, are good predictors for developing AKI in patients with sepsis, with IL-18 demonstrating the highest sensitivity [38]. The renal resistive index, an ultrasound-derived parameter, provides real-time perfusion data of the kidneys and can predict AKI [39]. Another retrospective study, which included patients with both bacterial and viral sepsis, concluded that IL-18 can be found in a wide range of elevated plasma concentrations. Mortality, AKI, and acute respiratory distress syndrome (ARDS) were correlated with IL-18 levels in both groups of sepsis [40]. Interleukin-18 serum levels rise after 6 h in the ICU, showing a significant difference between AKI and non-AKI septic patients. Nevertheless, the combination of IL-18 and NGAL performs better for AKI diagnosis, with a sensitivity of 77.9% and specificity of 94.6% [41]. Similar results were observed regarding IL-18 and the NLRP3 inflammasome, which were upregulated in septic patients compared to the control group and further increased in AKI patients versus non-AKI [42]. A study conducted on pregnant women, of which only 44% had a positive quick SOFA score on admission, concluded that IL-18 was not a good predictor for developing AKI [43]. Therefore, IL-18 could be a potential biomarker for predicting sepsis-associated AKI but not for other related causes.

Serum concentrations of IL-18 alongside IL-1β rise in a time-dependent manner in ALF models. After inhibiting pyroptosis proteins, survival rates greatly improved, liver damage was attenuated, and IL-18 concentration decreased significantly [44]. In patients with acute-on-chronic liver failure (ACLF) complicated with sepsis, serum IL-18 is significantly raised when compared to patients with ACLF with or without systemic inflammation. The authors of this study also noted that the five patients with signs of systemic inflammation and increasing IL-18 concentrations within 24 h of admission also developed sepsis [45]. IL-18 is a reliable predictor for the occurrence of hepato-biliary dysfunction (HBD) and DIC in septic patients, with an area under the curve of 0.78. A multiparametric approach, which also included IL-18BP, sCD163, soluble CD25 (sCD25), ferritin, IL-10, and other biomarkers, leads to an increase in the area under the curve to 0.93 [46]. The main key findings related to IL-18, as well as hepcidin and ferritin, can be found in Table 1.

Table 1. Summary of advantages and limitations for IL-18, hepcidin, and ferritin.

	Advantages	Limitations
IL-18	- Higher concentrations in septic patients - Correlated with sepsis mortality - Good predictive value for SA-AKI in multiple studies - High concentration in HBD + DIC	- Elevated in other inflammatory conditions - Studies with small study population
Hepcidin	- Levels correlate with sepsis diagnosis - Hepcidin treatment lowers mortality rates (preclinical studies) - Correlated with mortality for AKI patients	- Elevated in hereditary hemochromatosis and some cancers - Predictive value for SA-AKI is improved by combining with other biomarkers - Mortality for AKI patients is not specific for SA-AKI.

Table 1. *Cont.*

	Advantages	Limitations
Ferritin	- Good prognostic value for adult and pediatric sepsis - Serum values linked with AKI risk in septic patients - FtH protects mice from hepatic injury in sepsis models - High concentration in HBD + DIC	- Not specific for sepsis inflammation - Few clinical studies related to sepsis associated with liver injury

4.2. Hepcidin

Hepcidin is a key molecule in iron homeostasis, primarily produced by the liver and in smaller quantities by the heart, kidneys, macrophages, and other cells. There are three isoforms, of which only hepcidin-25 is considered actively involved in iron metabolism, while hepcidin-22 and hepcidin-20 are regarded as products of degradation. Hepcidin binds with ferroportin to limit iron efflux, resulting in both anemia and reduced availability of iron for bacteria. Liver production of hepcidin is downregulated by increased erythropoiesis, while conditions of inflammation and infection promote its synthesis, especially through interleukin-6. Elevated serum hepcidin has been reported in various cancers, inflammatory disorders, and sepsis [47].

One study, which included a limited number of patients with septic shock, reported that median hepcidin values were elevated compared to normal values, with maximal concentration registered at the time of inclusion. Additionally, in five patients who developed secondary complications such as pleural effusion and pneumonia, a further increase in hepcidin levels was noted [48]. In a follow-up study, the authors concluded that hepcidin values were significantly higher in the sepsis group than in the non-sepsis control group. Hepcidin levels decreased in the subsequent days and did not correlate with 28-day mortality [49]. One paper reported that hepcidin has the potential to discriminate between survivors and non-survivors in cancer patients who develop sepsis [50]. Another research group examined hepcidin and ferritin in patients with septic shock, COVID-19, and those who had undergone surgery. Although plasma hepcidin levels did not differ substantially among these groups, the hepcidin-to-ferritin ratio was significantly lower in non-survivors compared to survivors, only in the septic shock cohort [51].

In mouse sepsis models, hepcidin exhibits a protective role against organ damage. Hepcidin knock-out animals displayed greater mortality rates and more severe organ damage. Hepatic injury was assessed by area of necrosis and transaminase levels, which were significantly higher in knock-out mice than in controls [52]. The protective role of hepcidin is further supported by findings in another preclinical study. The authors showed that hepcidin pretreatment in mice polymicrobial sepsis models is associated with better preserved renal function and reduced tubular injury [53]. One retrospective study involving 807 participants with severe AKI (of which 64% were diagnosed with sepsis) highlighted that low plasma concentrations of hepcidin are correlated with 60-day mortality. Further research is needed to establish if hepcidin could provide therapeutic benefits for critically ill patients [54].

Data from one study reveal that hepcidin is an independent predictor of persistent AKI in septic patients [55]. The same authors showed that serum hepcidin can be a good predictor of AKI occurrence within 7 days of admission for septic patients. Combining hepcidin with urinary NGAL leads to a sensitivity of 79.6% and a specificity of 78.3% for AKI occurrence in sepsis patients [56]. Contrasting results obtained by another research group indicated no correlation between hepcidin concentrations and the development of stage 2–3 AKI for hospitalized patients with either sepsis or non-septic conditions [57]. While hepcidin has been linked to safeguarding the organism from sepsis-associated organ damage, further clinical trials are required to establish hepcidin as a biomarker for SA-AKI.

4.3. Ferritin

Pertaining to iron homeostasis, ferritin is a ubiquitous protein that is pivotal in the storage of intracellular iron and can also act as an iron carrier. Serum concentrations of ferritin act as a tool to examine iron storage. In acute and chronic inflammation, serum ferritin is usually elevated; however, iron is sequestered as a defensive mechanism. Therefore, ferritin has been widely researched as a marker in various states of inflammation related to malignancies, chronic kidney disease, autoimmune disorders, and acute infections [58].

Serum ferritin has been demonstrated to have a good prognostic value in children hospitalized for sepsis or septic shock. Patients with median values between 200 and 500 ng/mL had the best outcome, while patients with concentrations exceeding 500 ng/mL had the highest mortality [59–61]. A large retrospective study demonstrated that for every 1000 ng/mL increase in serum ferritin values, there is a non-linear increase in mortality between 28 days and one year [62].

As a protein, ferritin is composed of heavy chains (FtH) and light chains (FtL), with its circulatory form mainly attributed to light chains. In deficient FtH mice, survival rates are significantly improved in cecal ligation puncture (CLP) models, possibly due to a compensatory increase in serum ferritin concentrations. In these mice, renal function was better preserved, and hepatic injury was limited [63]. However, light chain-deficient mice exhibit the same levels of AKI when compared to control mice; therefore, an overexpression of ferritin could protect from organ damage in sepsis, while the loss of light chains does not influence the extension of the disease [64].

Ferritin has been linked to renal recovery in patients with AKI; however, patients with sepsis-associated AKI were excluded from the study [65]. In a large retrospective cohort study, using the MIMIC-IV database, higher ferritin was associated with a longer hospital stay and higher mortality, higher SOFA, and an increased risk of AKI development. The authors noted that even in the normal range, an increase in serum ferritin is still linked with an enhanced risk of AKI compared with the low ferritin group [66]. Another study on the MIMIC-IV.2.2 database extrapolated only patients with SA-AKI. Patients with ferritin over 1056.2 ng/mL had the highest values for heart rate, temperature, creatinine, SOFA score, and in-hospital mortality [67].

Given that ferritin can be released from damaged hepatocytes, its role as a biomarker in liver injury has been investigated. Mice deficient in FtH have higher serum ferritin concentrations. Sepsis models in these mice have revealed better preservation of renal function and less damage to the liver and lungs [63]. One investigation revealed that the FtH protein could establish disease tolerance to sepsis by regulating glucose metabolism. The authors showed that both FtH-deficient mice and control mice had low blood glucose after CLP; however, the control group restored the blood glucose the following days and the FtH-deficient mice did not [68]. In clinical studies, patients with sepsis-induced liver injury displayed significantly higher levels of serum ferritin, iron, and total-iron binding capacity compared to septic patients without hepatic injury [69].

More recently, levels of ferritin have been associated with mortality in COVID-19 patients, with median values almost three times higher for non-survivors compared to survivors [70,71]. Although sepsis was present in all non-survivor cases, ferritin was not directly correlated with this outcome [70]. Ferritin can also be used as a diagnostic tool for hepatic injury in COVID-19 patients, and it has been correlated with viral clearance and hospital stay but not antibiotic use [72,73].

4.4. IL-27

Interleukin-27 is a cytokine with a complex role in the immune system, expressed primarily by macrophages, monocytes, dendritic cells, and other endothelial or epithelial cells. Through its receptor, it was initially believed to have a pro-inflammatory role, as it induces interferon-gamma production; however, it has been proven to also produce an anti-inflammatory response [74]. Studies on mice have demonstrated that blocking the IL-27 receptor (IL-27R) leads to a decrease in mortality in sepsis models [75]. Alveolar macrophage killing capacity is also higher in mice lacking IL-27R, as the inflammatory response in these mice offers better protection against *Pseudomonas aeruginosa* infection [76]. For human studies, a meta-analysis showed that IL-27 is a good diagnostic biomarker for sepsis both in pediatric and adult settings. With a sensitivity of 0.84 and a specificity of 0.71, it has similar accuracy to procalcitonin and presepsin [77].

Serum concentration of IL-27 has also been shown to be higher in patients with sepsis-related acute hepatic injury compared to septic patients without liver injury. The increase in IL-27 was not associated with ICU stay [78]. The same authors confirmed that IL-27R-deficient mice had less severe histological hepatic damage, therefore confirming its role as a pro-inflammatory cytokine in the process of sepsis-induced ALF [78]. Further research indicates that in mouse models with CLP-induced infection, IL-27 exacerbates liver injury. Both serum levels and hepatic expression of IL-27 are increased after LPS stimulation. Gadolinium chloride (which inhibits Kupffer cells) pretreatment can lead to reduced concentrations of IL-27, attenuating liver damage but not injury to other organs, such as the lungs and kidneys [79]. Similar results were obtained in a follow-up study, with IL-27 knock-out mice presenting fewer inflammatory factors and attenuated hepatic injury. The authors determined that IL-27 promotes macrophage pyroptosis, leading to aggravated ALF [80].

Mouse models with induced AKI demonstrate that IL-27 treatment can minimize kidney damage, expressed by less tubular injury, increased production of anti-inflammatory cytokines, and decreased production of TNF-alpha, IL-6, and IL-17A [81]. In the previous study, AKI was induced by ischemia reperfusion, which can be a pathophysiological mechanism by which sepsis causes AKI [22]. Serum concentrations are also higher in sepsis-associated myocardial dysfunction compared to the control group. However, mouse studies showed that for the myocardium, IL-27 plays an anti-inflammatory role, as pretreatment with IL-27 decreases myocardial injury biomarkers [82]. The main key findings related to IL-27, as well as the following biomarkers: IL-17A, IL-10, IL-33/ST2, high-mobility group box-1, proenkephalin (PENK), C-X-C Motif Chemokine Ligand 9 (CXCL9), soluble CD163, soluble CD25, can be found in Table 2.

Table 2. Summary of advantages and limitations for IL-27, IL-17A, IL-10, IL-33/ST2, HMGB1, Proenkephalin, CXCL9, sCD163, sCD25.

	Advantages	Limitations
IL-27	- Similar diagnostic capacity as procalcitonin - Correlated with sepsis-associated liver injury in both preclinical and clinical studies	- Not specific for liver, investigated for sepsis myocardial dysfunction
IL-17A	- Targeted therapy leads to reduced renal injury in septic conditions	- Not sufficient clinical studies to sustain preclinical data

Table 2. *Cont.*

	Advantages	Limitations
IL-10	- Associated with hepatic dysfunction in septic patients	- Not sufficiently specific - Reflects immune response and not direct injury
IL-33 and ST2	- Linked with metabolic liver disease in septic patients - Correlated with mortality in AKI patients	- Mostly studied in relation to heart failure - Not specific for SA-AKI
HMGB1	- Targeted therapy leads to reduced renal and hepatic injury in mice sepsis models	- Not validated in large clinical trials
Proenkephalin	- Good predictive value for SA-AKI severity and function recovery	- Not yet established to provide better diagnosis over validated biomarkers
CXCL9	- Potential to define a new sepsis endotype	- Not enough data for organ-specific injury
sCD163	- Urinary concentrations display diagnostic capacities for SA-AKI	- Not yet validated in large clinical trials
sCD25	- Similar diagnosis ability as NGAL for SA-AKI	- Further validation needed

4.5. IL-17A

The Interleukin-17 family is a group of molecules that play a role in the inflammatory response against infection. They have the ability to stimulate macrophages, dendritic cells, and others to produce chemokines, cytokines, and matrix metalloproteinases. The most common protein from this group is IL-17A, mainly produced by a subset of CD4 T cells called Th17 cells [83].

Considering the newer hypothesis regarding SA-AKI pathogenesis, IL-17A has been studied in septic mice to observe its role in renal function. Data show that IL-17A knock-out mice have a better survival rate than wild-type mice under sepsis conditions. Histological changes pertain to ameliorated tissue damage and a lower tubular injury score [84]. Therefore, IL-17A could become a novel target for managing SA-AKI therapy. Another study on mice divided into a multiple organ dysfunction (MODS) group, LPS-challenged group, and sham-operated group, indicated that IL-17 levels decreased in the MODS group, gradually over time, possibly being consumed by the kidney. The same study included patients hospitalized with sepsis, and results expressed that IL-17 levels are higher in SA-AKI compared to sepsis associated with chronic renal failure [85].

One paper highlights the importance of the Th17 ratio to regulatory T cells in septic patients with and without AKI. The authors found that the Th17/Treg ratio could be used as a predictive factor for SA-AKI development and that IL-17 concentrations were higher in the group with acute kidney injury [86]. Similar results were obtained by another research team, where IL-17A levels were proportionately higher as the AKI stage was worse [87].

In patients with ACLF complicated with sepsis, IL-17 serum concentrations are highest when compared to patients with ACLF or liver cirrhosis. There is a significant difference between patients with ACLF and patients with cirrhosis, which could indicate that IL-17 plays a role in acute liver injury [88].

4.6. IL-10

The interleukin-10 molecule is part of the IL-10 superfamily, mainly produced by monocytes, macrophages, and T cells, with other immune cells capable of synthesizing this cytokine. Although many cytokines have pro-inflammatory roles, IL-10 is one of the most potent anti-inflammatory and immunosuppressive molecules. It can decrease or inhibit antigen presentation, phagocytosis, the expression of major histocompatibility complex (MHC) class II, and the production of IL-1 or TNF-alpha [89]. IL-10 can suppress IL-6 secretion from Kupffer cells when the hepatic cells are stimulated with endotoxin [90]. IL-10 plays a substantial role in the cytokine storm during sepsis. IL-10-deficient mice exhibit prolonged signs of illness and higher mortality after undergoing CLP. In septic patients, NK cells increase their IL-10 production [91].

As mentioned in Chapter 4.1, IL-10 levels are elevated in patients with liver impairment (Figure 3). In the subset of septic patients with HBP and DIC, IL-10 correlated with ferritin and IL-18, in contrast, with septic patients without HBD and DIC [46]. In the previously noted study regarding patients with ACLF and sepsis, the serum concentration of IL-10 was significantly increased compared to patients with ACLF or liver cirrhosis [88]. In pediatric septic patients, IL-10 could be used to differentiate children with organ dysfunction from those with a hyperinflammatory state. The sensitivity of diagnosis for IL-10 was 89.6% for concentrations >18.4 picograms (pg)/mL. The most common types of organ dysfunction in this study were low platelets and high bilirubin, indicating liver impairment [92].

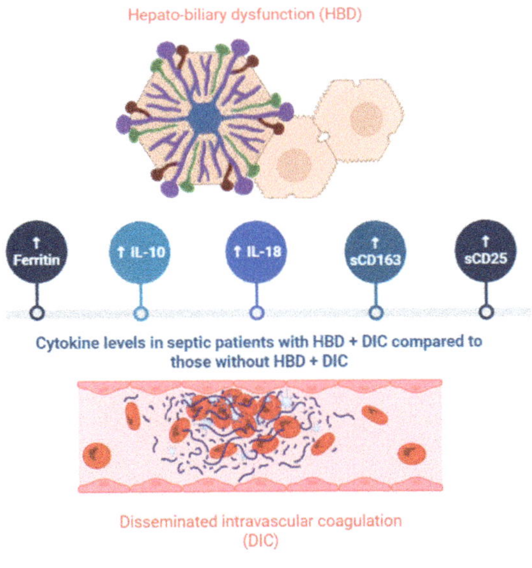

Figure 3. Levels of biomarkers in septic patients with and without liver impairment. Created in BioRender. Pasare, A. (2025) https://BioRender.com/g7vqax2. Accessed on 11 May 2025.

In mice, IL-10 plays a crucial role in the development of the anti-inflammatory response in septic AKI. In the first hours after inducing sepsis conditions, there is an increase in pro-inflammatory response, and at 24 h, there is an increase in IL-10. For ischemic AKI, cytokine levels were lower, and there was no peak in IL-10 levels [93]. Findings highlight that IL-10 levels are higher in patients with septic AKI compared to sepsis patients without AKI, and the receiver operating characteristic curve (ROC) analysis for predicting AKI was nearly as good as NGAL [94].

4.7. IL-33 and ST2

Interleukin-33 is part of the IL-1 superfamily, and it binds to Interleukin 1 receptor-like 1 (ST2), also part of the IL-1 receptor superfamily. IL-33 is produced mainly by endothelial and epithelial cells, stromal cells such as fibroblasts, and smooth muscle cells. When tissue damage happens, IL-33 is released into the extracellular space and acts as an alarmin, alerting immune cells [95,96]. ST2 has been especially studied as a marker for myocardial fibrosis with good predictive value for mortality in heart failure patients. However, it could also play a role in distinguishing the presence or absence of sepsis [97,98].

In septic mice, IL-33 treatment reduces mortality compared to control group mice. In the same experiment, pretreated mice showed a marked increase in neutrophil migration to the infection site, which led to an improvement in bacterial clearance [99]. IL-33 also promotes NK cells' activation in septic mice, and IL-33 treatment has a beneficial role in the early stages of sepsis but not in the late phases [100].

One study aimed to investigate the differences in the cytokine profile between septic patients with and without metabolic liver disease. Patients with liver disease had higher concentrations of IL-17 and IL-33 both on day 1 and day 5 of hospitalization. Patients in the metabolic disease group also had a significant increase in serum IL-33 between admission and day 5 and a decrease in IL-10. In the same category, IL-33 had a negative correlation with sepsis severity [101].

IL-33 plays a role in AKI, as its inhibition through ST2 can provide protection against functional and histological changes in mice induced with cisplatin [102]. In a hospital setting, patients with AKI who survived showed lower serum ST2 concentrations; therefore, the IL-33 receptor could act as a prognostic marker. Although the most common cause of AKI was sepsis, ST-2 could not distinguish between the different etiologies of AKI [103].

4.8. HMGB1

High-mobility group box-1 is part of a group of chromosomal proteins that play an essential role in sustaining life. As a nuclear protein, it binds deoxyribonucleic acid (DNA) and enhances transcription, replication, and repair. However, when released in the extracellular space, it acts as a potent pro-inflammatory mediator [104]. Due to its dual intra- and extracellular activity, HMGB1 has been studied in relation to different types of cancers, correlating to poor prognosis, and to sepsis. In murine polymicrobial sepsis models, HMGB1 levels usually peak late, associating with death [105]. Early clinical studies concluded that in sepsis patients, HMGB1 also peaks late and associates with the severity of organ dysfunction, but it cannot distinguish between survivors and non-survivors [106,107]. Nevertheless, academics revealed that late peaks of HMGB1 associated with inflammatory disease in infectious patients act as a strong risk factor for mortality [108].

HMGB1 sustains a pro-inflammatory loop in mice with induced acute liver failure by LPS and D-galactosamine hydrochloride (D-gal). When antibodies were used to neutralize HMGB1, levels of alanine transaminase were back to normal, and liver histology was similar to the control group [109]. HMGB1 accentuates liver injury by pyroptosis of macrophages in murine CLP models [110]. Comparable results were obtained by another group of authors on ALF and AKI animal models. After inhibiting the TNF-alpha pathway, serum concentrations of HMGB1, IL-1, and IL-18 decreased, and liver and renal function were drastically improved [111].

In CLP models, HMGB1 can also localize in renal tubular epithelial cells and pass into urine, unlike in healthy settings. In these conditions, HMGB1 can interact with TECs and promote active secretion of IL-1 and IL-6, which can aggravate sepsis and SA-AKI [112].

4.9. Proenkephalin

Proenkephalin and other biologically active enkephalins are a result of preproenkephalin A cleavage. This family of molecules act as endogenous opioids. PENK has gained interest due to the fact that the second highest density of opioid receptors is found in the kidney. Depending on the type of receptor, enkephalins can influence diuresis and natriuresis, and reduce kidney inflammation. PENK has been mostly studied in relation to AKI and septic AKI, as it can be freely filtered through the renal glomerulus [113,114].

In one study (preprint) that included 529 patients with sepsis or septic shock, AKI was diagnosed in 44% of subjects. PENK levels on admission were correlated with AKI severity, resulting in 72% sensitivity and 83% specificity to diagnose AKI in the first 48 h [115]. In the ALBIOS trial, 28% of patients developed AKI within 48 h, from a total of 895 patients. PENK concentrations were notably elevated in patients with AKI than in those without. Among those with AKI, PENK was lower in patients who improved renal function than in those who did not; therefore, PENK could be a candidate for predicting renal function recovery [116]. One meta-analysis, which included 11 studies, concluded that PENK shows an area under the curve of 0.77 for early AKI diagnosis. From the included studies, only four comprised sepsis-associated AKI [117].

PENK also shows promising value for predicting sepsis severity and mortality, as concentrations were significantly higher in non-survivors compared to survivors [118,119].

4.10. C-X-C Motif Chemokine Ligand 9

Chemokines are key drivers for chemotaxis, differentiation, and multiplication of leukocytes. C-X-C motif chemokine ligand 9, alongside CXCL10 and -11, determines the recruitment of cytotoxic lymphocytes, natural killers, and macrophages. Immune cells release CXCL9 in response to IFNγ [120]. One group of authors proposed IFN-driven sepsis (IDS) as a new sepsis endotype, besides immuno-paralysis and MALS. They demonstrated that almost 20% of sepsis patients, from a cohort of 5503, display IDS characteristics. As IFNγ is the sole trigger for CXCL9, this marker had higher values in the IDS category compared to MALS. Although the greatest mortality rate was registered in the MALS category, IDS is independently associated with 28-day mortality. Serum ferritin and IL-18 displayed the highest concentration in the MALS group, followed by the IDS and immuno-paralysis groups [121].

CXCL9 has been proven to distinguish between acute interstitial nephritis and other causes of AKI, but none were related to sepsis. It has also been associated with tubular inflammation, and low urinary levels can exclude kidney injury related to infection [122,123]. To the best of our knowledge, CXCL9 has not yet been linked to SA-AKI.

C-X-C motif chemokine receptor 3 (CXCR3) is the ligand for CXCL9, and in response to IFN, hepatocytes secrete CXCR3. In ischemia reperfusion models in mice, levels of CXCL9 are increased, leading to T cell infiltration. Blocking the interaction between CXCL9 and CXCR3 increases survival, and hepatocellular damage is reduced [124].

4.11. Soluble CD163

CD163 acts as a receptor for the hemoglobin–haptoglobin complexes, and it is expressed on the surface of macrophages, monocytes, and lymphocytes. After pathogen recognition, monocyte activation determines an increase in sCD163, with the role of depleting iron sources for bacteria. In the later phases of sepsis, sCD163 has been shown to lead to the release of IL-10 [125]. In small clinical settings, sCD163 levels were higher in septic patients compared to controls and correlated with IL-10. sCD163 was also statistically significantly higher in non-survivors, as patients with better outcomes displayed gradually declining serum levels [126–128]. Another group of authors showed that sCD163 is markedly increased in septic shock, and the sCD163/IL-18 ratio in septic and septic shock patients is significantly lower than in controls. For every 1 unit increase in this ratio, there was a 3.9-fold increase in the odds of death, but the results were not statistically significant [129].

Urinary sCD163 has been proposed as a diagnostic tool for SA-AKI, with a sensitivity of 80% and a specificity of 56%. The authors correlated urine sCD163 levels with serum sCD163 and discovered good concordance [130]. sCD163 concentrations have been linked to mortality in patients with acute liver failure of different etiologies [131]. In cirrhotic patients, median sCD163 levels are significantly elevated in those with acute decompensation and infection compared to those without infection [132].

4.12. Soluble CD25

The IL-2/IL-2 receptor (IL-2R) pathway plays a complex role in the immune system, establishing immune tolerance. IL-2R is composed of multiple chains, of which the α chain (CD25) is shed from T cells upon activation. Soluble CD25 has been researched as an indicator of immune-mediated disorders [133].

As a sepsis biomarker, sCD25 has been shown to display higher serum concentrations compared to controls, alongside sCD163 and IL-18; however, the author did not perform any multiparameter analysis [134].

Concerning SA-AKI, sCD25 has been investigated together with IL-10 and NGAL. Results showed that sCD25 was significantly elevated in septic AKI compared to both sepsis without AKI and AKI of other causes. In this context, sCD25 performed closely to NGAL regarding SA-AKI diagnosis, and their combination had the highest performance [94].

5. Future Directions and Study Limitations

Future directions regarding the integration of biomarkers in sepsis classification, diagnosis, and prognosis relate to the use of machine learning, a multiparametric approach, and personalized therapy. Machine learning utilizes large data sets to generate prediction algorithms and uncover hidden patterns. Data may take the form of biomarkers, metabolomics, and gene expression, which help create sepsis profiles, assess mortality prognosis, and support treatment decisions [135]. Specificity and sensitivity for sepsis-related organ injury can be significantly enhanced by using multi-biomarker panels, as they represent various aspects of the immune response. However, this approach faces limitations due to its cost, availability, and lack of standardization [136]. In addition to diagnosis and prognosis, biomarkers may also be used for personalized therapy in the form of agonists or antagonists. For example, hepcidin agonists could maintain renal function in septic conditions, and using antibodies against HMGB1 prevents ALF [53,109].

This review has several limitations. First, we limited our search to articles published in the English language, which may have led to the exclusion of pertinent studies in other languages. Second, the studies included in our review displayed considerable heterogeneity regarding study design and patient demographics, limiting our ability to draw uniform conclusions. Third, much of the presented evidence is derived from small-scale studies, which hinders the predictive validity of biomarkers. Fourth, we found limited data evaluating multiparametric approaches, which could improve diagnostic accuracy.

6. Conclusions

Sepsis is not only a heavy burden on the individual but on the medical society as well. While every organ can be gravely impacted by sepsis, acute kidney injury remains the most frequent organ dysfunction, increasing mortality risk, and liver damage can vastly influence the inflammatory response and modulate injury in other organs. While consecrated molecules such as C-reactive protein, procalcitonin, and presepsin perform well in practice, there is still a need for more specific diagnostic and predictive biomarkers for sepsis and related organ dysfunction. The biomarkers described in this review have multiple functions and could potentially be used in either AKI or ALF settings. IL-18, hepcidin, PENK, and sCD25 are good candidates for SA-AKI diagnosis. The sensitivity and specificity of IL-18 and hepcidin are enhanced by combining with NGAL. PENK also displays prognostic value for renal recovery, and ST-2 and IL-17 could be predictive of AKI severity and mortality. Liver injury is assessed by ferritin, IL-27, HMGB1, and CXCL9, mainly in preclinical studies, which leaves a gap in the knowledge regarding their abilities to act as biomarkers for SALI in clinical environments. We consider that biomarkers hold great potential for characterizing the complexity of sepsis syndrome, as various phenotypes display different biomarker serum levels and associate with different types of organ dysfunction. Further research is needed to establish the utility and practicality of novel biomarkers in clinical settings, with the goal of enhancing diagnostic accuracy and improving therapeutic choices.

Author Contributions: Conceptualization, M.-A.P. and I.-L.M.; writing—original draft preparation, M.-A.P., C.S.P. and M.G.G.; writing—review and editing, I.-L.M. and E.G.M.; supervision, E.G.M. All authors have read and agreed to the published version of the manuscript.

Funding: This research received no external funding.

Conflicts of Interest: The authors declare no conflicts of interest.

Abbreviations

ACLF: Acute-On-Chronic Liver Failure; AKI: Acute Kidney Injury; ALF: Acute Liver Failure; ARDS: Acute Respiratory Distress Syndrome; CD: Cluster Of Differentiation; COVID-19: Coronavirus disease; CLP: Cecal Ligation Puncture; CXCL: C-X-C Motif Chemokine Ligand; CXCR: C-X-C Motif Chemokine Receptor; DAMPs: damage-associated molecular patterns; D-Gal: D-Galactosamine Hydrochloride; DIC: Disseminated Intravascular Coagulation; DNA: Deoxyribonucleic Acid; eGFR: Estimated Glomerular Filtration Rate; FtH: Ferritin Heavy Chain; FtL: Ferritin Light Chain; HLA: Human Leucocyte Antigen; HBD: Hepato-Biliary Dysfunction; HMGB1: high-mobility group box-1; ICU: Intensive Care Unit; Ig: Immunoglobulin; IL: Interleukin; IL-18BP: IL-18 Binding Protein; IL-2R: IL-2 receptor; IL-27R: IL-27 receptor; IFN: Interferon; IDS: IFN-driven sepsis; KDIGO: Kidney Disease: Improving Global Outcomes; KIM-1: Kidney Injury Molecule 1; LPS: Lipopolysaccharide; MALS: Macrophage Activation-Like Syndrome; ml: milliliter; MHC: Major Histocompatibility Complex; MODS: Multiple Organ Dysfunction Syndrome; ng: nanograms; NGAL: Neutrophil Gelatinase-Associated Lipocalin; NK: Natural Killer; NLRP3: NOD-, LRR-, and Pyrin Domain-Containing Protein 3; NO: Nitric Oxide; PAI-1: Plasminogen Activator Inhibitor 1; PAMPs: pathogen-derived molecular patterns; PENK: Proenkephalin; pg: picograms; SA-AKI: Sepsis-Associated Acute Kidney Injury; SALI: Sepsis-Associated Liver Injury; SIC: Sepsis-Induced Coagulopathy; SBP: Systolic Blood Pressure; SOFA: Sequential Organ Failure Assessment; sCD25: soluble CD25; sCD163: soluble CD163; TECs: renal tubular epithelial cells; ROC: receiver operating characteristic curve; TF: Tissue Factor; TGFβ-1: transforming growth factor beta 1; Th: T helper; TNF: tumor necrosis factor.

References

1. Singer, M.; Deutschman, C.S.; Seymour, C.W.; Shankar-Hari, M.; Annane, D.; Bauer, M.; Bellomo, R.; Bernard, G.R.; Chiche, J.-D.; Coopersmith, C.M.; et al. The Third International Consensus Definitions for Sepsis and Septic Shock (Sepsis-3). *JAMA* **2016**, *315*, 801. [CrossRef]
2. Lambden, S.; Laterre, P.F.; Levy, M.M.; Francois, B. The SOFA score—Development, utility and challenges of accurate assessment in clinical trials. *Crit. Care* **2019**, *23*, 374. [CrossRef] [PubMed]

3. Rudd, K.E.; Kissoon, N.; Limmathurotsakul, D.; Bory, S.; Mutahunga, B.; Seymour, C.W.; Angus, D.C.; West, T.E. The global burden of sepsis: Barriers and potential solutions. *Crit. Care* **2018**, *22*, 232. [CrossRef] [PubMed]
4. Miftode, R.-S.; Costache, I.-I.; Constantinescu, D.; Mitu, O.; Timpau, A.-S.; Hancianu, M.; Leca, D.-A.; Miftode, I.-L.; Jigoranu, R.-A.; Oancea, A.-F.; et al. Syndecan-1: From a Promising Novel Cardiac Biomarker to a Surrogate Early Predictor of Kidney and Liver Injury in Patients with Acute Heart Failure. *Life* **2023**, *13*, 898. [CrossRef] [PubMed]
5. La Via, L.; Sangiorgio, G.; Stefani, S.; Marino, A.; Nunnari, G.; Cocuzza, S.; La Mantia, I.; Cacopardo, B.; Stracquadanio, S.; Spampinato, S.; et al. The Global Burden of Sepsis and Septic Shock. *Epidemiologia* **2024**, *5*, 456–478. [CrossRef]
6. Karakike, E.; Giamarellos-Bourboulis, E.J.; Kyprianou, M.; Fleischmann-Struzek, C.; Pletz, M.W.; Netea, M.G.; Reinhart, K.; Kyriazopoulou, E. Coronavirus Disease 2019 as Cause of Viral Sepsis: A Systematic Review and Meta-Analysis*. *Crit. Care Med.* **2021**, *49*, 2042–2057. [CrossRef]
7. Jarczak, D.; Kluge, S.; Nierhaus, A. Sepsis—Pathophysiology and Therapeutic Concepts. *Front. Med.* **2021**, *8*, 628302. [CrossRef]
8. Strnad, P.; Tacke, F.; Koch, A.; Trautwein, C. Liver—guardian, modifier and target of sepsis. *Nat. Rev. Gastroenterol. Hepatol.* **2017**, *14*, 55–66. [CrossRef]
9. Bellomo, R.; Kellum, J.A.; Ronco, C.; Wald, R.; Martensson, J.; Maiden, M.; Bagshaw, S.M.; Glassford, N.J.; Lankadeva, Y.; Vaara, S.T.; et al. Acute kidney injury in sepsis. *Intensive Care Med.* **2017**, *43*, 816–828. [CrossRef]
10. Gotts, J.E.; Matthay, M.A. Sepsis: Pathophysiology and clinical management. *BMJ* **2016**, *353*, i1585. [CrossRef]
11. Poston, J.T.; Koyner, J.L. Sepsis associated acute kidney injury. *BMJ* **2019**, *364*, k4891. [CrossRef] [PubMed]
12. Nesseler, N.; Launey, Y.; Aninat, C.; Morel, F.; Mallédant, Y.; Seguin, P. Clinical review: The liver in sepsis. *Crit. Care* **2012**, *16*, 235. [CrossRef]
13. Saxena, J.; Das, S.; Kumar, A.; Sharma, A.; Sharma, L.; Kaushik, S.; Kumar Srivastava, V.; Jamal Siddiqui, A.; Jyoti, A. Biomarkers in sepsis. *Clin. Chim. Acta* **2024**, *562*, 119891. [CrossRef] [PubMed]
14. Bhavani, S.V.; Wolfe, K.S.; Hrusch, C.L.; Greenberg, J.A.; Krishack, P.A.; Lin, J.; Lecompte-Osorio, P.; Carey, K.A.; Kress, J.P.; Coopersmith, C.M.; et al. Temperature Trajectory Subphenotypes Correlate With Immune Responses in Patients With Sepsis. *Crit. Care Med.* **2020**, *48*, 1645–1653. [CrossRef]
15. Leijte, G.P.; Kox, M.; Pickkers, P. Fever in Sepsis: Still a Hot Topic. *Am. J. Respir. Crit. Care Med.* **2019**, *200*, 263–264. [CrossRef]
16. Papathanakos, G.; Andrianopoulos, I.; Xenikakis, M.; Papathanasiou, A.; Koulenti, D.; Blot, S.; Koulouras, V. Clinical Sepsis Phenotypes in Critically Ill Patients. *Microorganisms* **2023**, *11*, 2165. [CrossRef] [PubMed]
17. Seymour, C.W.; Kennedy, J.N.; Wang, S.; Chang, C.-C.H.; Elliott, C.F.; Xu, Z.; Berry, S.; Clermont, G.; Cooper, G.; Gomez, H.; et al. Derivation, Validation, and Potential Treatment Implications of Novel Clinical Phenotypes for Sepsis. *JAMA* **2019**, *321*, 2003. [CrossRef]
18. Baghela, A.; Pena, O.M.; Lee, A.H.; Baquir, B.; Falsafi, R.; An, A.; Farmer, S.W.; Hurlburt, A.; Mondragon-Cardona, A.; Rivera, J.D.; et al. Predicting sepsis severity at first clinical presentation: The role of endotypes and mechanistic signatures. *eBioMedicine* **2022**, *75*, 103776. [CrossRef]
19. Leventogiannis, K.; Kyriazopoulou, E.; Antonakos, N.; Kotsaki, A.; Tsangaris, I.; Markopoulou, D.; Grondman, I.; Rovina, N.; Theodorou, V.; Antoniadou, E.; et al. Toward personalized immunotherapy in sepsis: The PROVIDE randomized clinical trial. *Cell Rep. Med.* **2022**, *3*, 100817. [CrossRef]
20. Kyriazopoulou, E.; Leventogiannis, K.; Norrby-Teglund, A.; Dimopoulos, G.; Pantazi, A.; Orfanos, S.E.; Rovina, N.; Tsangaris, I.; Gkavogianni, T.; Botsa, E.; et al. Macrophage activation-like syndrome: An immunological entity associated with rapid progression to death in sepsis. *BMC Med.* **2017**, *15*, 172. [CrossRef]
21. Umbro, I.; Gentile, G.; Tinti, F.; Muiesan, P.; Mitterhofer, A.P. Recent advances in pathophysiology and biomarkers of sepsis-induced acute kidney injury. *J. Infect.* **2016**, *72*, 131–142. [CrossRef]
22. Peerapornratana, S.; Manrique-Caballero, C.L.; Gómez, H.; Kellum, J.A. Acute kidney injury from sepsis: Current concepts, epidemiology, pathophysiology, prevention and treatment. *Kidney Int.* **2019**, *96*, 1083–1099. [CrossRef] [PubMed]
23. Manrique-Caballero, C.L.; Del Rio-Pertuz, G.; Gomez, H. Sepsis-Associated Acute Kidney Injury. *Crit. Care Clin.* **2021**, *37*, 279–301. [CrossRef]
24. Fattahi, F.; Zetoune, F.S.; Ward, P.A. Complement as a Major Inducer of Harmful Events in Infectious Sepsis. *Shock* **2020**, *54*, 595–605. [CrossRef] [PubMed]
25. Kramer, L.; Jordan, B.; Druml, W.; Bauer, P.; Metnitz, P.G.H. Incidence and prognosis of early hepatic dysfunction in critically ill patients—A prospective multicenter study. *Crit. Care Med.* **2007**, *35*, 1099-e7. [CrossRef]
26. Yao, Y.; Wang, D.; Yin, Y. Advances in sepsis-associated liver dysfunction. *Burn. Trauma* **2014**, *2*, 97. [CrossRef] [PubMed]
27. Tsantes, A.G.; Parastatidou, S.; Tsantes, E.A.; Bonova, E.; Tsante, K.A.; Mantzios, P.G.; Vaiopoulos, A.G.; Tsalas, S.; Konstantinidi, A.; Houhoula, D.; et al. Sepsis-Induced Coagulopathy: An Update on Pathophysiology, Biomarkers, and Current Guidelines. *Life* **2023**, *13*, 350. [CrossRef]
28. Kaplanski, G. Interleukin-18: Biological properties and role in disease pathogenesis. *Immunol. Rev.* **2018**, *281*, 138–153. [CrossRef]
29. Yasuda, K.; Nakanishi, K.; Tsutsui, H. Interleukin-18 in Health and Disease. *Int. J. Mol. Sci.* **2019**, *20*, 649. [CrossRef]

30. Kinoshita, M.; Kuranaga, N.; Matsumoto, A.; Ono, S.; Shinomiya, N.; Hiraide, H.; Seki, S. Multiple interleukin-18 injections promote both mouse Th1 and Th2 responses after sublethal *Escherichia coli* infection. *Clin. Exp. Immunol.* **2005**, *143*, 41–49. [CrossRef]
31. Kinoshita, M.; Shinomiya, N.; Ono, S.; Tsujimoto, H.; Kawabata, T.; Matsumoto, A.; Hiraide, H.; Seki, S. Restoration of Natural IgM Production from Liver B Cells by Exogenous IL-18 Improves the Survival of Burn-Injured Mice Infected with *Pseudomonas aeruginosa*. *J. Immunol.* **2006**, *177*, 4627–4635. [CrossRef]
32. Priori, R.; Colafrancesco, S.; Alessandri, C.; Minniti, A.; Perricone, C.; Iaiani, G.; Palazzo, D.; Valesini, G. Interleukin 18: A Biomarker for Differential Diagnosis Between Adult-onset Still's Disease and Sepsis. *J. Rheumatol.* **2014**, *41*, 1118–1123. [CrossRef]
33. Mierzchala-Pasierb, M.; Krzystek-Korpacka, M.; Lesnik, P.; Adamik, B.; Placzkowska, S.; Serek, P.; Gamian, A.; Lipinska-Gediga, M. Interleukin-18 serum levels in sepsis: Correlation with disease severity and inflammatory markers. *Cytokine* **2019**, *120*, 22–27. [CrossRef] [PubMed]
34. Eidt, M.V.; Nunes, F.B.; Pedrazza, L.; Caeran, G.; Pellegrin, G.; Melo, D.A.S.; Possuelo, L.; Jost, R.T.; Dias, H.B.; Donadio, M.V.F.; et al. Biochemical and inflammatory aspects in patients with severe sepsis and septic shock: The predictive role of IL-18 in mortality. *Clin. Chim. Acta* **2016**, *453*, 100–106. [CrossRef] [PubMed]
35. Nisula, S.; Yang, R.; Poukkanen, M.; Vaara, S.T.; Kaukonen, K.M.; Tallgren, M.; Haapio, M.; Tenhunen, J.; Korhonen, A.M.; Pettilä, V.; et al. Predictive value of urine interleukin-18 in the evolution and outcome of acute kidney injury in critically ill adult patients. *Br. J. Anaesth.* **2015**, *114*, 460–468. [CrossRef]
36. Puthumana, J.; Ariza, X.; Belcher, J.M.; Graupera, I.; Ginès, P.; Parikh, C.R. Urine Interleukin 18 and Lipocalin 2 Are Biomarkers of Acute Tubular Necrosis in Patients With Cirrhosis: A Systematic Review and Meta-analysis. *Clin. Gastroenterol. Hepatol.* **2017**, *15*, 1003–1013.e3. [CrossRef] [PubMed]
37. Zarbock, A.; Gomez, H.; Kellum, J.A. Sepsis-induced acute kidney injury revisited: Pathophysiology, prevention and future therapies. *Curr. Opin. Crit. Care* **2014**, *20*, 588–595. [CrossRef]
38. Shaker, A.M.; Mohamed, M.F.; Thabet, K.K.; Ramzy, T.; Abdelhamid, Y.M. Serum Interleukin-18, Kidney Injury Molecule-1, and the Renal Resistive Index for Predicating Acute Kidney Injury in Critically Ill Patients with Sepsis. *Saudi J. Kidney Dis. Transplant.* **2023**, *34*, S153–S160. [CrossRef]
39. Cuttone, G.; Geraci, G.; La Via, L.; Sorbello, M.; Pappalardo, F.; Carollo, C. Exploring the Utility of Renal Resistive Index in Critical Care: Insights into ARDS and Cardiac Failure. *Biomedicines* **2025**, *13*, 519. [CrossRef]
40. Qu, H.-Q.; Snyder, J.; Connolly, J.; Glessner, J.; Kao, C.; Sleiman, P.; Hakonarson, H. Circulating LIGHT (TNFSF14) and Interleukin-18 Levels in Sepsis-Induced Multi-Organ Injuries. *Biomedicines* **2022**, *10*, 264. [CrossRef]
41. Liu, Y.; Li, C.; Yang, X.; Guo, S.; Cui, Z.; Kang, H.; Ma, Z.; Wang, H. Neutrophil Gelatinase-Associated Lipocalin and Interleukin-18 in the Prediction of Acute Kidney Injury in Sepsis Patients. *Int. J. Gen. Med.* **2024**, *17*, 6335–6341. [CrossRef] [PubMed]
42. Zhou, J.; Ye, Y.; Chen, Z.; Liu, Y.; Wu, B.; Huang, H. Upregulation of Peripheral Blood NLRP3 and IL-18 in Patients With Acute Kidney Injury in Sepsis and Its Clinical Significance. *Immun. Inflamm. Dis.* **2024**, *12*, e70113. [CrossRef] [PubMed]
43. Naqvi, R.; Hossain, N.; Butt, S.; Bhellar, Z.; Fatima, E.; Imtiaz, S.; Ghulam Moosa, P.; Abbas, K.; Jafri, S.B.; Khan, S. Efficacy of multiple Biomarkers: NGAL, KIM1, Cystatin C and IL18 in predicting pregnancy related acute kidney injury. *Pak. J. Med. Sci.* **2022**, *39*, 34. [CrossRef]
44. Chen, Y.-L.; Xu, G.; Liang, X.; Wei, J.; Luo, J.; Chen, G.-N.; Yan, X.-D.; Zhong, M.; Lv, X. Inhibition of hepatic cells pyroptosis attenuates CLP-induced acute liver injury. *Am. J. Transl. Res.* **2016**, *8*, 5685. [PubMed]
45. Yadav, P.; Trehanpati, N.; Maiwall, R.; Sehgal, R.; Singh, R.; Islam, M.; Jagdish, R.K.; Vijayaraghavan, R.; Maheshwari, D.; Bhat, S.; et al. Soluble factors and suppressive monocytes can predict early development of sepsis in acute-on-chronic liver failure. *Hepatol. Commun.* **2022**, *6*, 2105–2120. [CrossRef]
46. Anderko, R.R.; Gómez, H.; Canna, S.W.; Shakoory, B.; Angus, D.C.; Yealy, D.M.; Huang, D.T.; Kellum, J.A.; Carcillo, J.A. Sepsis with liver dysfunction and coagulopathy predicts an inflammatory pattern of macrophage activation. *Intensive Care Med. Exp.* **2022**, *10*, 6. [CrossRef]
47. Kali, A.; Charles, M.V.; Seetharam, R.S. Hepcidin—A novel biomarker with changing trends. *Pharmacogn. Rev.* **2015**, *9*, 35. [CrossRef]
48. Olinder, J.; Ehinger, D.; Liljenborg, E.; Herwald, H.; Rydén, C. Plasma Levels of Hepcidin and Reticulocyte Haemoglobin during Septic Shock. *J. Innate Immun.* **2020**, *12*, 448–460. [CrossRef]
49. Olinder, J.; Börjesson, A.; Norrman, J.; West, T.; Carlström, J.; Gustafsson, A.; Annborn, M.; Herwald, H.; Rydén, C. Hepcidin discriminates sepsis from other critical illness at admission to intensive care. *Sci. Rep.* **2022**, *12*, 14857. [CrossRef]
50. Suastika, N.K.W.; Suega, K. The Role of Hepcidin Level as a Predictor for Mortality in Cancer Patients with Sepsis. *Open Access Maced. J. Med. Sci.* **2022**, *10*, 2599–2602. [CrossRef]
51. Hortová-Kohoutková, M.; Skotáková, M.; Onyango, I.G.; Slezáková, M.; Panovský, R.; Opatřil, L.; Slanina, P.; De Zuani, M.; Mrkva, O.; Andrejčinová, I.; et al. Hepcidin and ferritin levels as markers of immune cell activation during septic shock, severe COVID-19 and sterile inflammation. *Front. Immunol.* **2023**, *14*, 1110540. [CrossRef] [PubMed]

52. Zeng, C.; Chen, Q.; Zhang, K.; Chen, Q.; Song, S.; Fang, X. Hepatic Hepcidin Protects against Polymicrobial Sepsis in Mice by Regulating Host Iron Status. *Anesthesiology* **2015**, *122*, 374–386. [CrossRef] [PubMed]
53. Scindia, Y.; Wlazlo, E.; Leeds, J.; Loi, V.; Ledesma, J.; Cechova, S.; Ghias, E.; Swaminathan, S. Protective Role of Hepcidin in Polymicrobial Sepsis and Acute Kidney Injury. *Front. Pharmacol.* **2019**, *10*, 615. [CrossRef] [PubMed]
54. Leaf, D.E.; Rajapurkar, M.; Lele, S.S.; Mukhopadhyay, B.; Boerger, E.A.S.; Mc Causland, F.R.; Eisenga, M.F.; Singh, K.; Babitt, J.L.; Kellum, J.A.; et al. Iron, Hepcidin, and Death in Human AKI. *J. Am. Soc. Nephrol.* **2019**, *30*, 493–504. [CrossRef]
55. Qiu, Z.-L.; Yan, B.-Q.; Xu, D.-W.; Zhao, R.; Shen, K.; Lu, S.-Q. Mortality and serum hepcidin are associated with persistent and transient acute kidney injury in septic patients. *Clin. Nephrol.* **2021**, *95*, 303–311. [CrossRef]
56. Qiu, Z.-L.; Yan, B.-Q.; Zhao, R.; Xu, D.-W.; Shen, K.; Deng, X.; Lu, S.-Q. Combination of hepcidin with neutrophil gelatinase-associated lipocalin for prediction of the development of sepsis-induced acute kidney injury. *Clin. Chim. Acta* **2021**, *523*, 38–44. [CrossRef]
57. Olinder, J.; Stjernqvist, M.J.; Lindén, A.; Salomonsson, E.T.; Annborn, M.; Herwald, H.; Rydén, C. Hepcidin, in contrast to heparin binding protein, does not portend acute kidney injury in patients with community acquired septic shock. *PLoS ONE* **2024**, *19*, e0299257. [CrossRef]
58. Wang, W.; Knovich, M.A.; Coffman, L.G.; Torti, F.M.; Torti, S.V. Serum ferritin: Past, present and future. *Biochim. Biophys. Acta (BBA)-Gen. Subj.* **2010**, *1800*, 760–769. [CrossRef]
59. Garcia, P.C.R.; Longhi, F.; Branco, R.G.; Piva, J.P.; Lacks, D.; Tasker, R.C. Ferritin levels in children with severe sepsis and septic shock. *Acta Paediatr.* **2007**, *96*, 1829–1831. [CrossRef]
60. Tonial, C.T.; Costa, C.A.D.; Andrades, G.R.H.; Crestani, F.; Einloft, P.R.; Bruno, F.; Miranda, A.P.; Fiori, H.H.; Garcia, P.C.R. Prediction of Poor Outcomes for Septic Children According to Ferritin Levels in a Middle-Income Setting*. *Pediatr. Crit. Care Med.* **2020**, *21*, e259–e266. [CrossRef]
61. Sarkar, M.; Roychowdhury, S.; Uz Zaman, M.; Raut, S.; Bhakta, S.; Nandy, M. Can serum ferritin be employed as prognostic marker of pediatric septic shock and severe sepsis? *J. Pediatr. Crit. Care* **2021**, *8*, 20. [CrossRef]
62. He, L.; Guo, C.; Su, Y.; Ding, N. The relationship between serum ferritin level and clinical outcomes in sepsis based on a large public database. *Sci. Rep.* **2023**, *13*, 8677. [CrossRef] [PubMed]
63. Zarjou, A.; Black, L.M.; McCullough, K.R.; Hull, T.D.; Esman, S.K.; Boddu, R.; Varambally, S.; Chandrashekar, D.S.; Feng, W.; Arosio, P.; et al. Ferritin Light Chain Confers Protection Against Sepsis-Induced Inflammation and Organ Injury. *Front. Immunol.* **2019**, *10*, 131. [CrossRef] [PubMed]
64. Odum, J.D.; Akhter, J.; Verma, V.; Vollmer, G.; Davidson, A.; Hyndman, K.A.; Bolisetty, S. Myeloid-specific ferritin light chain deletion does not exacerbate sepsis-associated AKI. *Am. J. Physiol.-Ren. Physiol.* **2024**, *327*, F171–F183. [CrossRef]
65. Dimitrijevic, Z.M.; Salinger-Martinovic, S.S.; Jankovic, R.J.; Mitic, B.P. Elevated Serum Ferritin Levels Are Predictive of Renal Function Recovery among Patients with Acute Kidney Injury. *Tohoku J. Exp. Med.* **2019**, *248*, 63–71. [CrossRef]
66. Fang, Y.-P.; Zhang, H.-J.; Guo, Z.; Ren, C.-H.; Zhang, Y.-F.; Liu, Q.; Wang, Z.; Zhang, X. Effect of Serum Ferritin on the Prognosis of Patients with Sepsis: Data from the MIMIC-IV Database. *Emerg. Med. Int.* **2022**, *2022*, 2104755. [CrossRef] [PubMed]
67. Zhang, X.; Luo, T.; Luo, Y.; Lu, M.; Xie, Y. Association Between Serum Ferritin and In-hospital Mortality in Critical Ills with Sepsis-Associated Acute Kidney Injury: A Retrospective Cohort Study. *Mod. Health Sci.* **2025**, *8*, p58. [CrossRef]
68. Weis, S.; Carlos, A.R.; Moita, M.R.; Singh, S.; Blankenhaus, B.; Cardoso, S.; Larsen, R.; Rebelo, S.; Schäuble, S.; Del Barrio, L.; et al. Metabolic Adaptation Establishes Disease Tolerance to Sepsis. *Cell* **2017**, *169*, 1263–1275.e14. [CrossRef]
69. Wang, T.-W.; Zhou, L.-L.; Yuan, J.; Zhou, W.-X.; Wang, H.-R.; Yu, T.-T.; Zhai, J.-C.; Tang, C.-B.; Jiang, W.; Yu, J.-Q.; et al. Study of the relationship between iron metabolism disorders and sepsis-associated liver injury: A prospective observational study. *World J. Gastroenterol.* **2025**, *31*, 104584. [CrossRef]
70. Zhou, F.; Yu, T.; Du, R.; Fan, G.; Liu, Y.; Liu, Z.; Xiang, J.; Wang, Y.; Song, B.; Gu, X.; et al. Clinical course and risk factors for mortality of adult inpatients with COVID-19 in Wuhan, China: A retrospective cohort study. *Lancet* **2020**, *395*, 1054–1062. [CrossRef]
71. Timpau, A.-S.; Miftode, R.-S.; Petris, A.O.; Costache, I.-I.; Miftode, I.-L.; Rosu, F.M.; Anton-Paduraru, D.-T.; Leca, D.; Miftode, E.G. Mortality Predictors in Severe COVID-19 Patients from an East European Tertiary Center: A Never-Ending Challenge for a No Happy Ending Pandemic. *J. Clin. Med.* **2021**, *11*, 58. [CrossRef] [PubMed]
72. Cao, P.; Wu, Y.; Wu, S.; Wu, T.; Zhang, Q.; Zhang, R.; Wang, Z.; Zhang, Y. Elevated serum ferritin level effectively discriminates severity illness and liver injury of coronavirus disease 2019 pneumonia. *Biomarkers* **2021**, *26*, 207–212. [CrossRef]
73. Timpau, A.-S.; Miftode, R.-S.; Costache, I.-I.; Petris, A.O.; Miftode, I.-L.; Gheorghe, L.; Timpau, R.; Miftode, I.D.; Prepeliuc, C.S.; Coman, I.; et al. An Overview of the Impact of Bacterial Infections and the Associated Mortality Predictors in Patients with COVID-19 Admitted to a Tertiary Center from Eastern Europe. *Antibiotics* **2023**, *12*, 144. [CrossRef] [PubMed]
74. Yoshida, H.; Hunter, C.A. The Immunobiology of Interleukin-27. *Annu. Rev. Immunol.* **2015**, *33*, 417–443. [CrossRef]
75. Wirtz, S.; Tubbe, I.; Galle, P.R.; Schild, H.J.; Birkenbach, M.; Blumberg, R.S.; Neurath, M.F. Protection from lethal septic peritonitis by neutralizing the biological function of interleukin 27. *J. Exp. Med.* **2006**, *203*, 1875–1881. [CrossRef]

76. Cao, J.; Xu, F.; Lin, S.; Song, Z.; Zhang, L.; Luo, P.; Xu, H.; Li, D.; Zheng, K.; Ren, G.; et al. IL-27 controls sepsis-induced impairment of lung antibacterial host defence. *Thorax* **2014**, *69*, 926–937. [CrossRef]
77. Wang, Y.; Zhao, J.; Yao, Y.; Zhao, D.; Liu, S. Interleukin-27 as a Diagnostic Biomarker for Patients with Sepsis: A Meta-Analysis. *BioMed Res. Int.* **2021**, *2021*, 5516940. [CrossRef] [PubMed]
78. Fan, J.; Zhang, Y.; Zheng, D.; Zhang, M.; Liu, H.; He, M.; Wu, Z. IL-27 is elevated in sepsis with acute hepatic injury and promotes hepatic damage and inflammation in the CLP model. *Cytokine* **2020**, *127*, 154936. [CrossRef]
79. Fan, J.; He, M.; Wang, C.-J.; Zhang, M. Gadolinium Chloride Inhibits the Production of Liver Interleukin-27 and Mitigates Liver Injury in the CLP Mouse Model. *Mediat. Inflamm.* **2021**, *2021*, 2605973. [CrossRef]
80. Ye, L.; Wang, L.; Kuang, G.; Zhang, Z.; Peng, Q.; He, M.; Fan, J. IL-27 aggravates acute hepatic injury by promoting macrophage M1 polarization to induce Caspase-11 mediated Pyroptosis in vitro and in vivo. *Cytokine* **2025**, *188*, 156881. [CrossRef]
81. Zhou, P.; Deng, B.; Wu, M.; Ding, F.; Wang, L. Interleukin-27 Ameliorates Renal Ischemia-Reperfusion Injury through Signal Transducers and Activators of Transcription 3 Signaling Pathway. *Kidney Blood Press. Res.* **2019**, *44*, 1453–1464. [CrossRef] [PubMed]
82. Gao, F.; Yang, Y.; Feng, X.; Fan, T.; Jiang, L.; Guo, R.; Liu, Q. Interleukin-27 is elevated in sepsis-induced myocardial dysfunction and mediates inflammation. *Cytokine* **2016**, *88*, 1–11. [CrossRef] [PubMed]
83. Wang, Y.; Zhang, Y.; Shou, S.; Jin, H. The role of IL-17 in acute kidney injury. *Int. Immunopharmacol.* **2023**, *119*, 110307. [CrossRef]
84. Luo, C.; Luo, F.; Zhang, L.; Xu, Y.; Cai, G.; Fu, B.; Feng, Z.; Sun, X.; Chen, X. Knockout of interleukin-17A protects against sepsis-associated acute kidney injury. *Ann. Intensive Care* **2016**, *6*, 56. [CrossRef] [PubMed]
85. Maravitsa, P.; Adamopoulou, M.; Pistiki, A.; Netea, M.G.; Louis, K.; Giamarellos-Bourboulis, E.J. Systemic over-release of interleukin-17 in acute kidney injury after septic shock: Clinical and experimental evidence. *Immunol. Lett.* **2016**, *178*, 68–76. [CrossRef] [PubMed]
86. Zhou, X.; Yao, J.; Lin, J.; Liu, J.; Dong, L.; Duan, M. Th17/Regulatory T-Cell Imbalance and Acute Kidney Injury in Patients with Sepsis. *J. Clin. Med.* **2022**, *11*, 4027. [CrossRef]
87. Jin, H.; Wei, W.; Zhao, Y.; Ma, A.; Sun, K.; Lin, X.; Liu, Q.; Shou, S.; Zhang, Y. The roles of interleukin-17A in risk stratification and prognosis of patients with sepsis-associated acute kidney injury. *Kidney Res. Clin. Pract.* **2023**, *42*, 742–750. [CrossRef]
88. Li, L.; Chen, L.; Lin, F.; Mu, J.; Wang, D.; Zhang, W.; Mi, L.; Qin, Y.; Zhou, Y. Study of the Expression of Inflammatory Factors IL-4, IL-6, IL-10, and IL-17 in Liver Failure Complicated by Coagulation Dysfunction and Sepsis. *J. Inflamm. Res.* **2021**, *14*, 1447–1453. [CrossRef]
89. Sabat, R. IL-10 family of cytokines. *Cytokine Growth Factor Rev.* **2010**, *21*, 315–324. [CrossRef]
90. Knolle, P.A.; Löser, E.; Protzer, U.; Duchmann, R.; Schmitt, E.; Zum Büschenfelde, K.-H.M.; Rose-John, S.; Gerken, G. Regulation of endotoxin-induced IL-6 production in liver sinusoidal endothelial cells and Kupffer cells by IL-10. *Clin. Exp. Immunol.* **2003**, *107*, 555–561. [CrossRef]
91. Jensen, I.J.; McGonagill, P.W.; Butler, N.S.; Harty, J.T.; Griffith, T.S.; Badovinac, V.P. NK Cell–Derived IL-10 Supports Host Survival during Sepsis. *J. Immunol.* **2021**, *206*, 1171–1180. [CrossRef] [PubMed]
92. Zeng, G.; Chen, D.; Zhou, R.; Zhao, X.; Ye, C.; Tao, H.; Sheng, W.; Wu, Y. Combination of C-reactive protein, procalcitonin, IL -6, IL -8, and IL -10 for early diagnosis of hyperinflammatory state and organ dysfunction in pediatric sepsis. *Clin. Lab. Anal.* **2022**, *36*, e24505. [CrossRef]
93. Lee, S.-Y.; Lee, Y.-S.; Choi, H.-M.; Ko, Y.-S.; Lee, H.-Y.; Jo, S.-K.; Cho, W.-Y.; Kim, H.-K. Distinct pathophysiologic mechanisms of septic acute kidney injury: Role of immune suppression and renal tubular cell apoptosis in murine model of septic acute kidney injury. *Crit. Care Med.* **2012**, *40*, 2997–3006. [CrossRef] [PubMed]
94. Cho, E.; Lee, J.H.; Lim, H.J.; Oh, S.W.; Jo, S.K.; Cho, W.Y.; Kim, H.; Lee, S.Y. Soluble CD25 is increased in patients with sepsis-induced acute kidney injury. *Nephrology* **2014**, *19*, 318–324. [CrossRef] [PubMed]
95. Xu, H.; Turnquist, H.R.; Hoffman, R.; Billiar, T.R. Role of the IL-33-ST2 axis in sepsis. *Mil. Med. Res.* **2017**, *4*, 3. [CrossRef]
96. Zhou, Y.; Xu, Z.; Liu, Z. Role of IL-33-ST2 pathway in regulating inflammation: Current evidence and future perspectives. *J. Transl. Med.* **2023**, *21*, 902. [CrossRef]
97. Hur, M.; Kim, H.; Kim, H.J.; Yang, H.S.; Magrini, L.; Marino, R.; Cardelli, P.; Somma, S.D.; Network, O.B.O.G. Soluble ST2 Has a Prognostic Role in Patients With Suspected Sepsis. *Ann. Lab. Med.* **2015**, *35*, 570–577. [CrossRef]
98. Cepoi, M.-R.; Duca, S.T.; Chetran, A.; Costache, A.D.; Spiridon, M.R.; Afrăsânie, I.; Leancă, S.A.; Dmour, B.-A.; Matei, I.T.; Miftode, R.S.; et al. Chronic Kidney Disease Associated with Ischemic Heart Disease: To What Extent Do Biomarkers Help? *Life* **2023**, *14*, 34. [CrossRef]
99. Alves-Filho, J.C.; Sônego, F.; Souto, F.O.; Freitas, A.; Verri, W.A.; Auxiliadora-Martins, M.; Basile-Filho, A.; McKenzie, A.N.; Xu, D.; Cunha, F.Q.; et al. Interleukin-33 attenuates sepsis by enhancing neutrophil influx to the site of infection. *Nat. Med.* **2010**, *16*, 708–712. [CrossRef]
100. Bao, Q.; Lv, R.; Lei, M. IL-33 attenuates mortality by promoting IFN-γ production in sepsis. *Inflamm. Res.* **2018**, *67*, 531–538. [CrossRef]

101. Vrsaljko, N.; Radmanic Matotek, L.; Zidovec-Lepej, S.; Vince, A.; Papic, N. The Impact of Steatotic Liver Disease on Cytokine and Chemokine Kinetics During Sepsis. *Int. J. Mol. Sci.* **2025**, *26*, 2226. [CrossRef] [PubMed]
102. Akcay, A.; Nguyen, Q.; He, Z.; Turkmen, K.; Won Lee, D.; Hernando, A.A.; Altmann, C.; Toker, A.; Pacic, A.; Ljubanovic, D.G., et al. IL-33 Exacerbates Acute Kidney Injury. *J. Am. Soc. Nephrol.* **2011**, *22*, 2057–2067. [CrossRef]
103. Erfurt, S.; Hoffmeister, M.; Oess, S.; Asmus, K.; Patschan, S.; Ritter, O.; Patschan, D. Soluble IL-33 receptor predicts survival in acute kidney injury. *J. Circ. Biomark.* **2022**, *11*, 28–35. [CrossRef] [PubMed]
104. Huang, W.; Tang, Y.; Li, L. HMGB1, a potent proinflammatory cytokine in sepsis. *Cytokine* **2010**, *51*, 119–126. [CrossRef]
105. Diener, K.R.; Al-Dasooqi, N.; Lousberg, E.L.; Hayball, J.D. The multifunctional alarmin HMGB1 with roles in the pathophysiology of sepsis and cancer. *Immunol. Cell Biol.* **2013**, *91*, 443–450. [CrossRef] [PubMed]
106. Gibot, S.; Massin, F.; Cravoisy, A.; Barraud, D.; Nace, L.; Levy, B.; Bollaert, P.-E. High-mobility group box 1 protein plasma concentrations during septic shock. *Intensive Care Med.* **2007**, *33*, 1347–1353. [CrossRef]
107. Sundén-Cullberg, J.; Norrby-Teglund, A.; Rouhiainen, A.; Rauvala, H.; Herman, G.; Tracey, K.J.; Lee, M.L.; Andersson, J.; Tokics, L.; Treutiger, C.J. Persistent elevation of high mobility group box-1 protein (HMGB1) in patients with severe sepsis and septic shock*. *Crit. Care Med.* **2005**, *33*, 564–573. [CrossRef]
108. Karakike, E.; Adami, M.-E.; Lada, M.; Gkavogianni, T.; Koutelidakis, I.M.; Bauer, M.; Giamarellos-Bourboulis, E.J.; Tsangaris, I. Late Peaks of HMGB1 and Sepsis Outcome: Evidence For Synergy With Chronic Inflammatory Disorders. *Shock* **2019**, *52*, 334–339. [CrossRef]
109. Wang, W.; Sun, L.; Deng, Y.; Tang, J. Synergistic effects of antibodies against high-mobility group box 1 and tumor necrosis factor-α antibodies on D-(+)-galactosamine hydrochloride/lipopolysaccharide-induced acute liver failure. *FEBS J.* **2013**, *280*, 1409–1419. [CrossRef]
110. Huang, Y.; Zang, K.; Shang, F.; Guo, S.; Gao, L.; Zhang, X. HMGB1 mediates acute liver injury in sepsis through pyroptosis of liver macrophages. *Int. J. Burn. Trauma* **2020**, *10*, 60.
111. Wang, Y.; Zhang, H.; Chen, Q.; Jiao, F.; Shi, C.; Pei, M.; Lv, J.; Zhang, H.; Wang, L.; Gong, Z. TNF-α/HMGB1 inflammation signalling pathway regulates pyroptosis during liver failure and acute kidney injury. *Cell Prolif.* **2020**, *53*, e12829. [CrossRef] [PubMed]
112. Zheng, S.; Pan, Y.; Wang, C.; Liu, Y.; Shi, M.; Ding, G. HMGB1 Turns Renal Tubular Epithelial Cells into Inflammatory Promoters by Interacting with TLR4 During Sepsis. *J. Interferon Cytokine Res.* **2016**, *36*, 9–19. [CrossRef]
113. Khorashadi, M.; Beunders, R.; Pickkers, P.; Legrand, M. Proenkephalin: A New Biomarker for Glomerular Filtration Rate and Acute Kidney Injury. *Nephron* **2020**, *144*, 655–661. [CrossRef]
114. Beunders, R.; Struck, J.; Wu, A.H.B.; Zarbock, A.; Di Somma, S.; Mehta, R.L.; Koyner, J.L.; Nadim, M.K.; Maisel, A.S.; Murray, P.T.; et al. Proenkephalin (PENK) as a Novel Biomarker for Kidney Function. *J. Appl. Lab. Med.* **2017**, *2*, 400–412. [CrossRef]
115. Schulte, J.; Dépret, F.; Hartmann, O.; Pickkers, P.; Laterre, P.-F.; Uhle, F. AdrenOSS-1 study investigators. Clinical performance of proenkephalin A 119–159 for the early diagnosis of acute kidney injury in patients with sepsis or septic shock. *medRxiv* **2024**. [CrossRef]
116. Caironi, P.; Latini, R.; Struck, J.; Hartmann, O.; Bergmann, A.; Bellato, V.; Ferraris, S.; Tognoni, G.; Pesenti, A.; Gattinoni, L.; et al. Circulating Proenkephalin, Acute Kidney Injury, and Its Improvement in Patients with Severe Sepsis or Shock. *Clin. Chem.* **2018**, *64*, 1361–1369. [CrossRef] [PubMed]
117. Lin, L.-C.; Chuan, M.-H.; Liu, J.-H.; Liao, H.-W.; Ng, L.L.; Magnusson, M.; Jujic, A.; Pan, H.-C.; Wu, V.-C.; Forni, L.G. Proenkephalin as a biomarker correlates with acute kidney injury: A systematic review with meta-analysis and trial sequential analysis. *Crit. Care* **2023**, *27*, 481. [CrossRef]
118. Verras, C.; Bezati, S.; Bistola, V.; Ventoulis, I.; Matsiras, D.; Tsiodras, S.; Parissis, J.; Polyzogopoulou, E. Point-of-Care Serum Proenkephalin as an Early Predictor of Mortality in Patients Presenting to the Emergency Department with Septic Shock. *Biomedicines* **2024**, *12*, 1004. [CrossRef]
119. Kim, H.; Hur, M.; Struck, J.; Bergmann, A.; Somma, S.D.; GREAT Network. Proenkephalin Predicts Organ Failure, Renal Replacement Therapy, and Mortality in Patients With Sepsis. *Ann. Lab. Med.* **2020**, *40*, 466–473. [CrossRef] [PubMed]
120. Tokunaga, R.; Zhang, W.; Naseem, M.; Puccini, A.; Berger, M.D.; Soni, S.; McSkane, M.; Baba, H.; Lenz, H.-J. CXCL9, CXCL10, CXCL11/CXCR3 axis for immune activation—A target for novel cancer therapy. *Cancer Treat. Rev.* **2018**, *63*, 40–47. [CrossRef]
121. Giamarellos-Bourboulis, E.J.; Antonelli, M.; Bloos, F.; Kotsamidi, I.; Psarrakis, C.; Dakou, K.; Thomas-Rüddel, D.; Montini, L.; Briegel, J.; Damoraki, G.; et al. Interferon-gamma driven elevation of CXCL9: A new sepsis endotype independently associated with mortality. *eBioMedicine* **2024**, *109*, 105414. [CrossRef]
122. Moledina, D.G.; Obeid, W.; Smith, R.N.; Rosales, I.; Sise, M.E.; Moeckel, G.; Kashgarian, M.; Kuperman, M.; Campbell, K.N.; Lefferts, S.; et al. Identification and validation of urinary CXCL9 as a biomarker for diagnosis of acute interstitial nephritis. *J. Clin. Investig.* **2023**, *133*, e168950. [CrossRef] [PubMed]
123. Yang, H.; Chen, Y.; He, J.; Li, Y.; Feng, Y. Advances in the diagnosis of early biomarkers for acute kidney injury: A literature review. *BMC Nephrol.* **2025**, *26*, 115. [CrossRef] [PubMed]

124. Saiman, Y.; Friedman, S.L. The Role of Chemokines in Acute Liver Injury. *Front. Physiol.* **2012**, *3*, 213. [CrossRef]
125. Plevriti, A.; Lamprou, M.; Mourkogianni, E.; Skoulas, N.; Giannakopoulou, M.; Sajib, M.S.; Wang, Z.; Mattheolabakis, G.; Chatzigeorgiou, A.; Marazioti, A.; et al. The Role of Soluble CD163 (sCD163) in Human Physiology and Pathophysiology. *Cells* **2024**, *13*, 1679. [CrossRef] [PubMed]
126. Feng, L.; Zhou, X.; Su, L.-X.; Feng, D.; Jia, Y.-H.; Xie, L.-X. Clinical Significance of Soluble Hemoglobin Scavenger Receptor CD163 (sCD163) in Sepsis, a Prospective Study. *PLoS ONE* **2012**, *7*, e38400. [CrossRef]
127. Gaïni, S.; Pedersen, S.S.; Koldkjær, O.G.; Pedersen, C.; Moestrup, S.K.; Møller, H.J. New immunological serum markers in bacteraemia: Anti-inflammatory soluble CD163, but not proinflammatory high mobility group-box 1 protein, is related to prognosis. *Clin. Exp. Immunol.* **2008**, *151*, 423–431. [CrossRef]
128. Abdelrahman, R.; Wagih, A.; Elbarbary, A. The diagnostic value of serum level of soluble hemoglobin scavenger receptor CD163 for sepsis in the ICU. *Tanta Med. J.* **2015**, *43*, 9. [CrossRef]
129. Mierzchała-Pasierb, M.; Lipińska-Gediga, M.; Lewandowski, Ł.; Krzystek-Korpacka, M. Alterations in Serum Concentration of Soluble CD163 within Five Study Days from ICU Admission Are Associated with In-Hospital Mortality of Septic Patients—A Preliminary Study. *Int. J. Environ. Res. Public Health* **2023**, *20*, 2263. [CrossRef]
130. Su, L.; Feng, L.; Liu, C.; Jiang, Z.; Li, M.; Xiao, K.; Yan, P.; Jia, Y.; Feng, D.; Xie, L. Diagnostic value of urine sCD163 levels for sepsis and relevant acute kidney injury: A prospective study. *BMC Nephrol.* **2012**, *13*, 123. [CrossRef]
131. Møller, H.J.; Grønbæk, H.; Schiødt, F.V.; Holland-Fischer, P.; Schilsky, M.; Munoz, S.; Hassanein, T.; Lee, W.M. Soluble CD163 from activated macrophages predicts mortality in acute liver failure. *J. Hepatol.* **2007**, *47*, 671–676. [CrossRef]
132. Tornai, T.; Vitalis, Z.; Sipeki, N.; Dinya, T.; Tornai, D.; Antal-Szalmas, P.; Karanyi, Z.; Tornai, I.; Papp, M. Macrophage activation marker, soluble CD 163, is an independent predictor of short-term mortality in patients with cirrhosis and bacterial infection. *Liver Int.* **2016**, *36*, 1628–1638. [CrossRef] [PubMed]
133. Damoiseaux, J. The IL-2—IL-2 receptor pathway in health and disease: The role of the soluble IL-2 receptor. *Clin. Immunol.* **2020**, *218*, 108515. [CrossRef] [PubMed]
134. Garcia-Obregon, S.; Azkargorta, M.; Seijas, I.; Pilar-Orive, J.; Borrego, F.; Elortza, F.; Boyano, M.D.; Astigarraga, I. Identification of a panel of serum protein markers in early stage of sepsis and its validation in a cohort of patients. *J. Microbiol. Immunol. Infect.* **2018**, *51*, 465–472. [CrossRef] [PubMed]
135. Komorowski, M.; Green, A.; Tatham, K.C.; Seymour, C.; Antcliffe, D. Sepsis biomarkers and diagnostic tools with a focus on machine learning. *eBioMedicine* **2022**, *86*, 104394. [CrossRef]
136. He, R.-R.; Yue, G.-L.; Dong, M.-L.; Wang, J.-Q.; Cheng, C. Sepsis Biomarkers: Advancements and Clinical Applications—A Narrative Review. *Int. J. Mol. Sci.* **2024**, *25*, 9010. [CrossRef]

International Journal of
Molecular Sciences

Review

The Role of Scavenger Receptor BI in Sepsis

Dan Hao [1], Jian-Yao Xue [1], Qian Wang [2], Ling Guo [2] and Xiang-An Li [1,2,3,4,*]

[1] Department of Pharmacology and Nutritional Sciences, University of Kentucky College of Medicine, Lexington, KY 40536, USA
[2] Saha Cardiovascular Research Center, University of Kentucky, Lexington, KY 40536, USA
[3] Lexington VA Healthcare System, Lexington, KY 40502, USA
[4] Department of Physiology, University of Kentucky, Lexington, KY 40536, USA
* Correspondence: xli2@email.uky.edu

Abstract: Sepsis is a life-threatening condition resulting from a dysregulated host response to infection. Currently, there is no effective therapy for sepsis due to an incomplete understanding of its pathogenesis. Scavenger receptor BI (SR-BI) is a high-density lipoprotein (HDL) receptor that plays a key role in HDL metabolism by modulating the selective uptake of cholesteryl ester from HDL. Recent studies, including those from our laboratory, indicate that SR-BI protects against sepsis through multiple mechanisms: (1) preventing nitric oxide-induced cytotoxicity; (2) promoting hepatic lipopolysaccharide (LPS) clearance and regulating cholesterol metabolism in the liver; (3) inhibiting LPS-induced inflammatory signaling in macrophages; and (4) mediating the uptake of cholesterol from HDL for inducible glucocorticoid (iGC) synthesis in the adrenal gland, which controls systemic inflammatory response. In this article, we review the roles of SR-BI in sepsis.

Keywords: scavenger receptor BI; SR-BI; HDL; sepsis; adrenal stress response; glucocorticoid; precision medicine

1. Introduction

Sepsis is a major health issue, affecting 49 million people annually [1]. Sepsis results from a dysregulated host response to infection [2]. Upon infection (Figure 1), pattern recognition receptors (PRRs) on immune cells recognize and bind to the molecular structures of the invading microorganism, known as pathogen- or damage-associated molecular patterns (PAMPs and DAMPs). These trigger the activation of the innate immune system, leading to the release of cytokines, chemokines, nitric oxide, and oxygen radicals, and complement system activation. Concurrently, coagulation is triggered by endothelial damage and amplified by pro-inflammatory cytokines. The complement system and coagulation cascades cause vascular instability, microvascular occlusion, coagulation, fever, and capillary leakage, ultimately contributing to the development of multiple-organ failure [3–5]. Despite extensive efforts, hundreds of sepsis therapies have proven to be unsuccessful. An incomplete understanding of the pathogenesis of sepsis may contribute to these failed efforts.

Scavenger receptor BI (SR-BI) is a 75 kDa cell surface glycoprotein that is highly expressed in various tissues, including the liver, endothelial cells, macrophages, and steroidogenic tissues [6–8]. It was initially identified by Dr. Krieger's group as a receptor that binds to acetylated low-density lipoprotein (LDL), oxidized LDL, and native LDL in vivo [9]. Two years later, their research revealed that SR-BI also binds to high-density lipoprotein (HDL) and facilitates the selective uptake of cholesteryl esters from HDL particles into cells. This remarkable function led to its designation as "the HDL receptor" [10–14]. SR-BI-mediated uptake of cholesteryl ester from HDL is essential for reverse cholesterol transport in the liver, where HDL collects cholesterol from peripheral tissues and transfers it to hepatic SR-BI for disposal in bile. Mice deficient in SR-BI have elevated HDL levels, female infertility, and autoimmune disorders with aging [15], and are susceptible to atherosclerosis [16–20].

Similarly, humans with loss-of-function mutations in SR-BI exhibit impaired uptake of cholesteryl esters from HDL, elevated HDL levels, and an increased risk of coronary heart disease [21,22]. This indicates that SR-BI has similar functions in both humans and rodents (please refer to SR-BI reviews [23–25]).

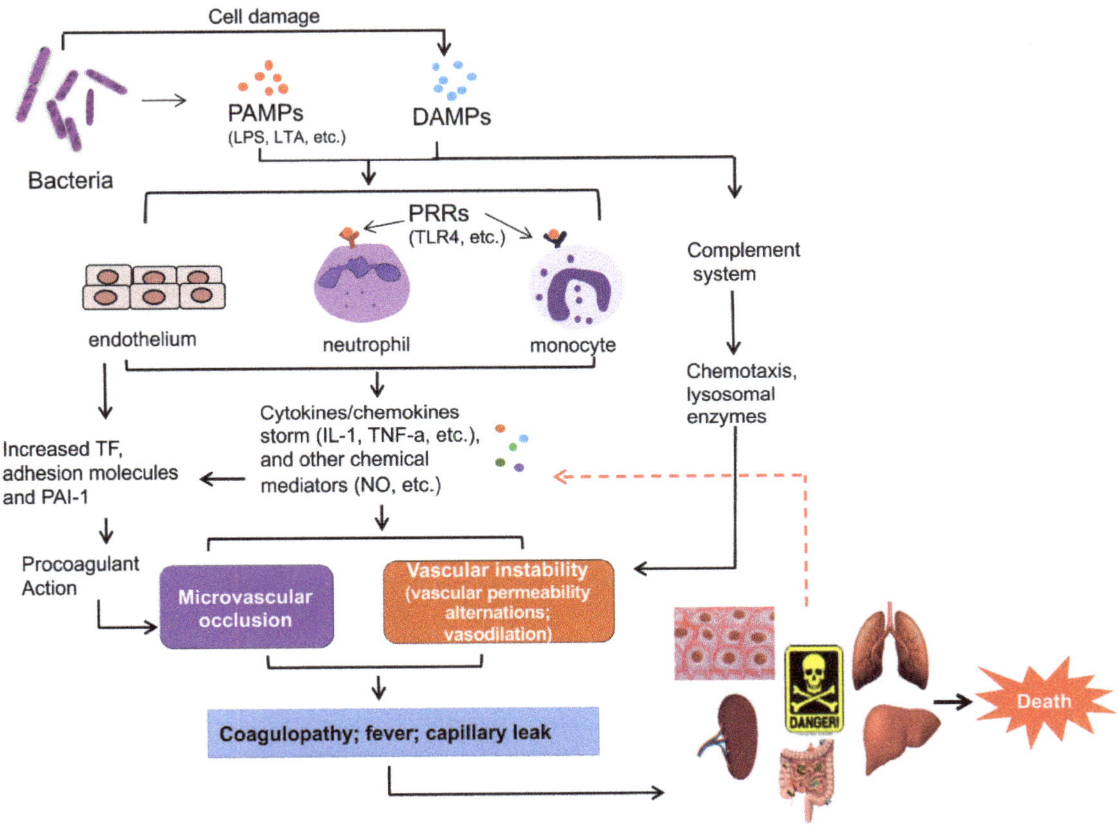

Figure 1. The pathogenesis of sepsis. Upon infection, pattern recognition receptors (PRRs) on immune cells recognize and bind to specific microbial structures known as PAMPs or DAMPs. The activation of the innate immune system results in the release of cytokines/chemokines, nitric oxide, and oxygen radicals, and complement system activation. This process leads to coagulation due to endothelial damage and the rapid release of pro-inflammatory cytokines. The complement system and coagulation cascades subsequently reduce vascular stability and cause microvascular blockages, resulting in coagulation, fever, capillary leakage, and ultimately multiple-organ failure. These factors drive the typical inflammatory response underlying sepsis' pathophysiology. LPS, lipopolysaccharide; LTA, lipoteichoic acid; PAMPs, pathogen-associated molecular patterns; DAMPs, damage-associated molecular patterns; TLR4, toll-like receptor 4; TF, tissue factor; PAI-1, plasminogen activator inhibitor-1; IL-1, interleukin-1; TNF-1α, tumor necrosis factor-1 alpha; NO, nitric oxide.

Dr. Li's laboratory first reported the protective effect of SR-BI against sepsis. They found that SR-BI-null mice have significantly higher mortality in LPS-induced sepsis (90% mortality in SR-BI-null mice versus 0% in wild-type mice) [26]. Using a cecal ligation and puncture (CLP)-induced sepsis model, they confirmed the protective role of SR-BI in sepsis [27]. Subsequent research from a number of laboratories has elucidated various mechanisms through which SR-BI exerts its protective functions, which will be explored in the following discussion.

2. Scavenger Receptor BI Protects Against Nitric-Oxide-Induced Cytotoxicity

It has been shown that HDL can enhance endothelial function and nitric oxide (NO)-dependent relaxation in aortas. However, this beneficial effect is not observed in the aortas of SR-BI-null mice, emphasizing the crucial role of SR-BI in this process. Further investigation has shown that HDL activates eNOS through SR-BI [28–31]. NO is a highly reactive molecule produced by nitric oxide synthase (NOS). It defends against pathogens but can become cytotoxic in excess [32]. It reacts with superoxide to form the hazardous peroxynitrite, leading to nitrotyrosine formation and cytotoxicity [33]. This process, called nitric oxidative stress, underlies diseases like septic shock [34], atherosclerosis [35], Alzheimer's disease [36], and diabetes [37]. Using Chinese Hamster Ovary (CHO) cell lines expressing wild-type or mutant SR-BI, Dr. Li's laboratory demonstrated SR-BI's protection against NO-induced cytotoxicity [26]. Using SR-BI-null mice, they found that SR-BI significantly reduces protein tyrosine nitration in the aorta and liver. To further investigate the physiological and pathological significance of SR-BI's protection against NO-induced cytotoxicity, they used a lipopolysaccharide (LPS) challenge as a model. When challenged with a low dose of LPS, 90% of SR-BI-knockout mice died, whereas none of the wild-type littermates died. An LPS challenge induces endotoxemia and serves as a model of sepsis. These findings establish SR-BI's protective role against sepsis.

3. Scavenger Receptor BI Mediates Lipopolysaccharide Clearance

SR-BI also functions as a receptor for LPS, a key factor in septic shock, and it is highly expressed in the liver, the primary site for LPS clearance. It is therefore considered pivotal in facilitating LPS clearance by the liver. Evidence shows that SR-BI binds and internalizes LPS in HeLa cells and macrophages, facilitating LPS clearance into hepatocytes and reducing the LPS burden [38]. Guo et al. demonstrated the role of SR-BI in LPS recruitment and clearance in CLP-induced sepsis [27]. Cai et al. found that SR-BI-null mice exhibited reduced plasma LPS clearance into the liver and hepatocytes [39], further emphasizing the crucial function of SR-BI in facilitating LPS clearance. Hepatic SR-BI is crucial for LPS clearance during sepsis, as observed in mice with hepatic SR-BI deficiency (Scarb1^{I179N} mice), experiencing a three-fold increase in serum LPS levels during CLP-induced sepsis compared to control mice [40]. These findings highlight the significant role of SR-BI in promoting LPS clearance during sepsis.

4. Scavenger Receptor BI-Mediated Cholesterol Metabolism Is Required for Protection Against Sepsis

Lipid metabolism often goes haywire in septic patients, leading to complications. Increased lipolysis releases free fatty acids (FFAs) into the bloodstream, but their utilization is impaired due to mitochondrial dysfunction and reduced enzyme activity. The systemic inflammatory response inhibits lipoprotein lipase (LPL), altering lipoprotein profiles and exacerbating inflammation. Oxidative stress further contributes to lipid peroxidation, damaging cell membranes and worsening lipid metabolism. These disruptions contribute to the pathophysiology of sepsis and affect patient outcomes [41,42].

Reverse cholesterol transport (RCT) plays a vital role in managing cholesterol levels in the bloodstream. During RCT, HDL gathers cholesterol from peripheral tissues and delivers it to the liver's SR-BI receptors. SR-BI then facilitates the uptake of cholesteryl esters from HDL, which are eventually excreted via bile. In a recent study by Wang et al., researchers used liver-specific SR-BI-null (AlbCreSR-BI$^{fl/fl}$) mice, which have impaired RCT, to explore how this process affects sepsis [43]. They discovered that these mice were much more vulnerable to CLP-induced polymicrobial sepsis, with a survival rate of only 14.3% compared to 80% in their SR-BI$^{fl/fl}$ littermates. Mechanistically, sepsis disrupted cholesterol metabolism in these mice, leading to a 4.8-fold increase in free cholesterol (FC) levels and a 4-fold increase in the FC/cholesteryl ester (CE) ratio compared to the control group. This disruption resulted in hemolysis and death. Interestingly, when the cholesterol-lowering drug probucol was administered, it normalized FC levels and the FC/CE ratio, significantly improving survival rates in the CLP-AlbCreSR-BI$^{fl/fl}$ mice. However, probucol treatment had the opposite effect in CLP-LDLR-knockout mice, which had elevated CE levels and a low FC/CE ratio, reducing their survival. These findings underscore that elevated FC levels and a high FC/CE ratio are significant risk factors for sepsis. Therefore, targeting these elevated FC levels and the FC/CE ratio could be a promising therapeutic strategy for managing sepsis.

5. Scavenger Receptor BI Regulates Inflammatory Response

Macrophages are a major cell type responsible for cytokine production, and SR-BI appears to regulate their inflammatory signaling. The expression of SR-BI suppresses inflammatory cytokine production in LPS-stimulated macrophages by modulating the TLR4-NF-κB pathway. Further study demonstrated that the regulation of SR-BI involves JNK and P38 signaling pathways [44]. Hematopoietic SR-BI deficiency leads to increased cytokine production in response to LPS, indicating its role in controlling in vivo inflammation. The inhibitory effects of SR-BI on the macrophage inflammation protect against septic death, exemplified by SR-BIC323G overexpression (a mutant SR-BI deficient in glucocorticoid generation but capable of suppressing TLR4-NF-κB signaling) significantly improving survival in SR-BI-deficient mice during a CLP challenge [27]. A recent bulk RNA-seq analysis found that adrenal SR-BI-knockout mice displayed hyperinflammatory responses during sepsis due to the transcriptional dysregulation of AP-1 and NK-κB. GC therapy effectively rescued these mice [45]. These findings underscore SR-BI's role in inflammation and its vital role in moderating inflammation for protection against sepsis-induced death.

Using the LPS model, Cai et al. confirmed that SR-BI-knockout mice are susceptible to LPS-induced endotoxic death, which is associated with a systemic hyperinflammatory response [39]. They further found that a deficiency in SR-BI leads to low levels of glucocorticoid (GC) production, which contributes to the uncontrolled inflammatory response (discussed further below).

6. Scavenger Receptor BI Regulates Adrenal Stress Response in Sepsis

In the adrenal gland, glucocorticoid (GC) production is markedly induced in response to septic stress and serves as potent inflammatory modulators during sepsis [46]. We refer to this stress-induced GC (iGC) as the adrenal stress response. GC is derived from intracellular cholesterol, which comes from three resources: (1) uptake from LDL through LDL receptors; (2) uptake from HDL through SR-BI; and (3) de novo synthesis. The SR-BI-HDL pathway appears to play a key role in iGC production. SR-BI-deficient mice maintain normal basal GC levels under physiological conditions, but cannot generate iGC under stress conditions induced by factors like LPS [39], adrenocorticotropic hormone (ACTH) stimulation [39], CLP [27,47,48], or long-term fasting [49,50]. SR-BI-null mice exhibit normal expression in key genes related to cholesterol de novo synthesis [39]. Given that rodents mainly have HDL with very low LDL levels in circulation, we generated humanized SR-BI-/- ApoBtg mice (SR-BI-null mice express with ApoB) with high LDL in circulation. The mice also failed to produce iGC in response to ACTH stimulation or under sepsis conditions [51]. Regarding the role of SR-BI in humans, an early study showed that human carriers' SR-BI P297S mutant, which has a 50% reduction in the uptake of cholesterol from HDL, displays a 50% reduction in iGC production to ACTH stimulation [22]. In contrast to SR-BI, a 50% reduction in LDL receptors in familial hypercholesterolemia patients does not hinder cholesterol delivery to the adrenal cortex [52]. These studies establish the SR-BI-HDL pathway as a key regulator of iGC production in sepsis.

7. Scavenger Receptor BI-Mediated Adrenal Stress Response Is an Essential Host Response for Protection Against Sepsis

SR-BI-null mice have a normal corticosterone level under physiologic conditions but lack iGC production during sepsis. This makes SR-BI-null mice a useful model to investigate the role of iGC in sepsis. Using whole-body SR-BI-null mice and the LPS endotoxemia model, Cai et al. showed that a lack of iGC production results in significantly elevated cytokine levels in circulation [39]. Using SF1CreHypoSR-BI$^{fl/fl}$ and the CLP sepsis model, Dr. Huby's group showed that these mice are more susceptible to CLP-induced septic death than control (HypoSR-BI$^{fl/fl}$) mice [47]. Using adrenal transplant-generated adrenal-specific SR-BI-null mice and the CLP sepsis model [48], Dr. Li's laboratory showed that mice deficient in adrenal SR-BI fail to produce iGC production in response to a CLP challenge and are more susceptible to CLP-induced septic death. Importantly, GC treatment two hours post CLP effectively rescued adrenal-specific SR-BI-null mice, but caused increased mortality in wild-type control mice. Since adrenal transplantation may disrupt catecholamine production by the adrenal gland, Dr. Li's laboratory generated new adrenal-specific SR-BI-null (SF1CreSR-BI$^{fl/fl}$) mice using floxed SR-BI mice [53,54]. They showed that adrenal SR-BI-specific knockout mice have impaired iGC production in response to ACTH stimulation and to CLP-induced sepsis. They demonstrated that while both wild-type and SF1CreSR-BI$^{fl/fl}$ mice exhibit a hyperinflammatory phenotype in the early stages of sepsis, iGC keeps the inflammatory response under control in wild-type mice. In contrast, SF1CreSR-BI$^{fl/fl}$ mice experience uncontrolled hyperinflammation due to the lack of iGC. These mice are more susceptible to CLP-induced sepsis. Supplementation with a low stress dose of GC in SF1CreSR-BI$^{fl/fl}$ mice controls the inflammatory response and rescues the mice. However, SR-BI$^{fl/fl}$ mice receiving GC treatment exhibited significantly less survival rates compared to SR-BI$^{fl/fl}$ mice without GC treatment.

Dr. Li's laboratory further assessed the importance of SR-BI-mediated iGC production in pediatric sepsis using 21-day-old mice [45]. Mice deficient in adrenal SR-BI were susceptible to both CLP and cecal slurry-induced septic death. SF1CreSRBI$^{fl/fl}$ mice featured persistent inflammatory responses, and were effectively rescued by administering GC two hours post CLP. GC treatment did not improve survival in CLP-challenged wild-type mice. Using an RNA-seq analysis, they found that the lack of iGC production in SF1CreSRBI$^{fl/fl}$ mice caused persistent inflammatory responses, primarily due to the transcriptional dysregulation of activator protein 1 (AP-1) and nuclear factor kappa B (NF-κB) [45]. In addition, they found that iGC functions to control cytokine-induced secondary inflammatory response [45].

It is of interest to discuss the effect of pretreatment of SR-BI KO mice with GC in LPS and CLP models. In an LPS endotoxemia model, Cai et al. [39] treated the mice with corticosterone via drinking water, 8 h prior to LPS injection, which effectively improved survival rates and physical condition in SR-BI-null mice. In a CLP-induced septic mice model [27], Guo et al. showed that corticosterone supplementation 8 h before CLP surgery does not rescue SR-BI-null mice from CLP-induced septic death. This may result from differences in the immune response between CLP-induced sepsis models and LPS-induced endotoxemia models. LPS injection simply triggers the release of inflammatory cytokines, which can be controlled by corticosterone supplementation; however, CLP-induced sepsis involves bacterial infection and necessary cytokine production for immune defense. Corticosterone given 8 h before CLP surgery could potentially leave the host vulnerable by suppressing the essential early immune response, making glucocorticoid pretreatment unfeasible for sepsis therapy. In another study, Leelahavanichkul et al. administered a high dose of dexamethasone to SR-BI KO and wild-type control mice 24 h before CLP, and found increased survival in SR-BI KO mice [55]. Unfortunately, the data did not support such a conclusion due to flaws in the experimental design [56]. For example, dexamethasone pretreatment completely eliminated SR-BI expression in the adrenal gland in wild-type control mice; the study used SR-BI-null mice on a C57BL/6/129 mixed background but used C57BL/6N mice as controls. Given that C57BL/6N mice are significantly more susceptible to sepsis than mice with a mixed background and that the adrenal SR-BI plays a key role in protection against sepsis, the increased survival in SR-BI KO mice is more likely due to the effect of GC pretreatment and the effect of the background. These early studies clearly showed that GC treatment to septic wild-type mice, especially pretreatment, is harmful.

8. Conclusions

SR-BI protects against sepsis through multiple mechanisms (Figure 2): (1) SR-BI protects against NO-induced cytotoxicity; (2) SR-BI mediates hepatic LPS clearance and cholesterol metabolism; (3) macrophage SR-BI inhibits LPS-induced inflammatory signaling; (4) adrenal SR-BI mediates the uptake of cholesterol from HDL for iGC synthesis, which controls the systemic inflammatory response.

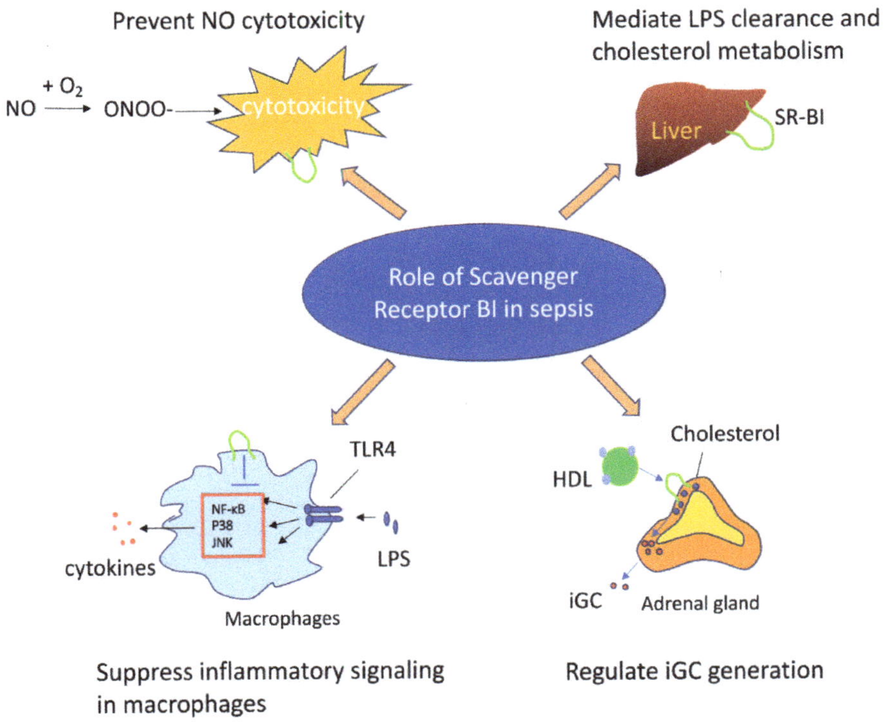

Figure 2. Summary of SR-BI protection against sepsis. SR-BI exerts its protective effect in sepsis through multiple mechanisms: (1) prevent NO-induced cytotoxicity; (2) mediate LPS clearance and cholesterol metabolism in liver; (3) suppress LPS-induced inflammatory signaling in macrophages; (4) mediate uptake of cholesterol from HDL for iGC synthesis in adrenal gland, which controls systemic inflammatory response.

9. Future Direction

Extensive clinical trials have failed to improve survival in septic patients [57]. A limitation is that these therapies were applied non-selectively to all septic patients. However, septic patients have heterogeneous clinical endotypes. Given the complexity of sepsis, emerging voices [58–60], including ours [45,48,53,61], have called for a precision medicine approach to sepsis therapy. Targeting a subgroup of patients with a specific endotype is a key component of a successful precision medicine approach [62,63].

Dysregulated lipid metabolism is common in septic patients [64], and statins have been tested as a sepsis therapy. However, the efficacy of statins is controversial [65–69]. A potential issue is that statins have been used indiscriminately in all septic patients, without accounting for variations in cholesterol metabolic subtypes. A mechanistic study using hepatic SR-BI-null mice as a model of dysregulated reverse cholesterol transport demonstrated that elevated free cholesterol, with a high free cholesterol/cholesteryl ester ratio, is a risk factor for sepsis [43]. Lowering cholesterol with probucol improved survival in hepatic SR-BI-null mice. Thus, probucol or statin treatment for septic patients with high free cholesterol levels and a high free cholesterol/cholesteryl ester ratio may offer an effective sepsis therapy.

Glucocorticoid (GC) therapy has been frequently used in septic patients, but its effectiveness remains hotly debated [70,71]. Current guidelines suggest GC therapy for septic patients experiencing shock [71]. While GC plays an important role in regulating blood pressure, this recommendation is largely based on clinical observations. Hypotension results from organ dysfunction. Given that hyperinflammation significantly contributes to organ injury, and mechanistic studies using adrenal SR-BI-null mice as an adrenal insufficiency model have demonstrated that GC functions control inflammation, and adrenal insufficiency is a risk factor for sepsis, we advocate for a precision medicine approach to guide GC therapy for sepsis—timely and selectively applying GC therapy to patients with adrenal insufficiency, not without.

Author Contributions: Conceptualization, D.H. and X.-A.L.; Original draft preparation, D.H. and X.-A.L. Writing—review and editing, D.H., L.G., J.-Y.X., Q.W. and X.-A.L.; Supervision, X.-A.L. Funding acquisition: X.-A.L. All authors have read and agreed to the published version of the manuscript.

Funding: This work was funded by the National Institutes of Health (R35GM141478), and the U.S. DEPARTMENT OF VETERANS AFFAIRS (VA) (VA 1I01BX004639 and VA 1I01BX006408).

Institutional Review Board Statement: Not applicable.

Informed Consent Statement: Not applicable.

Data Availability Statement: Not applicable.

Conflicts of Interest: The authors declare no conflicts of interest.

References

1. Rudd, K.E.; Johnson, S.C.; Agesa, K.M.; Shackelford, K.A.; Tsoi, D.; Kievlan, D.R.; Colombara, D.V.; Ikuta, K.S.; Kissoon, N.; Finfer, S.; et al. Global, regional, and national sepsis incidence and mortality, 1990–2017: Analysis for the Global Burden of Disease Study. *Lancet* **2020**, *395*, 200–211. [CrossRef]
2. Singer, M.; Deutschman, C.S.; Seymour, C.W.; Shankar-Hari, M.; Annane, D.; Bauer, M.; Bellomo, R.; Bernard, G.R.; Chiche, J.-D.; Coopersmith, C.M.; et al. The Third International Consensus Definitions for Sepsis and Septic Shock (Sepsis-3). *JAMA* **2016**, *315*, 801–810. [CrossRef] [PubMed]
3. Cohen, J. The immunopathogenesis of sepsis. *Nature* **2002**, *420*, 885–891. [CrossRef]
4. van der Poll, T.; Shankar-Hari, M.; Wiersinga, W.J. The immunology of sepsis. *Immunity* **2021**, *54*, 2450–2464. [CrossRef] [PubMed]
5. Jarczak, D.; Kluge, S.; Nierhaus, A. Sepsis—Pathophysiology and Therapeutic Concepts. *Front. Med.* **2021**, *8*. [CrossRef]
6. Chinetti, G.; Gbaguidi, F.G.; Griglio, S.; Mallat, Z.; Antonucci, M.; Poulain, P.; Chapman, J.; Fruchart, J.C.; Tedgui, A.; Najib-Fruchart, J.; et al. CLA-1/SR-BI is expressed in atherosclerotic lesion macrophages and regulated by activators of peroxisome proliferator-activated receptors. *Circulation.* **2000**, *101*, 2411–2417. [CrossRef]
7. Rhainds, D.; Brissette, L. The role of scavenger receptor class B type I (SR-BI) in lipid trafficking. *Int. J. Biochem. Cell Biol.* **2003**, *36*, 39–77. [CrossRef]
8. Krieger, M. Scavenger receptor class B type I is a multiligand HDL receptor that influences diverse physiologic systems. *J. Clin. Investig.* **2001**, *108*, 793–797. [CrossRef]
9. Acton, S.; Scherer, P.; Lodish, H.; Krieger, M. Expression cloning of SR-BI, a CD36-related class B scavenger receptor. *J. Biol. Chem.* **1994**, *269*, 21003–21009. [CrossRef]
10. Kozarsky, K.F.; Donahee, M.H.; Rigotti, A.; Iqbal, S.N.; Edelman, E.R.; Krieger, M. Overexpression of the HDL receptor SR-BI alters plasma HDL and bile cholesterol levels. *Nature* **1997**, *387*, 414–417. [CrossRef] [PubMed]
11. Rigotti, A.; Trigatti, B.L.; Penman, M.; Rayburn, H.; Herz, J.; Krieger, M. A targeted mutation in the murine gene encoding the high density lipoprotein (HDL) receptor scavenger receptor class B type I reveals its key role in HDL metabolism. *Proc. Natl. Acad. Sci. USA* **1997**, *94*, 12610–12615. [CrossRef]
12. Xu, S.; Laccotripe, M.; Huang, X.; Rigotti, A.; I Zannis, V.; Krieger, M. Apolipoproteins of HDL can directly mediate binding to the scavenger receptor SR-BI, an HDL receptor that mediates selective lipid uptake. *J. Lipid Res.* **1997**, *38*, 1289–1298. [CrossRef] [PubMed]

13. Thuahnai, S.T.; Lund-Katz, S.; Williams, D.L.; Phillips, M.C. Scavenger receptor class B, type I-mediated uptake of various lipids into cells: Influence of the nature of the donor particle interaction with the receptor. *J. Biol. Chem.* **2001**, *276*, 43801–43808. [CrossRef]
14. Acton, S.; Rigotti, A.; Landschulz, K.T.; Xu, S.; Hobbs, H.H.; Krieger, M. Identification of scavenger receptor SR-BI as a high density lipoprotein receptor. *Science* **1996**, *271*, 518–520. [CrossRef]
15. Feng, H.; Guo, L.; Wang, D.; Gao, H.; Hou, G.; Zheng, Z.; Ai, J.; Foreman, O.; Daugherty, A.; Li, X.-A.; et al. Deficiency of Scavenger Receptor BI Leads to Impaired Lymphocyte Homeostasis and Autoimmune Disorders in Mice. *Arter. Thromb. Vasc. Biol.* **2011**, *31*, 2543–2551. [CrossRef] [PubMed]
16. Arai, T.; Rinninger, F.; Varban, L.; Fairchild-Huntress, V.; Liang, C.-P.; Chen, W.; Seo, T.; Deckelbaum, R.; Huszar, D.; Tall, A.R. Decreased selective uptake of high density lipoprotein cholesteryl esters in apolipoprotein E knock-out mice. *Proc. Natl. Acad. Sci. USA* **1999**, *96*, 12050–12055. [CrossRef]
17. Braun, A.; Trigatti, B.L.; Post, M.J.; Sato, K.; Simons, M.; Edelberg, J.M.; Rosenberg, R.D.; Schrenzel, M.; Krieger, M. Loss of SR-BI Expression Leads to the Early Onset of Occlusive Atherosclerotic Coronary Artery Disease, Spontaneous Myocardial Infarctions, Severe Cardiac Dysfunction, and Premature Death in Apolipoprotein E–Deficient Mice. *Circ. Res.* **2002**, *90*, 270–276. [CrossRef] [PubMed]
18. Kozarsky, K.F.; Donahee, M.H.; Glick, J.M.; Krieger, M.; Rader, D.J. Gene Transfer and Hepatic Overexpression of the HDL Receptor SR-BI Reduces Atherosclerosis in the Cholesterol-Fed LDL Receptor–Deficient Mouse. *Arter. Thromb. Vasc. Biol.* **2000**, *20*, 721–727. [CrossRef] [PubMed]
19. Yu, H.; Zhang, W.; Yancey, P.G.; Koury, M.J.; Zhang, Y.; Fazio, S.; Linton, M.F. Macrophage Apolipoprotein E Reduces Atherosclerosis and Prevents Premature Death in Apolipoprotein E and Scavenger Receptor–Class BI Double-Knockout Mice. *Arter. Thromb. Vasc. Biol.* **2006**, *26*, 150–156. [CrossRef] [PubMed]
20. Van Eck, M.; Twisk, J.; Hoekstra, M.; Van Rij, B.T.; Van der Lans, C.A.; Bos, I.S.T.; Kruijt, J.K.; Kuipers, F.; Van Berkel, T.J. Differential effects of scavenger receptor BI deficiency on lipid metabolism in cells of the arterial wall and in the liver. *J. Biol. Chem.* **2003**, *278*, .23699–23705. [CrossRef] [PubMed]
21. Zanoni, P.; Khetarpal, S.A.; Larach, D.B.; Hancock-Cerutti, W.F.; Millar, J.S.; Cuchel, M.; DerOhannessian, S.; Kontush, A.; Surendran, P.; Saleheen, D.; et al. Rare variant in scavenger receptor BI raises HDL cholesterol and increases risk of coronary heart disease. *Science* **2016**, *351*, 1166–1171. [CrossRef] [PubMed]
22. Vergeer, M.; Korporaal, S.J.; Franssen, R.; Meurs, I.; Out, R.; Hovingh, G.K.; Hoekstra, M.; Sierts, J.A.; Dallinga-Thie, G.M.; Motazacker, M.M.; et al. Genetic Variant of the Scavenger Receptor BI in Humans. *N. Engl. J. Med.* **2011**, *364*, 136–145. [CrossRef] [PubMed]
23. Zheng, Z.; Ai, J.; Li, X.-A. Scavenger receptor class B type I and immune dysfunctions. *Curr. Opin. Endocrinol. Diabetes* **2014**, *21*, 121–128. [CrossRef]
24. Mineo, C.; Shaul, P.W. Functions of scavenger receptor class B, type I in atherosclerosis. *Curr. Opin. Infect. Dis.* **2012**, *23*, 487–493. [CrossRef]
25. Krieger, M. Charting the fate of the "good cholesterol": Identification and characterization of the high-density lipoprotein receptor SR-BI. *Annu. Rev. Biochem.* **1999**, *68*, 523–558. [CrossRef] [PubMed]
26. Li, X.-A.; Guo, L.; Asmis, R.; Nikolova-Karakashian, M.; Smart, E.J. Scavenger Receptor BI Prevents Nitric Oxide–Induced Cytotoxicity and Endotoxin-Induced Death. *Circ. Res.* **2006**, *98*, e60-5. [CrossRef]
27. Guo, L.; Song, Z.; Li, M.; Wu, Q.; Wang, D.; Feng, H.; Bernard, P.; Daugherty, A.; Huang, B.; Li, X.-A. Scavenger Receptor BI Protects against Septic Death through Its Role in Modulating Inflammatory Response. *J. Biol. Chem.* **2009**, *284*, 19826–19834. [CrossRef] [PubMed]
28. Li, X.-A.; Titlow, W.B.; Jackson, B.A.; Giltiay, N.; Nikolova-Karakashian, M.; Uittenbogaard, A.; Smart, E.J. High Density Lipoprotein Binding to Scavenger Receptor, Class B, Type I Activates Endothelial Nitric-oxide Synthase in a Ceramide-dependent Manner. *J. Biol. Chem.* **2002**, *277*, 11058–11063. [CrossRef] [PubMed]
29. Yuhanna, I.S.; Zhu, Y.; Cox, B.E.; Hahner, L.D.; Osborne-Lawrence, S.; Lu, P.; Marcel, Y.L.; Anderson, R.G.; Mendelsohn, M.E.; Hobbs, H.H.; et al. High-density lipoprotein binding to scavenger receptor-BI activates endothelial nitric oxide synthase. *Nat. Med.* **2001**, *7*, 853–857. [CrossRef]
30. Mineo, C.; Yuhanna, I.S.; Quon, M.J.; Shaul, P.W. High Density Lipoprotein-induced Endothelial Nitric-oxide Synthase Activation Is Mediated by Akt and MAP Kinases. *J. Biol. Chem.* **2003**, *278*, 9142–9149. [CrossRef]
31. Gong, M.; Wilson, M.; Kelly, T.; Su, W.; Dressman, J.; Kincer, J.; Matveev, S.V.; Guo, L.; Guerin, T.; Li, X.A.; et al. HDL-associated estradiol stimulates endothelial NO synthase and vasodilation in an SR-BI–dependent manner. *J. Clin. Investig.* **2003**, *111*, 1579–1587. [CrossRef] [PubMed]
32. Pisoschi, A.M.; Pop, A.; Iordache, F.; Stanca, L.; Predoi, G.; Serban, A.I. Oxidative stress mitigation by antioxidants - an overview on their chemistry and influences on health status. *Eur. J. Med. Chem.* **2020**, *209*, 112891. [CrossRef] [PubMed]
33. Halliwell, B.; Zhao, K.; Whiteman, M. Nitric oxide and peroxynitrite. The ugly, the uglier and the not so good: A personal view of recent controversies. *Free Radic. Res.* **1999**, *31*, 651–669. [CrossRef] [PubMed]
34. Titheradge, M.A. Nitric oxide in septic shock. *Biochim. Biophys. Acta (BBA)-Bioenerg.* **1999**, *1411*, 437–455. [CrossRef]
35. Shaul, P.W. Endothelial nitric oxide synthase, caveolae and the development of atherosclerosis. *J. Physiol.* **2003**, *547*, 21–33. [CrossRef] [PubMed]

36. Ischiropoulos, H.; Beckman, J.S. Oxidative stress and nitration in neurodegeneration: Cause, effect, or association? *J. Clin. Investig.* **2003**, *111*, 163–169. [CrossRef] [PubMed]
37. Zou, M.-H.; Cohen, R.A.; Ullrich, V. Peroxynitrite and Vascular Endothelial Dysfunction in Diabetes Mellitus. *Endothelium* **2004**, *11*, 89–97. [CrossRef]
38. Vishnyakova, T.G.; Bocharov, A.V.; Baranova, I.N.; Chen, Z.; Remaley, A.T.; Csako, G.; Eggerman, T.L.; Patterson, A.P. Binding and Internalization of Lipopolysaccharide by Cla-1, a Human Orthologue of Rodent Scavenger Receptor B1. *J. Biol. Chem.* **2003**, *278*, 22771–22780. [CrossRef]
39. Cai, L.; Ji, A.; de Beer, F.C.; Tannock, L.R.; van der Westhuyzen, D.R. SR-BI protects against endotoxemia in mice through its roles in glucocorticoid production and hepatic clearance. *J. Clin. Investig.* **2008**, *118*, 364–375. [CrossRef]
40. Guo, L.; Zheng, Z.; Ai, J.; Huang, B.; Li, X.-A. Hepatic Scavenger Receptor BI Protects Against Polymicrobial-induced Sepsis through Promoting LPS Clearance in Mice. *J. Biol. Chem.* **2014**, *289*, 14666–14673. [CrossRef] [PubMed]
41. Bulut, O.; Kilic, G.; Domínguez-Andrés, J.; Netea, M.G. Overcoming immune dysfunction in the elderly: Trained immunity as a novel approach. *Int. Immunol.* **2020**, *32*, 741–753. [CrossRef]
42. Bulut, O.; Kilic, G.; Domínguez-Andrés, J. Immune Memory in Aging: A Wide Perspective Covering Microbiota, Brain, Metabolism, and Epigenetics. *Clin. Rev. Allergy Immunol.* **2021**, *63*, 499–529. [CrossRef]
43. Wang, Q.; Guo, L.; Hao, D.; Ito, M.; Mineo, C.; Shaul, P.W.; Li, X.-A. Elevated free cholesterol levels due to impaired reverse cholesterol transport are a risk factor for polymicrobial sepsis in mice. *J. Biol. Chem.* **2024**. [CrossRef]
44. Cai, L.; Wang, Z.; Meyer, J.M.; Ji, A.; van der Westhuyzen, D.R. Macrophage SR-BI regulates LPS-induced pro-inflammatory signaling in mice and isolated macrophages. *J. Lipid Res.* **2012**, *53*, 1472–1481. [CrossRef] [PubMed]
45. Hao, D.; Guo, L.; Wang, Q.; Ito, M.; Huang, B.; Mineo, C.; Shaul, P.W.; Li, X.-A. Relative adrenal insufficiency is a risk factor for pediatric sepsis – a proof-of-concept study. *J. Infect. Dis.* **2023**, *229*, 1166–1177. [CrossRef] [PubMed]
46. Petta, I.; Dejager, L.; Ballegeer, M.; Lievens, S.; Tavernier, J.; De Bosscher, K.; Libert, C. The Interactome of the Glucocorticoid Receptor and Its Influence on the Actions of Glucocorticoids in Combatting Inflammatory and Infectious Diseases. *Microbiol. Mol. Biol. Rev.* **2016**, *80*, 495–522. [CrossRef]
47. Gilibert, S.; Galle-Treger, L.; Moreau, M.; Saint-Charles, F.; Costa, S.; Ballaire, R.; Couvert, P.; Carrié, A.; Lesnik, P.; Huby, T. Adrenocortical Scavenger Receptor Class B Type I Deficiency Exacerbates Endotoxic Shock and Precipitates Sepsis-Induced Mortality in Mice. *J. Immunol.* **2014**, *193*, 817–826. [CrossRef] [PubMed]
48. Ai, J.; Guo, L.; Zheng, Z.; Wang, S.-X.; Huang, B.; Li, X.-A. Corticosteroid Therapy Benefits Septic Mice With Adrenal Insufficiency But Harms Septic Mice Without Adrenal Insufficiency*. *Crit. Care Med.* **2015**, *43*, e490–e498. [CrossRef]
49. Hoekstra, M.; Meurs, I.; Koenders, M.; Out, R.; Hildebrand, R.B.; Kruijt, J.K.; Van Eck, M.; Van Berkel, T.J.C. Absence of HDL cholesteryl ester uptake in mice via SR-BI impairs an adequate adrenal glucocorticoid-mediated stress response to fasting. *J. Lipid Res.* **2008**, *49*, 738–745. [CrossRef] [PubMed]
50. Hoekstra, M.; van der Sluis, R.J.; Van Eck, M.; Van Berkel, T.J. Adrenal-specific scavenger receptor BI deficiency induces glucocorticoid insufficiency and lowers plasma very-low-density and low-density lipoprotein levels in mice. *Arterioscler. Thromb. Vasc. Biol.* **2013**, *33*, e39–e46. [CrossRef]
51. Ito, M.; Ye, X.; Wang, Q.; Guo, L.; Hao, D.; Howatt, D.; Daugherty, A.; Cai, L.; Temel, R.; Li, X.A. SR-BI (Scavenger Receptor BI), Not LDL (Low-Density Lipoprotein) Receptor, Mediates Adrenal Stress Response—Brief Report. *Arterioscler. Thromb. Vasc. Biol.* **2020**, *40*, 1830–1837. [CrossRef] [PubMed]
52. Allen, J.M.; Thompson, G.R.; Myant, N.B. Normal Adrenocortical Response to Adrenocorticotrophic Hormone in Patients with Homozygous Familial Hypercholesterolaemia. *Clin. Sci.* **1983**, *65*, 99–101. [CrossRef]
53. Wu, C.-H.; Guo, L.; Hao, D.; Wang, Q.; Ye, X.; Ito, M.; Huang, B.; Mineo, C.; Shaul, P.W.; Li, X.-A. Relative adrenal insufficiency is a risk factor and endotype of sepsis—A proof-of-concept study to support a precision medicine approach to guide glucocorticoid therapy for sepsis. *Front. Immunol.* **2023**, *13*, 1110516. [CrossRef] [PubMed]
54. Huang, L.; Chambliss, K.L.; Gao, X.; Yuhanna, I.S.; Behling-Kelly, E.; Bergaya, S.; Ahmed, M.; Michaely, P.; Luby-Phelps, K.; Darehshouri, A.; et al. SR-B1 drives endothelial cell LDL transcytosis via DOCK4 to promote atherosclerosis. *Nature* **2019**, *569*, 565–569. [CrossRef] [PubMed]
55. Leelahavanichkul, A.; Bocharov, A.V.; Kurlander, R.; Baranova, I.N.; Vishnyakova, T.G.; Souza, A.C.P.; Hu, X.; Doi, K.; Vaisman, B.; Amar, M.; et al. Class B scavenger receptor types I and II and CD36 targeting improves sepsis survival and acute outcomes in mice. *J. Immunol.* **2012**, *188*, 2749–2758. [CrossRef]
56. Guo, L.; Zheng, Z.; Ai, J.; Huang, B.; Li, X.-A. Comment on "Class B Scavenger Receptor Types I and II and CD36 Targeting Improves Sepsis Survival and Acute Outcomes in Mice". *J. Immunol.* **2012**, *189*, 501. [CrossRef]
57. Marshall, J.C. Why have clinical trials in sepsis failed? *Trends Mol. Med.* **2014**, *20*, 195–203. [CrossRef]
58. Coopersmith, C.M.M.; De Backer, D.M.; Deutschman, C.S.M.; Ferrer, R.; Lat, I.; Machado, F.R.; Martin, G.S.M.; Martin-Loeches, I.; Nunnally, M.E.M.; Antonelli, M.; et al. Surviving Sepsis Campaign: Research Priorities for Sepsis and Septic Shock. *Crit. Care Med.* **2018**, *46*, 1334–1356. [CrossRef]
59. Buchman, T.G.; Billiar, T.R.; Elster, E.; Kirk, A.D.; Rimawi, R.H.; Vodovotz, Y.; Zehnbauer, B.A. Precision Medicine for Critical Illness and Injury. *Crit. Care Med.* **2016**, *44*, 1635–1638. [CrossRef]
60. Peters Van Ton, A.M.; Kox, M.; Abdo, W.; Pickkers, P. Precision immunotherapy for sepsis. *Front. Immunol.* **2018**, *9*, 1926. [CrossRef]

61. Guo, L.; Wang, W.; Wang, Q.; Hao, D.; Ito, M.; Huang, B.; Mineo, C.; Shaul, P.W.; Choi, J.; Huang, L.F.; et al. The adrenal stress response is an essential host response against therapy-induced lethal immune activation. *Sci. Signal.* **2023**, *16*, eadd4900. [CrossRef]
62. Mirnezami, R.; Nicholson, J.; Darzi, A. Preparing for Precision Medicine. *N. Engl. J. Med.* **2012**, *366*, 489–491. [CrossRef]
63. Collins, F.S.; Varmus, H. A new initiative on precision medicine. *N. Engl. J. Med.* **2015**, *372*, 793–795. [CrossRef] [PubMed]
64. Golucci, A.P.B.S.; Marson, F.A.L.; Ribeiro, A.F.; Nogueira, R.J.N. Lipid profile associated with the systemic inflammatory response syndrome and sepsis in critically ill patients. *Nutrition* **2018**, *55–56*, 7–14. [CrossRef] [PubMed]
65. Kruger, P.; Bailey, M.; Bellomo, R.; Cooper, D.J.; Harward, M.; Higgins, A.; Howe, B.; Jones, D.; Joyce, C.; Kostner, K.; et al. A Multicenter Randomized Trial of Atorvastatin Therapy in Intensive Care Patients with Severe Sepsis. *Am. J. Respir. Crit. Care Med.* **2013**, *187*, 743–750. [CrossRef] [PubMed]
66. Hackam, D.G.; Mamdani, M.; Li, P.; A Redelmeier, D. Statins and sepsis in patients with cardiovascular disease: A population-based cohort analysis. *Lancet* **2006**, *367*, 413–418. [CrossRef]
67. Gupta, R.; Plantinga, L.C.; Fink, N.E.; Melamed, M.L.; Coresh, J.; Fox, C.S.; Levin, N.W.; Powe, N.R. Statin use and sepsis events [corrected] in patients with chronic kidney disease. *JAMA* **2007**, *297*, 1455–1464. [CrossRef]
68. Deshpande, A.; Pasupuleti, V.; Rothberg, M.B. Statin Therapy and Mortality from Sepsis: A Meta-analysis of Randomized Trials. *Am. J. Med.* **2015**, *128*, 410–417.e1. [CrossRef]
69. Patel, J.M.; Snaith, C.; Thickett, D.R.; Linhartova, L.; Melody, T.; Hawkey, P.; Barnett, A.H.; Jones, A.; Hong, T.; Cooke, M.W.; et al. Randomized double-blind placebo-controlled trial of 40 mg/day of atorvastatin in reducing the severity of sepsis in ward patients (ASEPSIS Trial). *Crit. Care* **2012**, *16*, R231. [CrossRef]
70. Rhodes, A.; Evans, L.E.; Alhazzani, W.; Levy, M.M.; Antonelli, M.; Ferrer, R.; Kumar, A.; Sevransky, J.E.; Sprung, C.L.; Nunnally, M.E.; et al. Surviving sepsis campaign: International guidelines for management of sepsis and septic shock: 2016. *Intensive Care Med.* **2017**, *43*, 304–377. [CrossRef] [PubMed]
71. Chaudhuri, D.M.; Nei, A.M.P.; Rochwerg, B.M.; Balk, R.A.M.; Asehnoune, K.; Cadena, R.M.; Carcillo, J.A.; Correa, R.; Drover, K.B.; Esper, A.M.M.; et al. 2024 Focused Update: Guidelines on Use of Corticosteroids in Sepsis, Acute Respiratory Distress Syndrome, and Community-Acquired Pneumonia. *Crit. Care Med.* **2024**, *52*, e219–e233. [CrossRef]

International Journal of
Molecular Sciences

MDPI

Review

Neonatal Fungemia by Non-Candida Rare Opportunistic Yeasts: A Systematic Review of Literature

Alexandra Mpakosi [1,*], Vasileios Cholevas [2], Joseph Meletiadis [3], Martha Theodoraki [4] and Rozeta Sokou [4,5,*]

1 Department of Microbiology, General Hospital of Nikaia "Agios Panteleimon", 18454 Piraeus, Greece
2 School of Medicine, University of Bologna, 40125 Bologna, Italy; billcholevas34@gmail.com
3 Clinical Microbiology Laboratory, Attikon University Hospital, Medical School, National and Kapodistrian University of Athens, 12462 Athens, Greece; jmeletiadis@med.uoa.gr
4 Neonatal Intensive Care Unit, General Hospital of Nikaia "Agios Panteleimon", 18454 Piraeus, Greece; anastasiosmmr@yahoo.gr
5 Neonatal Department, Aretaieio Hospital, National and Kapodistrian University of Athens, 11528 Athens, Greece
* Correspondence: alexiabakossi@yahoo.gr or ampakosi@auth.gr (A.M.); sokourozeta@yahoo.gr or rosesok@med.uoa.gr (R.S.)

Abstract: Fungal colonization poses a significant risk for neonates, leading to invasive infections such as fungemia. While *Candida* species are the most commonly identified pathogens, other rare yeasts are increasingly reported, complicating diagnosis and treatment due to limited data on antifungal pharmacokinetics. These emerging yeasts, often opportunistic, underscore the critical need for early diagnosis and targeted therapy in neonates. This systematic review aims to comprehensively analyze all published cases of neonatal fungemia caused by rare opportunistic yeasts, examining geographical distribution, species involved, risk factors, treatment approaches, and outcomes. Searching two databases (PubMed and SCOPUS), 89 relevant studies with a total of 342 cases were identified in the 42-year period; 62% of the cases occurred in Asia. *Pichia anomala* (31%), *Kodamaea ohmeri* (16%) and *Malassezia furfur* (15%) dominated. Low birth weight, the use of central catheters, prematurity, and the use of antibiotics were the main risk factors (98%, 76%, 66%, and 65%, respectively). 22% of the cases had a fatal outcome (80% in Asia). The highest mortality rates were reported in *Trichosporon beigelii* and *Trichosporon asahii* cases, followed by *Dirkmeia churashimamensis* cases (80%, 71%, and 42% respectively). Low birth weight, the use of central catheters, the use of antibiotics, and prematurity were the main risk factors in fatal cases (84%, 74%, 70%, and 67%, respectively). 38% of the neonates received fluconazole for treatment but 46% of them, died. Moreover, the rare yeasts of this review showed high MICs to fluconazole and this should be taken into account when planning prophylactic or therapeutic strategies with this drug. In conclusion, neonatal fungemia by rare yeasts is a life-threatening and difficult-to-treat infection, often underestimated and misdiagnosed.

Keywords: neonatal fungemia; rare opportunistic yeasts; non-*Candida* infection; premature neonates; low birth weight; fluconazole prophylaxis

1. Introduction

In recent years, there have been increasing cases of invasive fungal infections caused by rare yeasts, which comprise non-*Candida* and non-*Cryptococcus* species. These yeasts, although ubiquitous in the environment, have been defined as rare because they are almost never associated with human infections. However, these emerging species are increasingly harming human health, alarming the global scientific community. In 2022, recognizing the seriousness of this global health issue, the World Health Organization (WHO) introduced its first list of fungal "priority pathogens": https://iris.who.int/bitstream/handle/10665/363682/9789240060241-eng.pdf, access on 31 July 2024. This important initiative highlights the urgent need for policy reforms and enhanced research efforts, especially in understanding the spread of fungal diseases, emerging patterns of antifungal resistance, and identifying the populations most at risk for these infections. A significant concern in the management of these infections is the increasing resistance to existing antifungal therapies. This trend complicates treatment and highlights the need for new and more effective antifungal agents. Additionally, there is growing recognition of the role of fungal infections in worsening outcomes, particularly in critically ill and immunocompromised patients, including neonates.

Neonates, especially premature infants, are vulnerable organisms, easily colonized by fungi due to their immature immune system, poor skin, insufficient mucosal barriers, and multiple risk factors favoring fungal prevalence against normal flora.

Invasive fungal infections (IFIs) are a significant contributor to morbidity and mortality among neonates in neonatal intensive care units (NICUs), particularly affecting preterm infants and those with very low birth weight (VLBW, <1500 g birth weight [BW]) [1]. These neonates are especially vulnerable due to their compromised immune systems, exposure to broad-spectrum antibiotics, immature epithelial barriers, and frequent need for invasive procedures, which collectively heighten their risk for opportunistic fungal infections. The bulk of IFIs are attributed to *Candida* species [2]. Notably, invasive candidiasis (IC) ranks as the third leading cause of late-onset sepsis in VLBW neonates and is a major factor in morbidity and mortality within the NICU [3–6]. The prevalence of IC in NICUs varies widely, ranging from 0.5% to 20%, and is significantly influenced by the specific center and patient demographics. It is inversely related to gestational age and birth weight, with the highest rates (5–20%) observed among neonates with extremely low birth weight (ELBW) [2,3]. Recently, a global change in the epidemiology of candidemia has been observed, marked by the emergence of resistant non-albicans *Candida* species. Among these, *C. auris* has been spreading globally, causing outbreaks in hospitals among both pediatric and adult patients, particularly in ICUs, and has been highlighted in the CDC's report on urgent threats https://www.cdc.gov/antimicrobial-resistance/?CDC_AAref_Val=https://www.cdc.gov/DrugResistance/Biggest-Threats, access on 30 July 2024.

Fungal colonization is an important risk factor facilitating invasion, dissemination and eventually causing fungemia. Although *Candida* is the most commonly identified species of fungemia in neonates, other yeasts are also sporadically reported worldwide raising concerns due to difficulties in identification, limited pharmacokinetic data of the available antifungals, and lack of sufficient clinical and microbiological information. These rare yeasts are emerging, opportunistic pathogens that may lead to underdiagnosis of fungemia, delayed initiation of antifungal therapy, and often have fatal outcomes [4]. Therefore, an early and specific diagnosis and targeted treatment are critical, especially for neonates. To the best of our knowledge, there are no previous reviews of neonatal fungemia cases by rare opportunistic yeasts. The present study aims to provide a systematic review of all neonatal fungemia cases by rare opportunistic yeasts published in the literature.

2. Methods

A research methodological protocol was developed based on the PRISMA guidelines (presented as a Supplementary Material) [7] to collect and evaluate studies related to the subject under investigation. This protocol is registered in the PROSPERO database (CRD 42024561133).

2.1. Formulation of the Research Question

In order to clearly formulate the research question and facilitate a literature review, the PICO (Population, Intervention, Comparison, Outcome) framework was used:

- Population: Neonates
- Intervention: Rare opportunistic yeasts
- Comparison: Not required for this review
- Outcome: Cases of neonatal fungemia

2.2. Development of the Review Protocol

Research question: To conduct a review of all cases of neonatal fungemia from non-*Candida* rare opportunistic yeasts that have been published in the international literature.

Inclusion Criteria:

- Case reports and case series studies reporting on cases of neonatal fungemia from non-*Candida* rare opportunistic yeasts.
- Study designs focused on non-*Candida* rare opportunistic yeast infections, mainly defined as positive cultures from blood in neonates.
- Exclusion Criteria:
- Studies referring to other forms of fungal infections.
- Cases not involving neonates.
- Duplicate publications of the same cases.
- Review articles, systematic reviews, and meta-analyses. Conference proceedings will be excluded.
- Neonatal fungemia by *Candida* species

Main Outcomes:

1. Clinical presentation of non-*Candida* rare yeasts infections in neonates
2. Risk factors and characteristics of the affected population
3. Outcomes of the infections, including mortality

2.3. Search Strategy-Data Sources

The systematic literature review was conducted from June 2024 to July 2024. A systematic review of the existing literature was performed by searching the electronic databases PubMed and Scopus, with a final search date of 1 July 2024. The literature review was conducted using the following keywords: "neonatal fungemia", "rare yeasts", "non-*Candida* species", "fungal infections", "fungemia", "fungaemia", "neonates", "preterm infants", "preterm neonate*", "infant*", "newborn*", "case report", "case series", "case", in combination with Boolean operators (AND, OR). Additionally, to minimize the risk of missing studies and fully cover the extent of available literature, a manual electronic search and review of the references of each selected study, as well as references from previous systematic reviews in the same research field, was conducted.

2.4. Conflict Resolution

Screening, data extraction, and quality assessment were conducted independently by two researchers (AM and RS), with conflicts resolved through discussion and consensus between the researchers or, if necessary, by a third researcher (JM).

2.5. Data Synthesis and Presentation

Data were recorded in tabular form according to the following criteria: type of opportunistic yeasts, day of life when the infection manifested, comorbidities, risk factors, prematurity, administration of total parenteral nutrition, placement of central catheters, mechanical ventilation, and prior administration of broad-spectrum antibiotics, number of participants, number of events, and other relevant criteria for grouping the study population (subpopulations of neonates: preterm neonates, very low birth weight neonates, cardiac surgery or other surgical cases, neonates with congenital anomalies, etc.), year of publication.

3. Results

From the electronic database search, a total of 1990 studies were retrieved. Among these, 142 duplicate entries were identified and subsequently removed using the duplicate removal tool in the reference management software (EndNote X8). After carefully reading the titles and abstracts of the remaining studies, 1704 studies were excluded either because their subject matter did not serve the purpose of the review or because they met some of the exclusion criteria already visible at the title and abstract level. The careful reading of the full text of the 144 remaining studies revealed that only 89 studies met all the inclusion criteria and were included in this review. In total, 342 cases of neonates with rare opportunistic yeast infections were recorded. The flow diagram is presented in Figure 1.

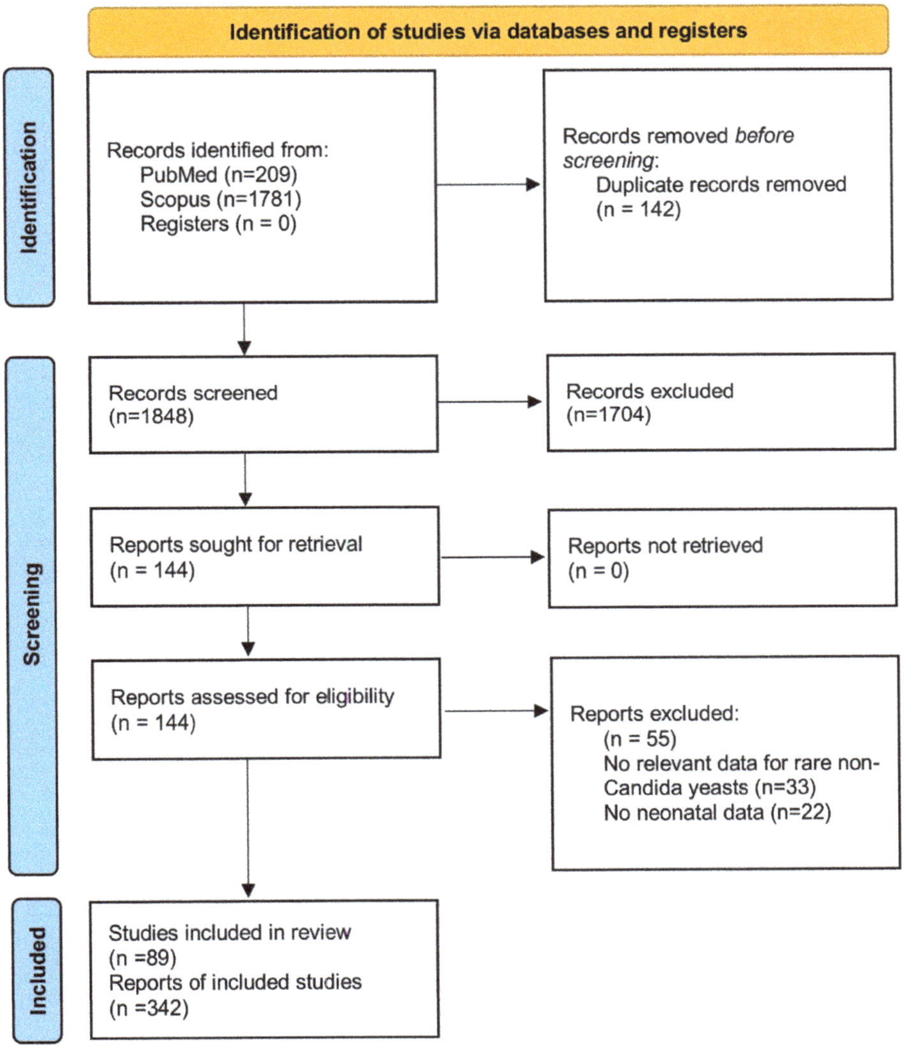

Figure 1. Flow diagram of the systematic review.

3.1. *Species Taxonomy and Geographical Distribution*

The first report of neonatal fungemia from rare non-*Candida* yeasts was in 1981. Since then, there have been several cases and studies examining the incidence, diagnosis, and treatment of these infections. Over the past 42 years, 342 cases of neonatal fungemia caused by rare non-*Candida* yeasts have been reported. (Tables 1 and 2, Figure 2)

Table 1. Neonatal fungemia cases by rare opportunistic yeasts published in literature, since 1981.

Location	Year	Cases	Yeast Species	Identification Method	Reference
USA	1981	1 case	*Malassezia furfur*	NA	[8]
USA	1984	4 cases	*Malassezia furfur*	NA	[9]
USA	1985	3 cases	*Malassezia furfur*	NA	[10]
UK	1986	7 cases	*Hansenula anomala*	API 20C	[11]
USA	1987	5 cases	*Malassezia furfur*	NA	[12]
USA	1987	6 cases	*Malassezia furfur*	NA	[13]
USA	1989	3 cases	*Malassezia furfur*	NA	[14]
BELGIUM	1989	6 cases	*Malassezia furfur*	NA	[15]
NY	1991	1 case	*Malassezia furfur*	NA	[16]
USA	1991	2 cases	*Malassezia furfur*	NA	[17]
FRANCE	1991	1 case	*Malassezia furfur*	NA	[18]
USA	1992	1 case	*Trichosporon beigelii*	NA	[19]
EUROPE	1992	1 case	*Trichosporon asteroides*	NA	[20]
NY	1993	2 cases	*Trichosporon beigelii*	BacT/Alert	[21]
ATLANTA	1994	5 cases	*Malassezia pachydermatis*	NA	[22]
USA	1997	2 cases	*Trichosporon beigelii*	NA	[23]
USA	1997	1 case	*Cryptococcus laurentii*	NA	[24]
USA	1998	8 cases	*Malassezia pachydermatis*	Molecular	[25]
UK	1998	1 case	*Trichosporon beigelii*	API 32 ATB	[26]
CHANDIGARH	1999	10 cases	*Pichia anomala*	NA	[27]
SPAIN	2000	2 case	*Saccharomyces cerevisiae*	Vitek 2 API 20C Molecular	[28]
TAIWAN	2000	1 case	*Hansenula anomala*	NA	[29]
MALAYSIA	2000	1 case	*Hansenula anomala*	NA	[30]
INDIA	2001	33 cases	*Pichia anomala*	Morphology Biochemical tests	[31]
BRAZIL	2001	4 cases	*Pichia anomala*	NA	[32]
TAIWAN	2001	1 case	*Cryptococcus laurentii*	Morphology India ink Vitek 2	[33]
SWEDEN	2001	8 cases	*Malassezia pachydermatis*	NA	[34]
EUROPE	2002	1 case	*Trichosporon asahii*	API ID 32C	[35]
TURKEY	2003	1 case	*Trichosporon asahii*	NA	[36]
TURKEY	2003	3 cases	*Trichosporon mucoides*	API AUX C	[37]
ARGENTINA	2003	1 case	*Hansenula anomala*	API ID 32C	[38]

Table 1. *Cont.*

Location	Year	Cases	Yeast Species	Identification Method	Reference
TURKEY	2004	1 case	*Pichia anomala*	API ID 32C	[39]
TURKEY	2005	1 case	*Saccharomyces cerevisiae*	NA	[40]
QATAR	2006	1 case	*Kodamaea ohmeri*	Vitek 2 API ID 32C Molecular	[41]
USA	2006	1 case	*Pichia fabianii*	Molecular	[42]
BRAZIL	2006	2 cases	*Pichia anomala*	Vitek 2	[43]
ITALY	2006	4 cases	*Rhodotorula mucilaginosa*	Vitek 2 API ID 32C	[44]
SOUTH KOREA	2007	1 case	*Kodamaea ohmeri*	Vitek 2 API20C	[45]
THAILAND	2008	1 case	*Cryptococcus neoformans*	NA	[46]
EUROPE	2008	1 case	*Trichosporon asahii*	Vitek 2	[47]
INDIA	2009	1 case	*Kodamaea ohmeri*	BacT/Alert 3D API ID 32C	[48]
BRAZIL	2009	1 case	*Trichosporon* spp.	Morphology	[49]
GREECE	2009	1 case	*Cryptococcus terreus*	Morphology MALDI-TOF MS Molecular	[50]
FRANCE	2010	1 case	*Pichia fabianii*	Molecular	[51]
INDIA	2011	1 case	*Rhodotorula mucilaginosa*	Morphology API 20C	[52]
ITALY	2011	1 case	*Malassezia furfur*	Morphology Molecular	[53]
KUWAIT	2011	1 case	*Kodamaea ohmeri*	Vitek 2 API 20C AUX Molecular	[54]
INDIA	2012	8 cases	*Trichosporon asahii*	Vitek 2	[55]
TAIWAN	2013	6 cases	*P. anomala (C. pelliculosa)*	API-32C Mini API Molecular	[56]
SOUTH AMERICA	2013	4 cases	*P. anomala (C. pelliculosa)*	Morphology Molecular	[57]
GREECE	2013	1 case	*Malassezia furfur*	Morphology MALDI-TOF MS Molecular	[50]
ITALY	2013	6 cases	*Malassezia furfur*	Vitek2 MALDI-TOF MS Molecular	[58]
TUNISIA	2013	1 case	*Saccharomyces cerevisiae*	NA	[59]
CHINA	2013	6 cases	*Pichia ohmeri*	Molecular	[60]
CHINA	2013	1 case	*Pichia fabianii*	API 20C AUX Molecular	[61]
CHINA	2013	1 case	*Kodamaea ohmeri*	API 20C AUX Vitek 2 Molecular	[62]
INDIA	2013	38 cases	*Kodamaea ohmeri*	Molecular	[63]
INDIA	2014	1 case	*Kodamaea ohmeri*	BacT/ALERT Vitek2	[64]

Table 1. *Cont.*

Location	Year	Cases	Yeast Species	Identification Method	Reference
INDIA	2014	1 case	*Pseudozyma aphidis*	API ID 32C Vitek 2 Molecular	[65]
KUWAIT	2014	1 case	*Malassezia pachydermatis*	Vitek 2 MALDI–TOF MS Molecular	[66]
INDIA	2015	2 cases	*Kodamaea ohmeri*	Vitek 2 Molecular	[67]
CROATIA	2015	2 cases	*Cyberlindnera fabianii*	Molecular	[68]
ASIA	2015	3 cases	*Trichosporon asahii*	NA	[69]
NIGERIA	2015	1 case	*Moesziomyces bullatus*	Molecular	[70]
COLOMBIA	2016	1 case	*Kodamaea ohmeri*	Vitek 2	[71]
TURKEY	2017	1 case	*Wickerhamomyces anomalus*	Vitek 2	[72]
INDIA	2017	9 cases	*Pichia kudriavzevii*	Molecular	[73]
INDIA	2017	4 cases	*Rhodotorula glutinis*	NA	[74]
INDIA	2017	8 cases	*Cyberlindnera fabianii*	Molecular	[75]
INDIA	2017	1 case	*Wickerhamomyces anomalus*	Molecular	[75]
INDIA	2017	2 cases	*Saccharomyces cerevisiae*	Molecular	[76]
INDIA	2018	1 case	*Cryptococcus laurentii*	Vitek 2	[77]
PORTUGAL	2018	1 case	*Malassezia furfur*	MALDI–TOF MS	[78]
ITALY	2018	9 cases	*Malassezia furfur*	BacT/Alert	[79]
KUWAIT	2019	10 cases	*Cyberlindnera fabianii*	Molecular	[80]
TAIWAN	2019	1 case	*Malassezia furfur*	BacT/Alert	[81]
TAIWAN	2020	4 cases	*Malassezia pachydermatis*	BD BACTEC FX	[82]
CALIFORNIA	2020	3 cases	*Malassezia pachydermatis*	Molecular	[83]
INDIA	2020	12 cases	*Dirkmeia churashimaensis*	Molecular	[84]
INDIA	2020	2 cases	*Cyberlindnera fabianii*	MALDI-TOF-MS	[85]
KUWAIT	2021	1 case	*Papiliotrema laurentii*	Vitek 2 Molecular	[86]
COLOMBIA	2021	1 case	*Malassezia sympodialis*	Molecular	[87]
CHINA	2021	1 case	*P. anomala (C. pelliculosa)*	Molecular	[88]
CHINA	2021	21 cases	*P. anomala (C. pelliculosa)*	Vitek MS	[89]
CHINA	2021	14 cases	*P. anomala (C. pelliculosa)*	Molecular	[90]
GREECE	2022	1 case	*Moesziomyces aphidis*	Vitek 2 Molecular	[91]
KUWAIT	2022	1 case	*Lodderomyces elongisporus*	Vitek 2 Molecular	[92]
BRAZIL	2023	1 case	*Lodderomyces elongisporus*	Molecular	[93]
NIGERIA	2023	1 case	*Cryptococcus laurentii*	Vitek 2	[94]
INDIA	2023	1 case	*Aureobasidium melanogenum*	Molecular	[95]
INDIA	2023	1 case	*Kodamaea ohmeri*	Vitek 2 MALDI–TOF	[96]

NA Not available, API Analytical Profile Index, MALDI-TOF Matrix-assisted laser desorption/ionization time-of-flight, MALDI-TOF MS matrix-assisted laser desorption ionization-time of flight mass spectrometry.

Table 2. Cases per decade.

Years	Cases
1981–1990	35
1991–2000	39
2001–2010	69
2011–2023	199

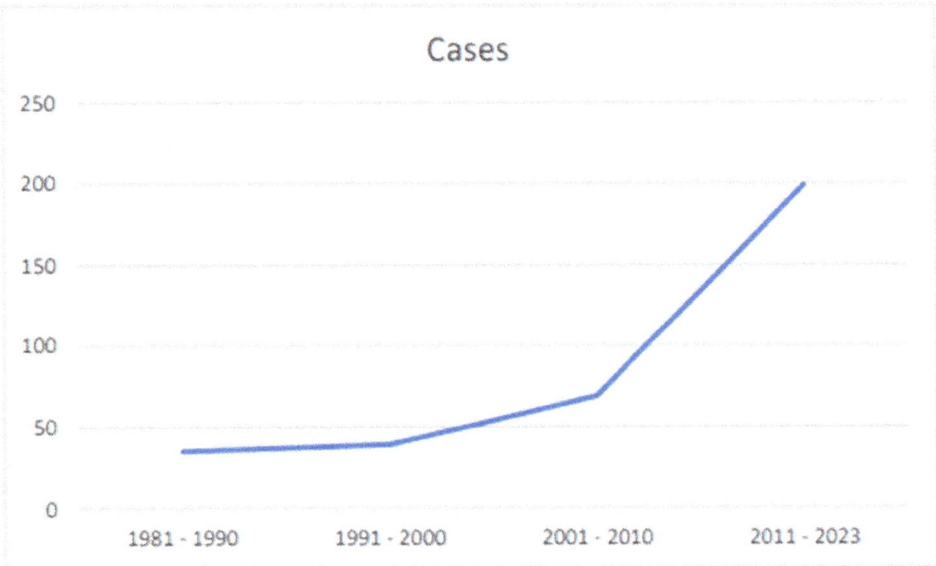

Figure 2. Published cases over the years.

Regarding the geographical distribution of all reported cases, 221 (65%) were from Asia, 55 (16%) from Europe, 48 (14%) from the USA, 15 (4%) from South America, and 3 (1%) from Africa (Figures 3 and 4). More specifically, *Pichia anomala* (synonyms: *Candida pelliculosa, Hansenula anomala, Wickerhamomyces anomalus*)was isolated in 108 (31%) cases (82% in Asia), *Kodamaea ohmeri* (previously known as *Pichia ohmeri*) in 54 (16%) cases (94% in Asia), *Malassezia furfur* in 51 (15%) cases (48% in USA, 48% in Europe), *Malassezia pachydermatis* in 29 (8%) cases (55% in USA), *Pichia fabianii* (synonym: *Cyberlindnera fabianii*) in 25 (7%) cases (84% in Asia), *Trichosporon asahii* in 14 (4%) cases (92% of the cases were in Asia), *Dirkmeia churashimaensis* in 12 (3%) cases (100% in Asia), *Pichia kudriavzevii* in 9 (3%) cases (100% in Asia), *Trichosporon beigelii* in 6 (2%) cases (83% in USA), *Saccharomyces cerevisiae* in 6 (2%) cases (67% in Asia), *Rhodotorula mucilaginosa* in 5 cases (1%) (80% in Europe), *Cryptococcus laurentii* (synonym: *Papiliotrema laurentii*) in 5 (1%) cases (75% in Asia), *Rhodotorula glutinis* in 4 (1%) cases (100% in Asia), *Trichosporon mucoides* in 3 cases (100% in Asia), *Moesziomyces (Pseudozyma) aphidis* in 2 cases (in Asia and in Europe), *Lodderomyces elongisporus* in 2 cases (in Latin America and in Asia), *Trichosporon* spp. in one case in Europe, *Malassezia sympodialis* in one case in South America, *Moesziomyces (Pseudozyma) bullatus* in one case in Africa, *Trichosporon asteroides* in one case in Europe, *Cryptococcus neoformans* in one case in Asia, *Aureobasidium melanogenum* in one case in Asia, and *Cryptococcus terreus* in one case in Europe (Figure 5).

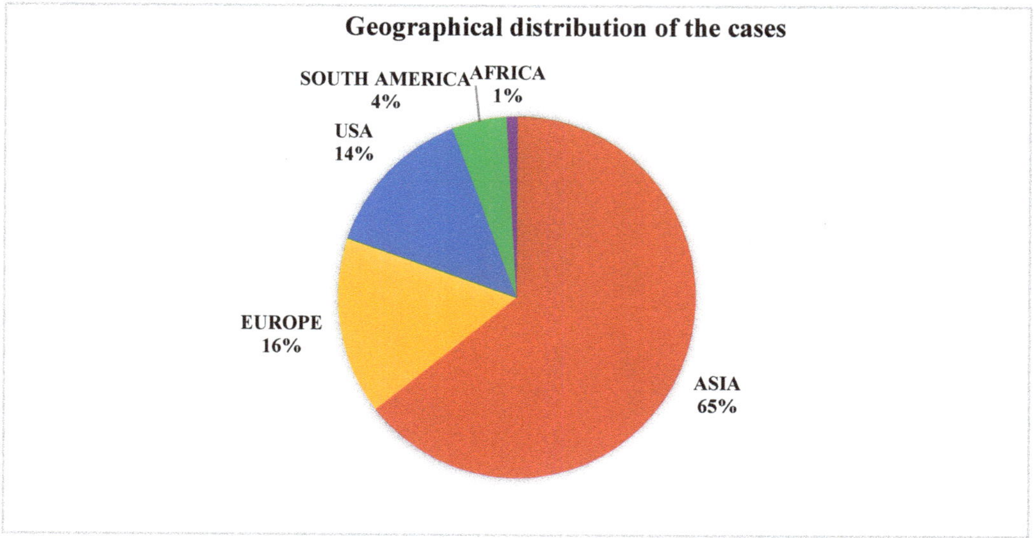

Figure 3. Geographical distribution of the cases.

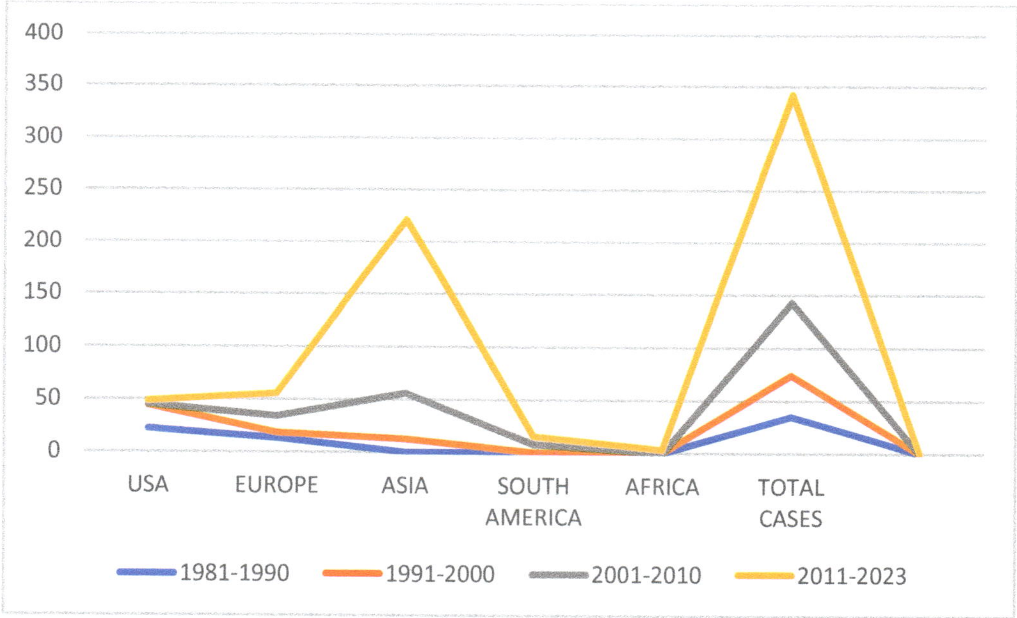

Figure 4. Geographical distribution of the cases over the decades.

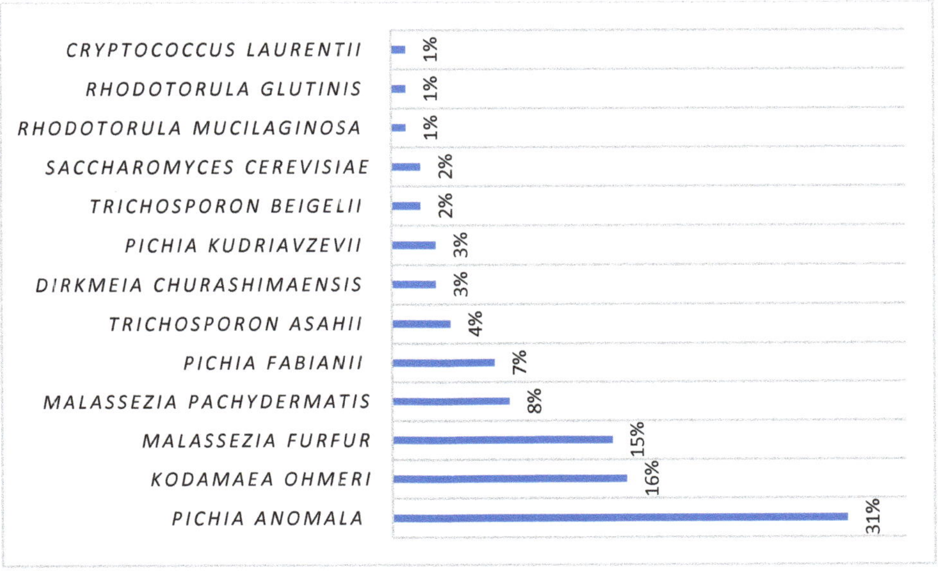

Figure 5. Neonatal fungemia by rare yeast species: Published data since 1981.

3.2. Risk Factors

Low birth weight, the use of central catheters, and prematurity are the three dominant risk factors for fungemia development (Figure 6).

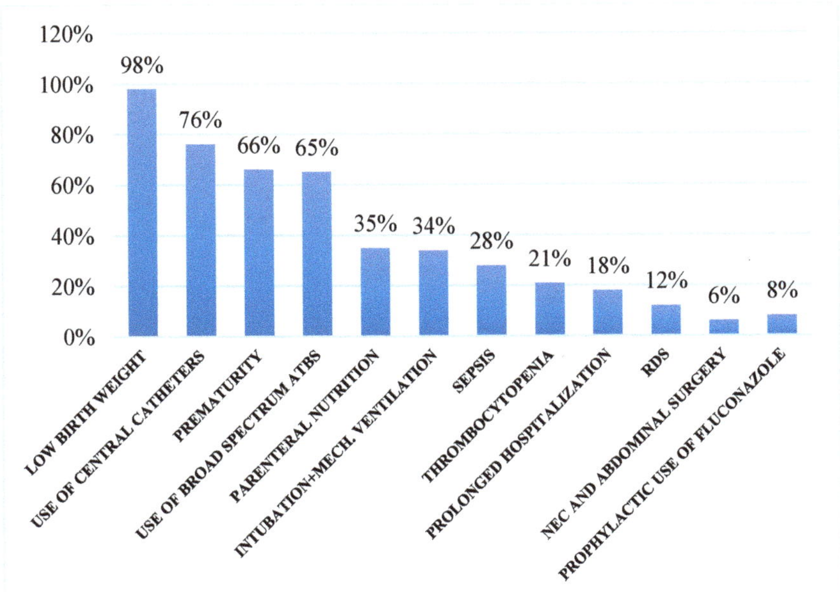

Figure 6. Reported risk factors. (Intubation + mech. Ventilation: Intubation + mechanical ventilation, RDS: Respiratory distress syndrome).

3.3. Outcome

In 12% of the cases, the outcome was not reported. Among the remaining cases, 22% of the neonates, died. Moreover, 80% of the cases with a fatal outcome were reported from Asia (Figure 7). The highest mortality rates were noted in cases of fungemia caused by the *Trichosporon* species (Figure 8).

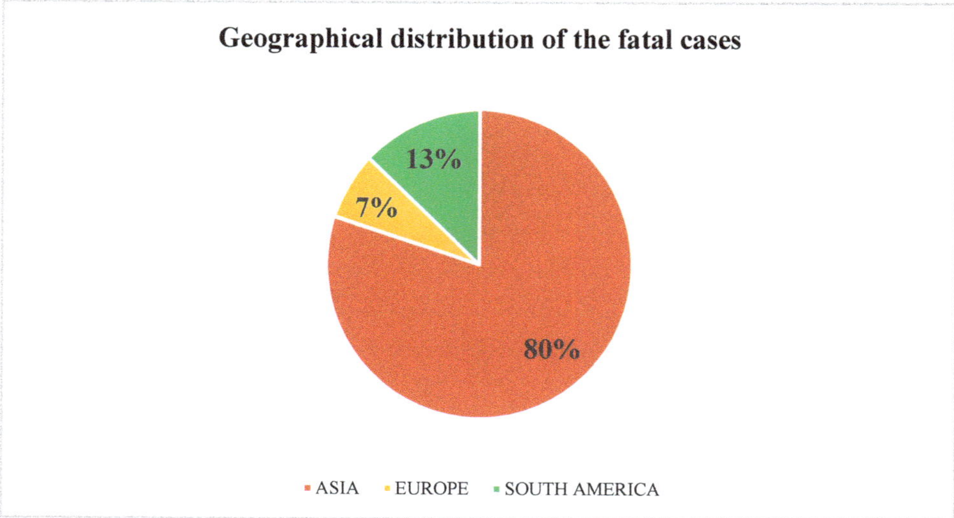

Figure 7. Mortality rates by continent.

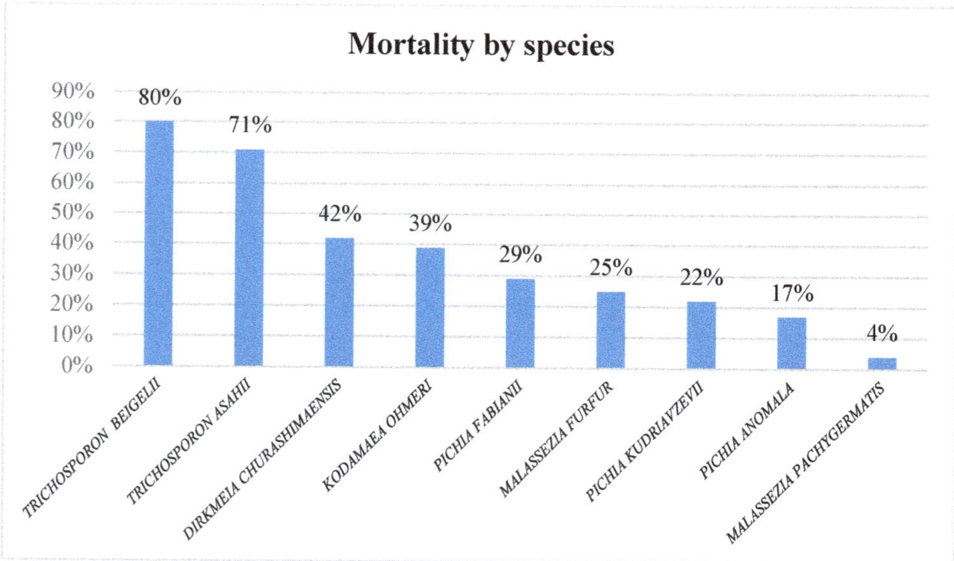

Figure 8. Mortality rates by species.

Neonates with Moesziomyces bullatus, Aureobasidium melanogenum, and Lodderomyces elongisporus fungemia also died.

The following risk factors were most commonly reported in total cases, compared to those associated with survival or exitus (Table 3).

Table 3. Risk factors (total cases/survival/exitus).

Risk Factors			
	Total Cases $n = 342$ **NA Outcome** $n = 41$	**Survival** $n = 235/301$ **(78 %)**	**Exitus** $n = 66/301$ **(22%)**
Low birth weight	335/342 (98%)	181/235 (77%)	55/66 (84%)
Central catheters	260/342 (76%)	178/235 (76%)	49/66 (74%)
Prematurity	226/342 (66%)	141/235 (60%)	44/66 (67%)
Broad spectrum antibiotics	222/342 (65%)	153/235 (65%)	46/66 (70%)
Parenteral nutrition	120/342 (35%)	89/235 (38%)	14/66 (21%)
Intubation/mechanical ventilation	116/342 (34%)	56/235 (24%)	43/66 (65%)
Sepsis	96/342 (28%)	63/235 (27%)	28/66 (43%)
Thrombocytopenia	72/342 (21%)	61/235 (26%)	14/66 (21%)
Prolonged hospitalization	61/342 (18%)	61/235 (26%)	28/66 (43%)
Respiratory distress syndrome	41/342 (12%)	28/235 (12%)	12/66 (19%)
Use of fluconazole	27/342 (8%)	9/235 (4%)	3/66 (5%)

NA (Not available) Outcome $n = 41$ (12%). Available Outcome $n = 301$ (88%).

3.4. *Antifungal Susceptibility*

Antifungal susceptibility testing was not reported in all cases. Nevertheless, the available data are presented in Table 4.

3.5. *Treatment*

The antifungal treatments varied notably among the cases, with Fluconazole and Amphotericin B being the most frequently administered medications. Timely removal (or replacement) of central venous catheters within 24 h of a positive blood culture is a crucial aspect of treatment. Conversely, delayed removal or replacement of central venous catheters in neonates with fungemia has been linked to higher mortality and morbidity. Our review and the available data indicated that only 18% of catheters were removed as part of the treatment intervention (Figure 9 and Table 5).

Table 4. Antifungal susceptibility testing of species. Minimum inhibitory concentrations in (mg/L).

Yeast	Number of Isolates	AMB	FLC	VRC	POS	ITC	ISA	5-FC	AFG	MFG	CAS	Method Used	References
Kodamaea ohmeri	1	0.064	32	NA	NA	0.25	NA	<0.002	NA	NA	NA	Etest	[41]
	1	0.023	4	0.047	0.012	0.125		0.032	0.064	0.125	0.25	Etest	[54]
	38	0.25–1	0.5–64	0.03–8	0.06–4	0.06–4	NA	NA	NA	NA	0.12–1	CLSI	[63]
	2	0.25	4	0.25	NA	NA	NA	1	NA	NA	0.25	VITEK2	[67]
	1	<0.5	NA	NA	NA	NA	NA	<1	NA	NA	<0.25	VITEK2	[64]
Cyberlindnera/Pichia fabianii	1	0.03	8	NA	NA	NA	NA	0.125	NA	NA	NA	NCCLS	[42]
	1	0.5	2	NA	NA	NA	NA	0.25	NA	NA	NA	Etest	[51]
	8	0.75–12	0.5–16	NA	NA	NA	NA	NA	NA	NA	NA	Etest	[75]
	1	1	≤1	0.125	NA	2	NA	≤4	NA	NA	NA	CLSI	[61]
	2	NA	NA	NA	NA	NA	NA	NA	0.016–0.064	1–4	0.125–0.19	EUCAST	[68]
Pichia anomala (Candida pelliculosa)	2	0.023–0.032	3–4	0.064–0.125	NA	NA	NA	NA	NA	NA	NA	Etest	[43]
	33	NA	Only one isolate >64	NA	NA	NA	NA	NA	NA	NA	NA	CLSI	[31]
	6	1–2	0.125	NA	2	NA	NA	NA	NA	0.25–0.5	2	CLSI	[56]
	21	<0.5	2–4	0.125–0.25	NA	0.125–0.25	NA	<4	NA	NA	NA	CLSI	[89]
Pichia kudriavzevii	9	1	2–16	0.25	0.25–1	0.25–0.5	NA	NA	0.25–0.5	0.25–0.5	0.25–0.5	CLSI	[73]
Moesziomyces (Pseudozyma) aphidis	1	2	<0.125	8	0.03	0.03	≤0.016	>64	>8	>8	>8	EUCAST	[91]
Moesziomyces (Pseudozyma) bullatus	1	1	128	0.03	0.03	0.12	NA	64	8	8	8	Sensititre YeastOne Y010 microdilution method	[70]
Dirkmeia (Pseudozyma) churashimaensis	12	0.198	1 to 4	0.03–0.125	0.03–0.25	0.03–0.25	0.03–0.125	0.157	>8	>8	>8	CLSI	[84]
Rhodotoroula mucilaginosa	4	0.25	>256	2	NA	2	NA	0.125	NA	NA	NA	NA	[44]
	1	1.5	>256	0.38	NA	NA	NA	NA	NA	NA	>16	Etest	[52]
Cryptococcus laurentii	1	0.25	4	NA	NA	NA	NA	NA	NA	NA	NA	NCCLS	[33]

Table 4. *Cont.*

Yeast	Number of Isolates	AMB	FLC	VRC	POS	ITC	ISA	5-FC	AFG	MFG	CAS	Method Used	References
	1	0.25	2	NA	NA	NA	NA	NA	NA	NA	NA	NA	[77]
Cryptococcus terreus	1	0.125–1.5	128–256	0.125–0.5	0.25–0.5	NA	1	8–32	8–32	8–32	8–32	broth microdilution method Micronaut-AM and E-test	[50]
Malassezia furfur	1	0.19	0.25	0.094	0.094	0.125	0.5	16	32	32	32	MIC method on modified RPMI 1640 agar	[50]
Malassezia pachydermatis	1	0.19	>256	0.012	0.016	NA	NA	>32	NA	NA	>32	Etest	[66]

AMB: Amphotericin B, FLC: Fluconazole, VRC: Voriconazole, POS: Posaconazole, ITC: Itraconazole, ISA: Isavuconazole, 5-FC: Flucytosine, AFG: Anidulafungin, MFG: Micafungin, CAS: Caspofungin, NA: Not available, MIC: minimum inhibitory concentration, CLSI: Clinical and Laboratory Standards Institute, NCCLS: National Committee for Clinical Laboratory Standards, EUCAST: European Committee on Antimicrobial Susceptibility Testing.

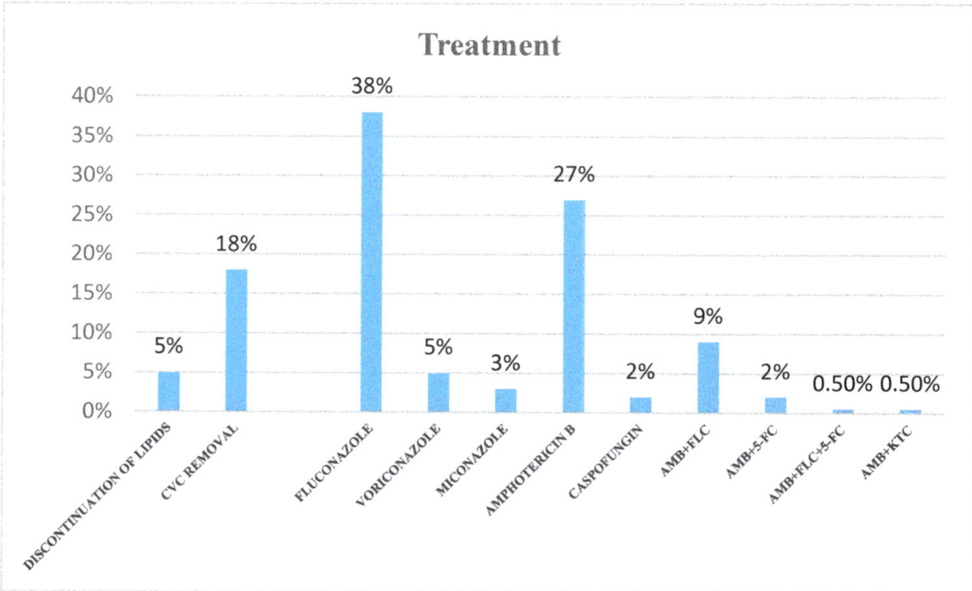

Figure 9. Treatment of fungemia cases (from available data). Amphotericin B (AmB), Fluconazole (FLC), Voriconazole (VOR), Miconazole (MIC), Caspofungin (CAS), 5-FC (5-flucytosine), KTC (ketoconazole).

Table 5. Treatment administered to neonates who survived and to whom died (survival/exitus). Amphotericin B (AmB), Fluconazole (FLC), Voriconazole (VOR), Miconazole (MIC), Caspofungin (CAS), 5-FC (5-flucytosine), KTC (ketoconazole).

Treatment	Survival	Exitus
CVC removal	21%	3%
Fluconazole (FLC)	30%	46%
Voriconazole (VOR)	5%	3%
Miconazole (MIC)	3%	2%
Caspofungin (CAS)	2%	0% or NA
Amphotericin B (AmB)	21%	33%
AmB + FLC	8%	10%
AmB + 5-FC (5-flucytosine)	4%	3%
AmB + FLC + 5-FC	4%	2%
AmB + KTC (ketoconazole)	1%	0% or NA

Most yeasts of this review have been recognized for decades as fungal contaminants but not as human pathogens. Systemic infections caused by them have been considered to be rare and most published studies to date are sporadic cases from all over the world. According to the data above, the majority of neonatal fungemia cases were reported in Asia, where developing countries often have low socio-economic conditions and living standards, with shortages in resources, infrastructure, and modern methods of diagnosing infections, as well as insufficient surveillance, legislation, infection control measures, and inadequately trained medical personnel who lack sufficient information about rare fungi [96]. To the best of our knowledge, from 1981 to 1990 no cases of neonatal fungemia from Asia were published and this is probably explained by the above.

Fluconazole prophylaxis is recommended worldwide in preterm infants < 1000gr from birth and until they no longer require central or peripheral catheters, as it is assumed to decrease mortality [96]. According to the respective guidelines, a third-generation cephalosporin therapy, duration of treatment with a systemic broad-spectrum antibiotic for more than 10 days, fungal colonization, and the use of a central venous catheter, are additional factors for prophylactic administration of fluconazole in such vulnerable organisms [97].

A previous systematic review and meta–analysis showed that prophylactic administration of fluconazole in different regimens may reduce mortality. Furthermore, prophylactic administration of the same regimens of fluconazole in ELBW neonates may reduce the incidence of mortality due to invasive fungal infections [98]. In addition, amphotericin B is not commercially available in 42 developing countries and is not licensed in 22 countries, making fluconazole an effective alternative therapy [96]. Nevertheless, the overuse of fluconazole in these countries, as a cheap prophylaxis in preterm low birth weight neonates, may contribute to infection development by fluconazole-resistant species [96,99]. The current study highlighted, in agreement with previous findings, the high fluconazole-resistant rates of rare yeast species such as *Pichia* spp., *Kodamaea ohmeri*, *Trichosporon* spp., *Rhodotorula* spp., *Saccharomyces cerevisiae*, etc. [100,101]. Therefore, the isolates of the present review showed elevated fluconazole MICs. This may explain why fluconazole was not the appropriate antifungal agent against those uncommon yeast species, despite the fact that it had been preferred as a treatment in 38% of all the fungemia cases. Unfortunately, 46% of the neonates who had received fluconazole therapy died. Therefore, the prophylactic use of fluconazole in neonatal intensive care units (NICUs) should be done with care to avoid resistance development and the subsequent selection of resistant species or species with reduced azole susceptibility [101]. Alternatively, nystatin is inexpensive, well-tolerated, safe, and so far with good results when prophylactically administered to preterm infants with risk factors [102,103].

4. Discussion

In our review the highest mortality was revealed in *Trichosporon* fungemia cases: 80% by *T. beigelii* and 71% by *T. asahii*. Previous studies have demonstrated that *Trichosporon* species were more competent than other basidiomycetes such as *Rhodotorula* spp. and *Cryptococcus* spp., to produce dense biofilms, resistant to triazoles or amphotericin B [104–106]. This seems to agree with our results in which all the neonatal fungemia cases by *Rhodotorula* spp. and *Cryptococcus* spp., showed zero mortality rates, despite their ability to produce biofilms on the medical devices. Previous research revealed the isolation of *Trichosporon* spp. from the hospital environment and the skin of premature neonates. Moreover, *T. beigelii* (*T. cutaneum*) was more often reported in these older studies as the causative organism of invasive infections. Nevertheless, *T. asahii* is now recognized as the dominant cause of invasive trichosporonosis threatening patients in immunosuppression and risk factors, such as neutropenia, prematurity, AIDS, extensive burns, use of catheters, broad-spectrum antibiotics or corticosteroids, mechanical ventilation, heart valve surgery, etc. Trichosporonosis is a difficult-to-treat infection due to the frequent resistance of yeast, as well as to amphotericin B, fluconazole, and combinations of the two. Nevertheless, voriconazole, posaconazole, and ravuconazole seem to act more effectively against *Trichosporon* species [105].

According to our data, *P. fabianii* fungemia cases demonstrated 29% mortality. *P. fabianii* (*Candida fabianii*, *Cyberlindnera fabianii*) is an opportunistic, emerging yeast species and may cause invasive bloodstream infections often with fatal outcomes, mainly due to its characteristic ability to produce biofilms causing resistance to antifungals [107]. Previous studies reported that *P. fabianii* may develop resistance to fluconazole, voriconazole, caspofungin, and amphotericin B [108,109].

P. anomala (*Wickerhamomyces anomalus*) is a plant pathogen and opportunistic cause of fungemia in both immunocompetent and immunocompromised patients. In our study, 17% of the cases had a fatal outcome. *Pichia anomala* has previously been shown to exhibit variable antifungal susceptibility with fluconazole resistance predominance [110,111]. This seems to agree with our findings and must be taken into account in NICUs for effective antifungal prophylactic and therapeutic strategies.

Fungemia by *P. kudriavzevii* (*Candida krusei*) is another life-threatening and difficult-to-treat infection due to its intrinsic resistance to fluconazole and the ability for rapid resistance development to other antifungal drugs. Vulnerable patients suffering from gastrointestinal diseases, who had previously received antibiotics, especially carbapenems, and prophylactic fluconazole, are at greater risk of developing invasive infection. In addition, whenever outbreaks occurred, sink traps and surfaces, intravenous dextrose multi-electrolyte infusion bottles, suction devices, pediatric emergency wards, and hands of health care personnel were reported as the most common sources of transmission [110]. Moreover, this species is able to produce a robust biofilm, formed by multiple layers of pseudohyphae in the polymer matrix [111]

All 12 of the neonatal fungemia cases by *Dirkmeia* occurred in the same NICU of a multispecialty hospital in Delhi with a 42% mortality rate (5/12). Surveillance cultures were obtained, but the source of infection was not identified. Infection control measures appeared to be effective as no further cases of *Dirkmeia* fungemia were reported [82]. All the twelve isolates of *Dirkmeia* had high minimum inhibitory concentrations for echinocandins and low minimum inhibitory concentrations for azoles, amphotericin B, and flucytosine.

39% of the neonates who developed fungemia by *K. ohmeri*, died. Chakrabarti et al. showed that prolonged hospitalization, piperacillin-tazobactam administration, endotracheal intubation, and mechanical ventilation, were major risk factors for the fungemia development by this rare yeast. They also demonstrated that the patients with *K. ohmeri* fungemia had significantly higher (50%) mortality than other groups of patients (some of them with *C. tropicalis* fungemia and others without fungemia), mainly due to the virulence mechanisms of the yeast species [61]. The identification of *K. ohmeri* in the laboratory is a challenge. On *Candida* chromogenic agar the color of *K. ohmeri* colonies changes from pink to blue within 48 h. Usually, species identification is performed by automated identification systems such as API 20C, Vitek 2 ID YST, and Microscan with molecular methods. For molecular identification PCR amplification is used followed by sequencing of 18S rRNA, the D1/D2 domains of 26SrRNA, the internal transcriber spacer 1/2 (ITS) of the ribosomal DNA,28SrRNA, and/or 5.8SrRNA. The pulsed field gel electrophoresis for karyotyping has been also used. Restriction endonuclease analysis of NotI-digested DNA (REAG-N) is used for genotyping of the clinical isolates of *K. ohmeri*. Fluorescent amplified fragment length polymorphism was used by Chakrabarti et al. for molecular typing. Moreover, in their study, *K. ohmeri* strains presented high fluconazole MICs [61].

Among all the *Malassezia* spp. fungemia cases, *M. furfur* dominated, from which 25% had a fatal outcome, followed by *M. pachydermatis*, with 4% mortality, and one case of *M. sympodialis* (the newborn survived). It was previously demonstrated that *M. furfur* presents high MICs to azoles. Therefore, the administration of prophylactic fluconazole in patients with risk factors such as prematurity, may lead to resistant strains and *M. furfur* colonization [112]. In catheter-related neonatal colonization by *M. furfur*, the removal of the catheter and discontinuation of intravenous lipid administration are usually sufficient and effective strategies. Furthermore, it is demonstrated that in life-threatening *M. furfur* fungemia, the preferred antifungal drug is amphotericin B [79]. In this review, *M. furfur* isolates showed elevated MICs for echinocandins.

This study also revealed the first case of neonatal fungemia due to *Aureobasidium melanogenum*. *Aureobasidium* species can survive in extreme ecological conditions, usually found in wet, oligotrophic environments, while their natural habitats are often subjected to osmotic stress and in many cases to solar radiation. *Aureobasidium* species can also survive on wet surfaces such as in bathrooms and saunas, in hospital environments, and can colonize organs and human skin [113]. Wang M et al. compared the two species *A. pullulans* and *A. melanogenum* and found that *Aureobasidium melanogenum* showed significantly better survival at 37 °C than *A. pullulans*, possibly due to its response to elevated temperatures with elevated melanin production which *A. pullulans* did not. This mechanism probably enhanced the virulence and pathogenicity of *A. melanogenum* [113]. This is why its accurate and timely identification is key to proper treatment as *A. melanogenum* also exhibits significant antifungal resistance. Unfortunately, *A. melanogenum* can be easily confused with *Candida* species on Gram-stained smears, while it cannot be easily identified by conventional diagnostic methods, such as VITEK 2 and MALDI-TOF MS, leaving molecular techniques as the only diagnostic selection [94].

It has recently been suggested that climate change and particularly global warming have affected the ecosystem microbiome with dramatic effects on human health. High temperatures and heat waves can lead to microbes adapting, making them thermotolerant and allowing them to survive at the human body temperature. This is particularly important for environmental fungi, most of which grow best below 37 °C. According to this view, more fungal species such as *Aureobasidium melanogenum* with resistance to environmental stress and increased pathogenicity will appear more and more frequently due to the global climate crisis threatening vulnerable organisms [114]. The same hypothesis has been made for *Candida auris*, which probably acquired the property of heat resistance due to global warming, which transformed it from an environmental species to an opportunistic human pathogen [115].

In this study, two fatal neonatal fungemia cases from another opportunistic yeast pathogen, *Lodderomyces elongisporus*, were also included. Its close relationship with *C. parapsilosis* confuses correct diagnosis, delaying treatment [92,93]. Clinical isolates of *L. elongisporus* have previously been misidentified as *C. parapsilosis* by conventional methods such as API 20C, ID 32C, and Vitek 2, while MALDI-TOF MS and molecular methods were required for correct identification [116]. However, it has been suggested that CHROMagar can be used as a preliminary identification method in laboratories where molecular methods are not available as on this agar isolates of *L. elongisporus* form turquoise blue colonies instead of the white to light pink colonies of *C. parapsilosis* [117]. This is particularly important for the timely selection of the correct antifungal therapy, as echinocandins appear to be quite effective for treating *L. elongisporus* infections but not for *C. parapsilosis* infections mainly due to the different amino acid sequence of beta-1,3 glucan synthase, which is the target of this class of antifungals [116].

This study, also showed that low birth weight, the use of central catheters, prematurity, and the use of broad-spectrum antibiotics constituted the strongest risk factors for neonatal fungemia cases as well as for the cases with fatal outcomes. It is, after all, recognized that birth weight is the major predictor of nosocomial infection development and our results are in accordance with this [118].

The birth process plays a major role in neonatal colonization by fungi. During the natural delivery, the neonatal skin is directly colonized from the maternal vaginal mycobiome. It has been previously shown that this mode of delivery is related to high colonization of *Malassezia* [119]. On the other hand, premature neonates, are mainly born via cesarian section and are thus colonized by maternal skin and the hospital environment. It has also been shown that the babies are immediately colonized by *Malassezia* species after birth with a predominance of *Malassezia furfur*, *Malassezia sympodialis*, and *Malassezia restricta* [119]. Moreover, it has been found that the neonatal gut mycobiome is already shaped at the age of 10 days with a prevalence of *Candida albicans* and *Malassezia* spp. Furthermore, *Saccharomyces cerevisiae* has been found to be the dominant fungal species in the gut mycobiome of both mothers and their 1–2-year-old babies [120]. In addition, the gut microbiome of a premature newborn contains a higher proportion of fungi than an adult's. Moreover, factors associated with prematurity, such as an immature gastrointestinal system and intestinal barrier, an underdeveloped immune response, administration of antibiotics, and antifungal prophylaxis, can cause hematogenous dissemination of fungi and fungemia [121,122]. The type of prophylactic antifungal drug plays an important role in the composition of the gut mycobiome: a prophylactic administration of azoles may lead to prevalence of *Candida glabrata* and other azole-resistant species, while a prophylactic echinocandin strategy may cause prevalence of *Candida parapsilosis* or other echinocandin resistant species [123,124].

Neonatal infections within 48 h of birth are therefore associated with pathogens transmitted from the mother's vagina. Other modes of transmission of microorganisms to neonates are by contact with a person or a contaminated source, droplets, or airborne transmission. Fungi are widely distributed in the environment and thus can be transmitted very easily by human agents or inanimate objects and threaten the lives of such vulnerable patients. In addition to the immature immune system, skin, or mucosal barriers, other risk factors for the development of life-threatening neonatal infections such as fungemia, include the use of catheters, invasive procedures, steroid administration, prolonged hospitalization, mechanical respiratory support, prolonged parenteral nutrition, necrotizing enterocolitis, etc. [118,121]. The colonization of the catheter or the skin at the insertion site, contamination of intravenous fluids, low frequency of catheter tubing changes, or catheter replacement may also predispose individuals to bloodstream infections. Removal of central venous catheters is therefore critical to the outcome of fungemia [123]. Moreover, it has been previously reported that the retention of a catheter is associated with increased mortality rates in *Candida* bloodstream infections [124]. The strong association between not removing the catheter and the fatal outcome was also revealed in the present review.

According to our findings, intubation and mechanical ventilation have been found in 34% of all the fungemia cases and in 65% of the fatal cases. Mechanical ventilation is recognized as a risk factor for bloodstream infections due to colonization of humidified air, or due to traumatism from the endotracheal tube and its suctioning [125]. Prolonged hospital stay also dominated in the cases with lethal outcomes (43%) compared with total cases (18%). This is understandable because a prolonged hospital stay means prolonged presence of indwelling catheters, performance of invasive procedures, and prolonged use of broad-spectrum antibiotics that favor the colonization of fungal pathogens [126]. Total parenteral nutrition and intralipids may also predispose to fungemia due to the risk of contamination or translocation of pathogens across the immature neonatal gastrointestinal mucosa and bloodstream dissemination [127]. Moreover, intralipids are predispose to infections by *Malassezia* spp. [118].

Regarding treatment management, our systematic review revealed that antifungal therapies varied significantly among cases, with Fluconazole and Amphotericin B being the most commonly administered medications. Timely removal (or replacement) of central venous catheters within 24 h of a positive blood culture is a critical component of effective treatment. Conversely, delayed removal or replacement of central venous catheters in neonates with fungemia has been associated with increased mortality and morbidity [128]. Our review and the available data showed that only 18% of catheters were removed as part of the treatment intervention. A multicenter prospective study involving 13 neonatal intensive care units was conducted in Italy to evaluate the incidence of bacterial sepsis and invasive fungal infections, fungal colonization, risk factors for sepsis and mortality rates in neonates and infants under 3 months old undergoing major surgery. They concluded that preventive measures, including early removal of vascular catheters and the use of fluconazole prophylaxis, should be implemented to mitigate the risk of bacterial and fungal infection in infants undergoing abdominal surgery, especially those with fungal colonization [129].

As mentioned above, fungal infections from fungi that were previously not considered pathogenic have been reported more and more frequently in recent years, which was also evident in our study. Given the rapid development of multidrug resistance of these emerging fungi, these infections are difficult to manage and are often associated with high mortality rates. Several studies have hypothesized an environmental pathway for this development of fungal drug resistance. For example, the widespread use of antifungals in agriculture may have caused rapid species evolution and selection of resistant strains [130]. Such opportunistic fungi can then especially threaten immunocompromised individuals including neonates.

Interestingly, our study revealed a steady increase in reported cases from 1991 to 2000, followed by a near tripling of cases from 2001 to 2023. The increase in neonatal fungemia is partially attributed to the enhanced survival rates of very low birth weight (VLBW) and extremely low birth weight (ELBW) infants. This progress has been achieved due to the regionalization of perinatal care, a better understanding of the pathophysiology of extremely premature neonates, the administration of antenatal steroids, and the critical use of postnatal surfactant therapy. Surfactant therapy has significantly improved outcomes in preterm infants by reducing the incidence and severity of neonatal respiratory distress syndrome (RDS), a common complication in very preterm infants. The introduction of surfactants has enhanced lung function, decreased the need for mechanical ventilation, and improved overall survival rates. Advances in surfactant formulations and administration techniques have further optimized its effectiveness [130]. Additionally, the use of intravenous nutrition and ongoing technological advancements have contributed to the overall improvement in preterm infant care.

Despite significant advances in perinatal medicine, caring for extremely preterm infants remains challenging due to their high mortality and morbidity risks. While survival rates have improved, these infants continue to face serious health issues. Effective management strategies, supported by meta-analyses and randomized controlled trials, are essential for reducing mortality and impairments. However, the efficacy and safety of some emerging strategies are still uncertain. Neonatal sepsis is a major concern, exacerbated by immature immune systems, prolonged hospitalizations, and frequent invasive procedures. Empiric broad-spectrum antibiotics are commonly used to treat sepsis, with therapy adjusted once pathogens are identified. Prophylactic maternal antibiotics and infection control measures, such as hand hygiene and central line care, are recommended. Nonetheless, overuse of antibiotics has led to increased rates of multidrug-resistant organisms and related complications, including bronchopulmonary dysplasia (BPD), necrotizing enterocolitis (NEC), and fungal infections. Furthermore, climate change, agricultural practices, occupational hazards, deforestation, human migration patterns, soil dispersion, patient immunosuppression, and advancements in infection detection and diagnostic testing all contribute to the rise of fungal diseases. The increasing rates of fungal morbidity and mortality are closely linked to antifungal resistance, drug tolerance, and biofilm formation [131]. Antifungal tolerance refers to the partial growth of fungi after 24 h of exposure to inhibitory drug concentrations, as evidenced in susceptibility tests. In contrast, antifungal resistance is characterized by the complete lack of a toxic effect on fungal pathogens despite treatment [132]. Current antifungal therapies are limited to a few drug classes, including polyenes, azoles, echinocandins, allylamines, and flucytosine. While allylamines are primarily used for superficial infections, the other four classes are highly effective against invasive mycosis. Moreover, evidence from randomized trials indicates that fluconazole prophylaxis may increase the risk of colonization with fluconazole-susceptible dose-dependent or resistant fungi. However, it does not significantly alter the risk of invasive infections caused by these fungi. The risk of breakthrough infections remains a concern and should be investigated further in large prospective studies [133]. Hence when managing a patient with or at risk for invasive fungal infections (IFI), clinicians must consider various factors to tailor therapy and optimize outcomes. Recent advancements have expanded antifungal options, each varying in spectrum, pharmacokinetics, indications, safety, cost, and usability. Matching these drug characteristics with patient-specific factors is crucial for effective treatment with minimal toxicity. Decision-making becomes especially complex for highly immunocompromised patients, such as ELBW neonates with rare IFIs, where a high level of suspicion is needed for early initiation of therapy. To achieve the best outcomes, extended antifungal treatment should be combined with addressing underlying risk factors and performing radical debridement of affected tissues.

5. Study Limitations

It is important to acknowledge the limitations of our study and interpret its findings with caution. The primary limitation is that our analysis relied exclusively on data from case reports and case series, which are known for their limited generalizability and validity, and their inability to establish causal relationships. Additionally, there may be significant biases related to publication, the retrospective nature of the study, and the focus on rare or atypical cases. However, some case reports and series can still provide valuable insights, especially in the absence of data from randomized controlled trials (RCTs) and observational studies. This is particularly relevant when a few studies suggest a significant and probable causal link in the context of an emerging epidemic or a newly introduced medication [134,135].

It should also be noted that due to the ongoing flux in the nomenclature of fungal agents, several *Candida* spp. have been renamed non-*Candida* genus, which are no longer considered causative agents for candidiasis. For example, *Candida pelliculosa* (now renamed to *Wickerhamomyces anomalus/Pichia anomala*) or *Candida norvegensis* (now renamed to *Pichia norvegensis*) [136].

In addition, significant neonatal risk factors were not available for all cases. There was also a lack of evidence on antifungal prophylaxis, antifungal susceptibility testing, and treatment administered. Moreover, fungemia-attributable mortality data was not available for all cases as well. Such gaps together with significant heterogeneity between review studies in recording baseline data were the main inhibiting factors for conducting a meta-analysis.

6. Conclusions

The present study has provided us with extended insight into the epidemiology of neonatal fungemia by non-*Candida* rare opportunistic yeasts among geographically different areas all over the world for an extended time period.

A rapid identification of these rare yeasts is a key element for adequate therapy and better outcomes for these vulnerable patients. Although recent advancements have paved the way with modern techniques and methodologies, fungemia by these opportunistic pathogens remains underestimated. Furthermore, it is obvious that the compliance of healthcare workers to general principles of hygiene is crucial in neonatal intensive care units. The problem is bigger in developing countries mainly due to a deficiency of resources.

Supplementary Materials: The following supporting information can be downloaded at: https://www.mdpi.com/article/10.3390/ijms25179266/s1, Reference [137] is cited in the supplementary materials.

Author Contributions: Conceptualization, A.M. and R.S.; methodology, A.M. and R.S.; investigation, A.M., R.S., V.C., J.M. and M.T.; data curation, A.M., R.S., J.M., V.C. and M.T.; writing—original draft preparation, A.M., R.S., J.M., V.C. and M.T.; writing—review and editing, A.M., R.S., J.M., V.C. and M.T.; supervision, A.M. and R.S. All authors have read and agreed to the published version of the manuscript.

Funding: This research received no external funding.

Institutional Review Board Statement: Not applicable.

Informed Consent Statement: Not applicable.

Data Availability Statement: Data are contained within the article.

Conflicts of Interest: The authors declare no conflicts of interest.

References

1. Stoll, B.J.; Hansen, N.; Fanaroff, A.A.; Wright, L.L.; Carlo, W.A.; Ehrenkranz, R.A.; Lemons, J.A.; Donovan, E.F.; Stark, A.R.; Tyson, J.E.; et al. Late-Onset Sepsis in Very Low Birth Weight Neonates: The Experience of the NICHD Neonatal Research Network. *Pediatrics* **2002**, *110*, 285–291. [CrossRef]
2. Weimer, K.E.D.; Smith, P.B.; Puia-Dumitrescu, M.; Aleem, S. Invasive fungal infections in neonates: A review. *Pediatr. Res.* **2021**, *91*, 404–412. [CrossRef] [PubMed]
3. Taliaka, P.K.; Tsantes, A.G.; Konstantinidi, A.; Houhoula, D.; Tsante, K.A.; Vaiopoulos, A.G.; Piovani, D.; Nikolopoulos, G.K.; Bonovas, S.; Iacovidou, N.; et al. Risk Factors, Diagnosis, and Treatment of Neonatal Fungal Liver Abscess: A Systematic Review of the Literature. *Life* **2023**, *13*, 167. [CrossRef]
4. Nelson, R. Emergence of resistant Candida auris. *Lancet Microbe* **2023**, *4*, e396. [CrossRef]
5. Sokou, R.; Palioura, A.E.; Kopanou Taliaka, P.; Konstantinidi, A.; Tsantes, A.G.; Piovani, D.; Tsante, K.A.; Gounari, E.A.; Iliodromiti, Z.; Boutsikou, T.; et al. Candida auris Infection, a Rapidly Emerging Threat in the Neonatal Intensive Care Units: A Systematic Review. *J. Clin. Med.* **2024**, *13*, 1586. [CrossRef] [PubMed]
6. Miceli, M.H.; Díaz, J.A.; Lee, S.A. Emerging opportunistic yeast infections. *Lancet Infect. Dis.* **2011**, *11*, 142–151. [CrossRef]
7. Moher, D.; Liberati, A.; Tetzlaff, J.; Altman, D.G. Preferred reporting items for systematic reviews and meta-analyses: The PRISMA statement. *J. Clin. Epidemiol.* **2009**, *62*, 1006–1012. [CrossRef]
8. Redline, R.W.; Dahms, B.B. Malassezia Pulmonary Vasculitis in an Infant on Long-Term Intralipid Therapy. *N. Engl. J. Med.* **1981**, *305*, 1395–1398. [CrossRef]
9. Powell, D.A.; Aungst, J.; Snedden, S.; Hansen, N.; Brady, M. Broviac catheter-related Malassezia furfur sepsis in five infants receiving intravenous fat emulsions. *J. Pediatr.* **1984**, *105*, 987–990. [CrossRef]
10. Redline, R.W.; Redline, S.S.; Boxerbaum, B.; Dahms, B.B. Systemic Malassezia furfur infections in patients receiving intralipid therapy. *Hum. Pathol.* **1985**, *16*, 815–822. [CrossRef]
11. Murphy, N.; Damjanovic, V.; Hart, C.A.; Buchanan, C.R.; Whitaker, R.; Cooke, R.W.I. Infection and colonisation of neonates by hansenula anomala. *Lancet* **1986**, *327*, 291–293. [CrossRef] [PubMed]
12. Dankner, W.M.; Spector, S.A.; Fierer, J.; Davis, C.E. Malassezia fungemia in neonates and adults: Complication of hyperalimentation. *Rev. Infect. Dis.* **1987**, *9*, 743–753. [CrossRef] [PubMed]
13. Alpert, G.; Bell, L.M.; Campos, J.M. Malassezia furfur fungemia in infancy. *Clin. Pediatr.* **1987**, *26*, 528–531. [CrossRef]
14. Shek, Y.H.; Tucker, M.C.; Viciana, A.L.; Manz, H.J.; Connor, D.H. Malassezia furfur--disseminated infection in premature infants. *Am. J. Clin. Pathol.* **1989**, *92*, 595–603. [CrossRef]
15. Surmont, I.; Gavilanes, A.; Vandepitte, J.; Devlieger, H.; Eggermont, E. Malassezia furfur fungaemia in infants receiving intravenous lipid emulsions. A rarity or just underestimated? *Eur. J. Pediatr.* **1989**, *148*, 435–438. [CrossRef]
16. Weiss Malassezia Furfur Fungemia Associated with Central Venous Catheter Lipid Emulsion Infusion—Αναζήτηση Google. Available online: https://www.google.com/search?q=weiss+Malassezia+furfur+fungemia+associated+with+central+venous+catheter+lipid+emulsion+infusion&sca_esv=578293274&ei=soJBZf2BAoyGxc8Pn--UgA0&udm=&ved=0ahUKEwj9ooTkraGCAxUMQ_EDHZ83BdAQ4dUDCBA&uact=5&oq=weiss+Malassezia+furf (accessed on 1 November 2023).
17. Hruszkewycz, V.; Holtrop, P.C.; Batton, D.G.; Morden, R.S.; Gibson, P.; Band, J.D. Complications associated with central venous catheters inserted in critically ill neonates. *Infect. Control Hosp. Epidemiol.* **1991**, *12*, 544–548. [CrossRef] [PubMed]
18. Masure, O.; Leostic, C.; Abalain, M.; Chastel, C.; Yakoub-Agha, I.; Berthou, C.; Briere, J. Malassezia furfur septicaemia in a child with leukaemia. *J. Infect.* **1991**, *23*, 335–336. [CrossRef]
19. Giacoia, G.P. Trichosporon beigelii: A Potential Cause of Sepsis in Premature Infants. *South. Med. J.* **1992**, *85*, 1247–1248. [CrossRef]
20. Herbrecht, R.; Waller, J.; Dufour, P.; Koenig, H.; Lioure, B.; Marcellin, L.; Oberling, F. Rare opportunistic fungal diseases in patients with organ or bone marrow transplantation. *Agressologie* **1992**, *33*, 77–80.
21. Fisher, D.J.; Christy, C.; Spafford, P.; Maniscalco, W.M.; Hardy, D.J.; Graman, P.S. Neonatal Trichosporon beigelii infection: Report of a cluster of cases in a neonatal intensive care unit. *Pediatr. Infect. Dis. J.* **1993**, *12*, 149–155. [CrossRef]
22. Welbel, S.F.; McNeil, M.M.; Pramanik, A.; Silberman, R.; Oberle, A.D.; Midgley, G.; Crow, S.; Jarvis, W.R. Nosocomial Malassezia pachydermatis bloodstream infections in a neonatal intensive care unit. *Pediatr. Infect. Dis. J.* **1994**, *13*, 104–108. [CrossRef] [PubMed]
23. Yoss, B.S.; Sautter, R.L.; Brenker, H.J. Trichosporon beigelii, a new neonatal pathogen. *Am. J. Perinatol.* **1997**, *14*, 113–117. [CrossRef] [PubMed]
24. Johnson, L.B.; Bradley, S.F.; Kauffman, C.A. Fungaemia due to Cryptococcus laurentii and a review of non-neoformans cryptococcaemia. *Mycoses* **1998**, *41*, 277–280. [CrossRef] [PubMed]
25. Chang, H.J.; Miller, H.L.; Watkins, N.; Arduino, M.J.; Ashford, D.A.; Midgley, G.; Aguero, S.M.; Pinto-Powell, R.; von Reyn, C.F.; Edwards, W.; et al. An epidemic of Malassezia pachydermatis in an intensive care nursery associated with colonization of health care workers' pet dogs. *N. Engl. J. Med.* **1998**, *338*, 706–711. [CrossRef]
26. Sweet, D.; Reid, M. Disseminated neonatal Trichosporon beigelii infection: Successful treatment with liposomal amphotericin B. *J. Infect.* **1998**, *36*, 120–121. [CrossRef]
27. Singh, K.; Chakrabarti, A.; Narang, A.; Gopalan, S. Yeast colonisation & fungaemia in preterm neonates in a tertiary care centre. *Indian J. Med. Res.* **1999**, *110*, 169.

28. Perapoch, J.; Planes, A.M.; Querol, A.; López, V.; Martínez-Bendayán, I.; Tormo, R.; Fernández, F.; Peguero, G.; Salcedo, S. Fungemia with Saccharomyces cerevisiae in two newborns, only one of whom had been treated with ultra-levura. *Eur. J. Clin. Microbiol. Infect. Dis.* **2000**, *19*, 468–470. [CrossRef]
29. Ma, J.S.; Chen, P.Y.; Chen, C.H.; Chi, C.S. Neonatal fungemia caused by Hansenula anomala: A case report. *J. Microbiol. Immunol. Infect.* **2000**, *33*, 267–270.
30. Wong, A.R.; Ibrahim, H.; Van Rostenberghe, H.; Ishak, Z.; Radzi, M.J. *Hansenula anomala* infection in a neonate. *J. Paediatr. Child. Health* **2000**, *36*, 609–610. [CrossRef]
31. Chakrabarti, A.; Singh, K.; Narang, A.; Singhi, S.; Batra, R.; Rao, K.L.; Ray, P.; Gopalan, S.; Das, S.; Gupta, V.; et al. Outbreak of Pichia anomala infection in the pediatric service of a tertiary-care center in Northern India. *J. Clin. Microbiol.* **2001**, *39*, 1702–1706. [CrossRef]
32. Aragão, P.A.; Oshiro, I.C.V.; Manrique, E.I.; Gomes, C.C.; Matsuo, L.L.; Leone, C.; Moretti-Branchini, M.L.; Levin, A.S. Pichia anomala outbreak in a nursery: Exogenous source? *Pediatr. Infect Dis. J.* **2001**, *20*, 843–848. [CrossRef] [PubMed]
33. Cheng, M.-F.; Chiou, C.C.; Liu, Y.-C.; Wang, H.-Z.; Hsieh, K.-S. *Cryptococcus laurentii* Fungemia in a Premature Neonate. *J. Clin. Microbiol.* **2001**, *39*, 1608–1611. [CrossRef]
34. Chryssanthou, E.; Broberger, U.; Petrini, B. Malassezia pachydermatis fungaemia in a neonatal intensive care unit. *Acta Paediatr.* **2007**, *90*, 323–327. [CrossRef]
35. Panagopoulou, P.; Evdoridou, J.; Bibashi, E.; Filioti, J.; Sofianou, D.; Kremenopoulos, G.; Roilides, E. Trichosporon asahii: An unusual cause of invasive infection in neonates. *Pediatr. Infect. Dis. J.* **2002**, *21*, 169–170. [CrossRef] [PubMed]
36. Yıldıran, A.; Kücüködük, Ş.; Saniç, A.; Belet, N.; Güvenli, A. Disseminated *Trichosporon asahii* Infection in a Preterm. *Am. J. Perinatol.* **2003**, *20*, 269–271. [CrossRef] [PubMed]
37. Gökahmetoğlu, S.; Nedret Koç, A.; Güneş, T.; Cetin, N. Case reports. Trichosporon mucoides infection in three premature newborns. *Mycoses* **2002**, *45*, 123–125. [CrossRef]
38. Baron, E.; Anaissie, E.; Dumphy, F.; McCredie, K.; Fainstein, V. Hansenula anomala fungemia. *Clin. Infect. Dis.* **1988**, *10*, 1182–1186. [CrossRef]
39. Bakır, M.; Çerikcioğlu, N.; Tırtır, A.; Berrak, S.; Özek, E.; Canpolat, C. Pichia anomala fungaemia in immunocompromised children. *Mycoses* **2004**, *47*, 231–235. [CrossRef] [PubMed]
40. Belet, N.; Dalgiç, N.; Oncel, S.; Ciftçi, E.; Ince, E.; Güriz, H.; Barlas, M.; Doğru, U. Catheter-related fungemia caused by Saccharomyces cerevisiae in a newborn. *Pediatr. Infect. Dis. J.* **2005**, *24*, 1125. [CrossRef]
41. Taj-Aldeen, S.J.; Doiphode, S.H.; Han, X.Y. Kodamaea (Pichia) ohmeri fungaemia in a premature neonate. *J. Med. Microbiol.* **2006**, *55*, 237–239. [CrossRef]
42. Bhally, H.S.; Jain, S.; Shields, C.; Halsey, N.; Cristofalo, E.; Merz, W.G. Infection in a neonate caused by Pichia fabianii: Importance of molecular identification. *Med. Mycol.* **2006**, *44*, 185–187. [CrossRef] [PubMed]
43. Paula, C.R.; Krebs, V.L.; Auler, M.E.; Ruiz, L.S.; Matsumoto, F.E.; Silva, E.H.; Diniz, E.M.; Vaz, F.A. Nosocomial infection in newborns by Pichia anomala in a Brazilian intensive care unit. *Med. Mycol.* **2006**, *44*, 479–484. [CrossRef] [PubMed]
44. Perniola, R.; Faneschi, M.L.; Manso, E.; Pizzolante, M.; Rizzo, A.; Damiani, A.S.; Longo, R. Rhodotorula mucilaginosa outbreak in neonatal intensive care unit: Microbiological features, clinical presentation, and analysis of related variables. *Eur. J. Clin. Microbiol. Infect. Dis.* **2006**, *25*, 193–196. [CrossRef] [PubMed]
45. Vivas, R.; Beltran, C.; Munera, M.I.; Trujillo, M.; Restrepo, A.; Garcés, C. Fungemia due to Kodamaea ohmeri in a young infant and review of the literature. *Med. Mycol. Case Rep.* **2016**, *13*, 5–8. [CrossRef]
46. Ngerncham, S.; Lapphra, K. Cryptococcus neoformans septicemia in an immunocompetent neonate: First case report in Thailand. *Southeast Asian J. Trop. Med. Public Health* **2008**, *39*, 697–700.
47. Téllez-Castillo, C.J.; Gil-Fortuño, M.; Centelles-Sales, I.; Sabater-Vidal, S.; Serrano, F.P. Trichosporon asahii fatal infection in a preterm newborn. *Rev. Chil. Infectología* **2008**, *25*, 213–215.
48. Poojary, A.; Sapre, G. Kodamaea ohmeri infection in a neonate. *Indian Pediatr.* **2009**, *46*, 629–631.
49. Pereira, D.N.; Nader, S.S.; Nader, P.; Martins, P.G.; Furlan, S.P.; Hentges, C.R. Disseminated *Trichosporon* spp infection in preterm newborns: A case report. *J. Pediatr.* **2009**, *85*, 459–461.
50. Noni, M.; Stathi, A.; Velegraki, A.; Malamati, M.; Kalampaliki, A.; Zachariadou, L.; Michos, A. Rare Invasive Yeast Infections in Greek Neonates and Children, a Retrospective 12-Year Study. *J. Fungi* **2020**, *6*, 194. [CrossRef]
51. Grenouillet, F.; Millon, L.; Chamouine, A.; Thiriez, G.; Schulze, O.; Leroy, J. Pichia fabianii Fungemia in a Neonate. *Pediatr. Infect. Dis. J.* **2010**, *29*, 191. [CrossRef]
52. Duggal, S.; Jain, H.; Tyagi, A.; Sharma, A.; Chugh, T.D. Rhodotorula fungemia: Two cases and a brief review. *Med. Mycol.* **2011**, *49*, 879–882. [PubMed]
53. Oliveri, S.; Trovato, L.; Betta, P.; Romeo, M.G.; Nicoletti, G. Malassezia furfur fungaemia in a neonatal patient detected by lysis-centrifugation blood culture method: First case reported in Italy. *Mycoses* **2011**, *54*, 638. [CrossRef]
54. Al-Sweih, N.; Khan, Z.U.; Ahmad, S.; Devarajan, L.; Khan, S.; Joseph, L.; Chandy, R. Kodamaea ohmeri as an emerging pathogen: A case report and review of the literature. *Med. Mycol.* **2011**, *49*, 766–770. [PubMed]
55. Vashishtha, V.M.; Mittal, A.; Garg, A. A fatal outbreak of Trichosporon asahii Sepsis in a neonatal intensive care unit. *Indian Pediatr.* **2012**, *49*, 745–747. [CrossRef]

56. Lin, H.-C.; Lin, H.-Y.; Su, B.-H.; Ho, M.-W.; Ho, C.-M.; Lee, C.-Y.; Lin, M.-H.; Hsieh, H.-Y.; Lin, H.-C.; Li, T.-C.; et al. Reporting an outbreak of Candida pelliculosa fungemia in a neonatal intensive care unit. *J. Microbiol. Immunol. Infect.* **2013**, *46*, 456–462. [CrossRef]
57. da Silva, C.M.; de Carvalho Parahym, A.M.; Leão, M.P.; de Oliveira, N.T.; de Jesus Machado Amorim, R.; Neves, R.P. Fungemia by Candida pelliculosa (Pichia anomala) in a neonatal intensive care unit: A possible clonal origin. *Mycopathologia* **2013**, *175*, 175–179. [CrossRef]
58. Iatta, R.; Cafarchia, C.; Cuna, T.; Montagna, O.; Laforgia, N.; Gentile, O.; Rizzo, A.; Boekhout, T.; Otranto, D.; Montagna, M.T. Bloodstream infections by Malassezia and Candida species in critical care patients. *Med. Mycol.* **2014**, *52*, 264–269. [CrossRef]
59. Chioukh, F.Z.; Ben Hmida, H.; Ben Ameur, K.; Toumi, A.; Monastiri, K. Saccharomyces cerevisiae fungemia in a premature neonate treated receiving probiotics. *Med. Mal. Infect.* **2013**, *43*, 359–360. [CrossRef]
60. Liu, C.X.; Yang, J.H.; Dong, L.; Mai, J.Y.; Zhang, L.; Zhu, J.H. Clinical features and homological analysis of Pichia ohmeri-caused hospital-acquired fungemia in premature infants. *Zhonghua Yi Xue Za Zhi* **2013**, *93*, 285–288.
61. Wu, Y.; Wang, J.; Li, W.; Jia, H.; Che, J.; Lu, J.; Liu, L.; Cheng, Y. Pichia fabianii blood infection in a premature infant in China: Case report. *BMC Res. Notes* **2013**, *6*, 77. [CrossRef] [PubMed]
62. Kodamaea Ohmeri as an Emerging Pathogen in Mainland China—Αναζήτηση Google. Available online: https://www.google.com/search?q=%0D%0AKodamaea+ohmeri+as+an+Emerging+Pathogen+in+Mainland+China&sca_esv=578502807&ei=aWtCZfutD86Rxc8PoKSAsAc&udm=&ved=0ahUKEwi7htvbi6OCAxXOSPEDHSASAHYQ4dUDCBA&uact=5&oq=%0D%0AKodamaea+ohmeri+as+an+Emerging+Pathogen+in+Mainland+China&gs_lp=Egxnd3Mtd2l6LXNlcnAiOgpLb2RhbWFlYSBvaG1lcmkgYXMgYW4gRW1lcmdpbmcgUGF0aG9nZW4gaW4gTWFpbmxhbmQgQ2hpbmFIwwtQnwhYnwhwAXgBkAEAmAEAoAEAqgEAuAEDyAEA-AEB-AECqAIA4gMEGAAgQYgGAQ&sclient=gws-wiz-serp (accessed on 1 November 2023).
63. Chakrabarti, A.; Rudramurthy, S.M.; Kale, P.; Hariprasath, P.; Dhaliwal, M.; Singhi, S.; Rao, K.L.N. Epidemiological study of a large cluster of fungaemia cases due to Kodamaea ohmeri in an Indian tertiary care centre. *Clin. Microbiol. Infect.* **2014**, *20*, O83–O89. [CrossRef] [PubMed]
64. Borade, A.; Kapdi, M.; Suryavanshi, K. Kodamaea Ohmeri—An Emerging Fungal Pathogen in Neonatal Intensive Care Unit. *Pediatr. Oncall* **2014**, *11*, 114–116. [CrossRef]
65. Prakash, A.; Wankhede, S.; Singh, P.K.; Agarwal, K.; Kathuria, S.; Sengupta, S.; Barman, P.; Meis, J.F.; Chowdhary, A. First neonatal case of fungaemia due to Pseudozyma aphidis and a global literature review. *Mycoses* **2014**, *57*, 64–68. [CrossRef]
66. Al-Sweih, N.; Ahmad, S.; Joseph, L.; Khan, S.; Khan, Z. Malassezia pachydermatis fungemia in a preterm neonate resistant to fluconazole and flucytosine. *Med. Mycol. Case Rep.* **2014**, *5*, 9–11. [CrossRef]
67. Biswal, D.; Sahu, M.; Mahajan, A.; Advani, S.H.; Shah, S. Kodameae ohmeri—An Emerging Yeast: Two Cases and Literature Review. *J. Clin. Diagn. Res.* **2015**, *9*, DD01. [CrossRef]
68. Mlinarić-Missoni, E.; Hatvani, L.; Kocsube, S.; Vágvölgyi, C.; Škarić, I.; Lukić-Grlić, A. Cyberlindnera fabianii in the neonatal and paediatric intensive care unit: Case reports. *JMM Case Rep.* **2015**, *2*, e000032. [CrossRef]
69. Basu, S.; Tilak, R.; Kumar, A. Multidrug-resistant *Trichosporon*: An unusual fungal sepsis in preterm neonates. *Ann. Trop. Med. Parasitol.* **2015**, *109*, 202–206. [CrossRef]
70. Okolo, O.M.; Van Diepeningen, A.D.; Toma, B.; Nnadi, N.E.; Ayanbimpe, M.G.; Onyedibe, I.K.; Sabitu, M.Z.; Banwat, B.E.; Groenewald, M.; Scordino, F.; et al. First report of neonatal sepsis due to Moesziomyces bullatus in a preterm low-birth-weight infant. *JMM Case Rep.* **2015**, *2*, e000011. [CrossRef]
71. Socarras, J.A.; Rojas Torres, J.P.; Vargas Soler, J.A.; Guerrero, C. Kodamaea ohmeri infection in a newborn with a mediastinal mass. *Arch. Argent. Pediatr.* **2016**, *114*, e319–e322.
72. Yılmaz-Semerci, S.; Demirel, G.; Taştekin, A. Wickerhamomyces anomalus blood stream infection in a term newborn with pneumonia. *Turk. J. Pediatr.* **2017**, *59*, 349–351. [CrossRef]
73. Nagarathnamma, T.; Chunchanur, S.K.; Rudramurthy, S.M.; Vineetha, K.R.; Ramamurthy, K.; Joseph, J.; Ambica, R. Outbreak of Pichia kudriavzevii fungaemia in a neonatal intensive care unit. *J. Med. Microbiol.* **2017**, *66*, 1759–1764. [CrossRef]
74. Kulkarni, V.; Manasa, B.M. Rhodotorula: An emerging pathogen in NICU. *Perinatology* **2017**, *18*, 77–80.
75. Kumar, A.; Roy, P.; Rai, G.; Das, S.; Ansari, M.A. Cyberlindnera fabianii and Wickerhamomyces anomalous fungemia in newborns: An experience from a North Indian tertiary-care centre. *Indian J. Med. Spéc.* **2017**, *8*, 131–133. [CrossRef]
76. Roy, U.; Jessani, L.G.; Rudramurthy, S.M.; Gopalakrishnan, R.; Dutta, S.; Chakravarty, C.; Jillwin, J.; Chakrabarti, A. Seven cases of *Saccharomyces* fungaemia related to use of probiotics. *Mycoses* **2017**, *60*, 375–380. [CrossRef] [PubMed]
77. Gupta, M.; Mishra, A.K.; Singh, S.K. Cryptococcus laurentii fungemia in a low birth weight preterm neonate: India. *J. Infect. Public. Health* **2018**, *11*, 896–897. [CrossRef] [PubMed]
78. Pedrosa, A.F.; Lisboa, C.; Rodrigues, A.G. *Malassezia* infections with systemic involvement: Figures and facts. *J. Dermatol.* **2018**, *45*, 1278–1282. [CrossRef] [PubMed]
79. Iatta, R.; Battista, M.; Miragliotta, G.; Boekhout, T.; Otranto, D.; Cafarchia, C. Blood culture procedures and diagnosis of Malassezia furfur bloodstream infections: Strength and weakness. *Med. Mycol.* **2017**, *56*, 828–833. [CrossRef]
80. Al-Sweih, N.; Ahmad, S.; Khan, S.; Joseph, L.; Asadzadeh, M.; Khan, Z. *Cyberlindnera fabianii* fungaemia outbreak in preterm neonates in Kuwait and literature review. *Mycoses* **2018**, *62*, 51–61. [CrossRef]

81. Chen, I.T.; Chen, C.C.; Huang, H.C.; Kuo, K.C. Malassezia furfur Emergence and Candidemia Trends in a Neonatal Intensive Care Unit During 10 Years: The Experience of Fluconazole Prophylaxis in a Single Hospital. *Adv. Neonatal Care* **2020**, *20*, E3–E8 [CrossRef]
82. Huang, C.-Y.; Peng, C.-C.; Hsu, C.-H.; Chang, J.-H.; Chiu, N.-C.; Chi, H. Systemic Infection Caused by Malassezia pachydermatis in Infants: Case Series and Review of the Literature. *Pediatr. Infect. Dis. J.* **2020**, *39*, 444–448. [CrossRef]
83. Chow, N.A.; Chinn, R.; Pong, A.; Schultz, K.; Kim, J.; Gade, L.; Jackson, B.R.; Beer, K.D.; Litvintseva, A.P. Use of whole-genome sequencing to detect an outbreak of Malassezia pachydermatis infection and colonization in a neonatal intensive care unit-California, 2015–2016. *Infect. Control. Hosp. Epidemiol.* **2020**, *41*, 851–853. [CrossRef] [PubMed]
84. Chowdhary, A.; Sharada, K.; Singh, P.K.; Bhagwani, D.K.; Kumar, N.; de Groot, T.; Meis, J.F. Outbreak of Dirkmeia churashimaensis Fungemia in a Neonatal Intensive Care Unit, India. *Emerg. Infect. Dis.* **2020**, *26*, 764. [CrossRef]
85. Pandey, N.; Paul, P.; Kumar, D.; Tilak, R. Case report of a rare yeast Cyberlindnera fabianii fungemia in preterm twin neonates from North India: Diagnostic and therapeutic challenge. *Indian J. Case Rep.* **2020**, *6*, 563–565. [CrossRef]
86. Al-Otaibi, H.; Asadzadeh, M.; Ahmad, S.; Al-Sweih, N.; Joseph, L. Papiliotrema laurentii fungemia in a premature, very low-birth-weight neonate in Kuwait successfully treated with liposomal amphotericin B. *J. Med. Mycol.* **2021**, *31*, 101123. [CrossRef]
87. Galvis-Marín, J.C.; Giraldo-Ospina, B.; Martínez-Ríos, J.B.; Echeverri-Peláez, S. Fungemia by malassezia sympodialis in a neonatal intensive care unit in Colombia. *Infectio* **2021**, *25*, 130–134. [CrossRef]
88. Cai, Z.; Wei, W.; Cheng, Z. Candida pelliculosa sepsis in a neonate: A casereport. *J. Int. Med. Res.* **2021**, *49*, 0300060520982804. [CrossRef] [PubMed]
89. Zhang, Z.; Cao, Y.; Li, Y.; Chen, X.; Ding, C.; Liu, Y. Risk factors and biofilm formation analyses of hospital-acquired infection of Candida pelliculosa in a neonatal intensive care unit. *BMC Infect. Dis.* **2021**, *21*, 620. [CrossRef]
90. Yang, Y.; Wu, W.; Ding, L.; Yang, L.; Su, J.; Wu, B. Two different clones of Candida pelliculosa bloodstream infection in a tertiary neonatal intensive care unit. *J. Infect. Dev. Ctries.* **2021**, *15*, 870–876. [CrossRef]
91. Mpakosi, A.; Siopi, M.; Demetriou, M.; Falaina, V.; Theodoraki, M.; Meletiadis, J. Fungemia due to Moesziomyces aphidis (*Pseudozyma aphidis*) in a premature neonate. Challenges in species identification and antifungal susceptibility testing of rare yeasts. *J. Med. Mycol.* **2022**, *32*, 101258. [CrossRef]
92. Asadzadeh, M.; Al-Sweih, N.; Ahmad, S.; Khan, S.; Alfouzan, W.; Joseph, L. Fatal Lodderomyces elongisporus Fungemia in a Premature, Extremely Low-Birth-Weight Neonate. *J. Fungi.* **2022**, *8*, 906. [CrossRef]
93. da Silva, C.M.; Jucá, M.B.; Melo AS de, A.; Lima, S.L.; Galvão, P.V.M.; Macêdo, D.P.C.; Neves, R.P. Neonatal fungemia caused by Lodderomyces elongisporus: First case report in Latin America. *Diagn. Microbiol. Infect. Dis.* **2023**, *107*, 116077. [CrossRef] [PubMed]
94. Davies, A.A.; Osuagwu, C.S.; Aikhomu, V.; Oladele, R.O.O. Cryptococcus laurentii fungaemia in a Tertiary Hospital in Nigeria: Case reports. *Microbes Infect. Dis.* **2023**, *4*, 1428–1434. [CrossRef]
95. Samaddar, A.; Sharma, A. First case of neonatal fungemia caused by Aureobasidium melanogenum. *J. Med. Mycol.* **2023**, *33*, 101334. [CrossRef] [PubMed]
96. Ashraf, A.A.; Karnaker, V.K.; Sreelatha, S.V.; Ramdas, S.; Nair, S.; Varma, S.R. A Rare Case of Fungaemia Due to Kodamaea ohmeri in a Neonate. *Online J. Health Allied Sci.* **2023**, *22*, 11.
97. Kaur, H.; Chakrabarti, A. Strategies to Reduce Mortality in Adult and Neonatal Candidemia in Developing Countries. *J. Fungi* **2017**, *3*, 41. [CrossRef]
98. McCrossan, B.; McHenry, E.; O'Neill, F.; Ong, G.; Sweet, D.G. Selective fluconazole prophylaxis in high-risk babies to reduce invasive fungal infection. *Arch. Dis. Child.-Fetal Neonatal Ed.* **2007**, *92*, F454–F458. [CrossRef]
99. Anaraki, M.R.; Nouri-Vaskeh, M.; Oskoei, S.A. Fluconazole prophylaxis against invasive candidiasis in very low and extremely low birth weight preterm neonates: A systematic review and meta-analysis. *Clin. Exp. Pediatr.* **2021**, *64*, 172–179. [CrossRef]
100. Bretagne, S.; Renaudat, C.; Desnos-Ollivier, M.; Sitbon, K.; Lortholary, O.; Dromer, F.; the Cochrane Adverse Effects Methods Group. Predisposing factors and outcome of uncommon yeast species-related fungaemia based on an exhaustive surveillance programme (2002–2014). *J. Antimicrob. Chemother.* **2017**, *72*, 1784–1793. [CrossRef]
101. Borman, A.M.; Muller, J.; Walsh-Quantick, J.; Szekely, A.; Patterson, Z.; Palmer, M.D.; Fraser, M.; Johnson, E.M. Fluconazole Resistance in Isolates of Uncommon Pathogenic Yeast Species from the United Kingdom. *Antimicrob. Agents Chemother.* **2019**, *63*, 10–1128. [CrossRef]
102. Lee, J.; Kim, H.-S.; Shin, S.H.; Choi, C.W.; Kim, E.-K.; Choi, E.H.; Kim, B.I.; Choi, J.-H. Efficacy and safety of fluconazole prophylaxis in extremely low birth weight infants: Multicenter pre-post cohort study. *BMC Pediatr.* **2016**, *16*, 67. [CrossRef]
103. Iosifidis, E.; Papachristou, S.; Roilides, E. Advances in the Treatment of Mycoses in Pediatric Patients. *J. Fungi.* **2018**, *4*, 115. [CrossRef]
104. Nunes, J.M.; Bizerra, F.C.; Carmona e Ferreira, R.; Colombo, A.L. Molecular Identification, Antifungal Susceptibility Profile, and Biofilm Formation of Clinical and Environmental Rhodotorula Species Isolates. *Antimicrob. Agents Chemother.* **2013**, *57*, 382–389. [CrossRef]
105. Martinez, L.R.; Casadevall, A. Cryptococcus neoformans Biofilm Formation Depends on Surface Support and Carbon Source and Reduces Fungal Cell Susceptibility to Heat, Cold, and UV Light. *Appl. Environ. Microbiol.* **2007**, *73*, 4592–4601. [CrossRef]

106. Iturrieta-González, I.A.; Padovan, A.C.B.; Bizerra, F.C.; Hahn, R.C.; Colombo, A.L. Multiple Species of Trichosporon Produce Biofilms Highly Resistant to Triazoles and Amphotericin B. *PLoS ONE* **2014**, *9*, e109553. [CrossRef]
107. Pfaller, M.A.; Diekema, D.J.; Merz, W.G. Infections caused by non-Candida, non-Cryptococcus yeasts. *Clin. Mycol.* **2009**, *10*, 251–270.
108. Jindal, N.; Arora, S.; Dhuria, N.; Arora, D. Cyberlindnera (Pichia) fabianii infection in a neutropenic child: Importance of molecular identification. *JMM Case Rep.* **2015**, *2*, e000033. [CrossRef]
109. Hamal, P.; Ostransky, J.; Dendis, M.; Horváth, R.; Ruzicka, F.; Buchta, V.; Vejsova, M.; Sauer, P.; Hejnar, P.; Raclavsky, V. A case of endocarditis caused by the yeast Pichia fabianii with biofilm production and developed in vitro resistance to azoles in the course of antifungal treatment. *Sabouraudia* **2008**, *46*, 601–605. [CrossRef] [PubMed]
110. Barchiesi, F.; Tortorano, A.M.; Di Francesco, L.F.; Cogliati, M.; Scalise, G.; Viviani, M.A. In-vitro activity of five antifungal agents against uncommon clinical isolates of *Candida* spp. *J. Antimicrob. Chemother.* **1999**, *43*, 295–299. [CrossRef]
111. Chitasombat, M.N.; Kofteridis, D.P.; Jiang, Y.; Tarrand, J.; Lewis, R.E.; Kontoyiannis, D.P. Rare opportunistic (non-Candida, non-Cryptococcus) yeast bloodstream infections in patients with cancer. *J. Infect.* **2012**, *64*, 68–75. [CrossRef]
112. Kaur, H.; Shankarnarayana, S.A.; Hallur, V.; Muralidharan, J.; Biswal, M.; Ghosh, A.K.; Ray, P.; Chakrabarti, A.; Rudramurthy, S.M. Prolonged Outbreak of *Candida krusei* Candidemia in Paediatric Ward of Tertiary Care Hospital. *Mycopathologia* **2020**, *185*, 257–268. [CrossRef] [PubMed]
113. Pannanusorn, S.; Fernandez, V.; Römling, U. Prevalence of biofilm formation in clinical isolates of *Candida* species causing bloodstream infection. *Mycoses* **2012**, *56*, 264–272. [CrossRef] [PubMed]
114. Rojas, F.D.; Sosa, M.d.L.A.; Fernández, M.S.; Cattana, M.E.; Córdoba, S.B.; Giusiano, G.E. Antifungal susceptibility of Malassezia furfur, Malassezia sympodialis, and Malassezia globosa to azole drugs and amphotericin B evaluated using a broth microdilution method. *Med. Mycol.* **2014**, *52*, 641–646. [CrossRef] [PubMed]
115. Wang, M.; Danesi, P.; James, T.Y.; Al-Hatmi, A.M.S.; Najafzadeh, M.J.; Dolatabadi, S.; Ming, C.; Liou, G.; Kang, Y.; de Hoog, S. Comparative pathogenicity of opportunistic black yeasts in *Aureobasidium*. *Mycoses* **2019**, *62*, 803–811. [CrossRef]
116. Smith, D.F.Q.; Casadevall, A. Disaster Microbiology—A New Field of Study. *mBio* **2022**, *13*, e0168022. [CrossRef] [PubMed]
117. Casadevall, A.; Kontoyiannis, D.P.; Robert, V. On the Emergence of Candida auris: Climate Change, Azoles, Swamps, and Birds. *mBio* **2019**, *10*, 10–1128. [CrossRef]
118. Wang, Y.; Xu, J. Lodderomyces elongisporus: An emerging human fungal pathogen. *PLoS Pathog.* **2023**, *19*, e1011613. [CrossRef]
119. Al-Obaid, K.; Ahmad, S.; Joseph, L.; Khan, Z. Lodderomyces elongisporus: A bloodstream pathogen of greater clinical significance. *New Microbes New Infect.* **2018**, *26*, 20–24. [CrossRef]
120. Heath, J.A.; Zerr, D.M. Infections Acquired in the Nursery: Epidemiology and Control. *Infect. Dis. Fetus Newborn Infant.* **2006**, *2006*, 1179–1205.
121. Hobi, S.; Cafarchia, C.; Romano, V.; Barrs, V.R. Malassezia: Zoonotic Implications, Parallels and Differences in Colonization and Disease in Humans and Animals. *J. Fungi.* **2022**, *8*, 708. [CrossRef]
122. Schei, K.; Avershina, E.; Øien, T.; Rudi, K.; Follestad, T.; Salamati, S.; Ødegård, R.A. Early gut mycobiota and mother-offspring transfer. *Microbiome. BioMed* **2017**, *5*, 107. [CrossRef]
123. Golubkova, A.; Hunter, C.J. Development of the Neonatal Intestinal Barrier, Microbiome, and Susceptibility to NEC. *Microorganisms* **2023**, *11*, 1247. [CrossRef] [PubMed]
124. Fan, Y.; Wu, L.; Zhai, B. The mycobiome: Interactions with host and implications in diseases. *Curr. Opin. Microbiol.* **2023**, *75*, 102361. [CrossRef]
125. O'Grady, N.P.; Alexander, M.; Burns, L.A.; Dellinger, E.P.; Garland, J.; Heard, S.O.; Lipsett, P.A.; Masur, H.; Mermel, L.A.; Pearson, M.L.; et al. Summary of Recommendations: Guidelines for the Prevention of Intravascular Catheter-related Infections. *Clin. Infect. Dis.* **2011**, *52*, 1087–1099. [CrossRef] [PubMed]
126. Fu, J.; Ding, Y.; Jiang, Y.; Mo, S.; Xu, S.; Qin, P. Persistent candidemia in very low birth weight neonates: Risk factors and clinical significance. *BMC Infect. Dis.* **2018**, *18*, 558. [CrossRef] [PubMed]
127. Saiman, L.; Ludington, E.; Pfaller, M.; Rangel-Frausto, S.; Wiblin, R.T.; Dawson, J.; Blumberg, H.M.; Patterson, J.E.; Rinaldi, M.; Edwards, J.E. Risk factors for candidemia in Neonatal Intensive Care Unit patients. The National Epidemiology of Mycosis Survey study group. *Pediatr. Infect. Dis. J.* **2000**, *19*, 319–324. [CrossRef] [PubMed]
128. De Rose, D.U.; Santisi, A.; Ronchetti, M.P.; Martini, L.; Serafini, L.; Betta, P.; Maino, M.; Cavigioli, F.; Cocchi, I.; Pugni, L.; et al. Invasive *Candida* Infections in Neonates after Major Surgery: Current Evidence and New Directions. *Pathogens* **2021**, *10*, 319. [CrossRef]
129. Auriti, C.; De Rose, D.; Santisi, A.; Martini, L.; Ronchetti, M.; Ravà, L.; Antenucci, V.; Bernaschi, P.; Serafini, L.; Catarzi, S.; et al. Incidence and risk factors of bacterial sepsis and invasive fungal infection in neonates and infants requiring major surgery: An Italian multicentre prospective study. *J. Hosp. Infect.* **2022**, *130*, 122–130. [CrossRef]
130. McPherson, C.; Wambach, J.A. Prevention and Treatment of Respiratory Distress Syndrome in Preterm Neonates. *Neonatal Netw.* **2018**, *37*, 169–177. [CrossRef]
131. Cosio, T.; Pica, F.; Fontana, C.; Pistoia, E.S.; Favaro, M.; Valsecchi, I.; Zarabian, N.; Campione, E.; Botterel, F.; Gaziano, R. *Stephanoascus ciferrii* Complex: The Current State of Infections and Drug Resistance in Humans. *J. Fungi* **2024**, *10*, 294. [CrossRef]
132. Garvey, M.; Rowan, N.J. Pathogenic Drug Resistant Fungi: A Review of Mitigation Strategies. *Int. J. Mol. Sci.* **2023**, *24*, 1584. [CrossRef]

133. Brion, L.P.; Uko, S.E.; Goldman, D.L. Risk of resistance associated with fluconazole prophylaxis: Systematic review. *J. Infect.* **2007**, *54*, 521–529. [CrossRef] [PubMed]
134. Loke, Y.K.; Price, D.; Herxheimer, A.; the Cochrane Adverse Effects Methods Group. Systematic reviews of adverse effects: Framework for a structured approach. *BMC Med. Res. Methodol.* **2007**, *7*, 32. [CrossRef]
135. Nambiema, A.; Sembajwe, G.; Lam, J.; Woodruff, T.; Mandrioli, D.; Chartres, N.; Fadel, M.; Le Guillou, A.; Valter, R.; Deguigne, M.; et al. A Protocol for the Use of Case Reports/Studies and Case Series in Systematic Reviews for Clinical Toxicology. *Front. Med.* **2021**, *8*, 708380. [CrossRef] [PubMed]
136. Sharma, M.; Chakrabarti, A. Candidiasis and Other Emerging Yeasts. *Curr. Fungal Infect. Rep.* **2023**, *17*, 15–24. [CrossRef]
137. Page, M.J.; McKenzie, J.E.; Bossuyt, P.M.; Boutron, I.; Hoffmann, T.C.; Mulrow, C.D.; Shamseer, L.; Tetzlaff, J.M.; Akl, E.A.; Brennan, S.E.; et al. The PRISMA 2020 statement: An updated guideline for reporting systematic reviews. *BMJ* **2021**, *372*, n71. [CrossRef]

MDPI AG
Grosspeteranlage 5
4052 Basel
Switzerland
Tel.: +41 61 683 77 34

International Journal of Molecular Sciences Editorial Office
E-mail: ijms@mdpi.com
www.mdpi.com/journal/ijms

www.ingramcontent.com/pod-product-compliance
Lightning Source LLC
Chambersburg PA
CBHW062040220926
51850CB00010B/2618
9783725872060